PAIN MANAGEMENT

Nursing Perspective

PAIN MANAGEMENT

Nursing Perspective

Judith H. Watt-Watson RN, BScN, MScN
Clinical Associate Professor
Faculty of Nursing
University of Toronto
Toronto, Ontario

Marilee Ivers Donovan, PhD, RN, FAAN
Associate Hospital Director, Nursing Services
Oregon Health Sciences University Hospitals and Clinic
Portland, Oregon

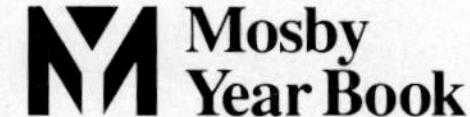

St. Louis Baltimore Boston Chicago London Philadelphia Sydney Toronto

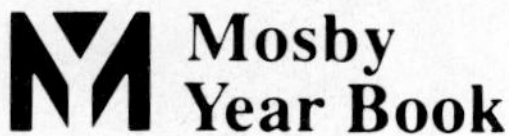

Dedicated to Publishing Excellence

Editor: Linda Duncan
Developmental Editor: Kathy Sartori
Project Manager: John Rogers
Production Editor: Chuck Furgason
Designer: Julie Taugner

A NOTE TO THE READER
The authors and publisher have made every attempt to check dosages and nursing content for accuracy. Because the science of pharmacology is continually advancing, our knowledge base continues to expand. Therefore we recommend that the reader always check product information for changes in dosage or administration before administering any medication. This is particularly important with new or rarely used drugs.

Printed in the United States of America

Mosby–Year Book, Inc.
11830 Westline Industrial Drive
St. Louis, MO 63146

Library of Congress Cataloging in Publication Data

Pain management: nursing perspective/[edited by] Judith H. Watt
—Watson, Marilee Ivers Donovan.
p. cm.
Includes bibliographical references and index.
ISBN 1-55664-251-2
1. Pain—Nursing. I. Watt-Watson, Judith H. II. Donvan. Marilee Ivers.
[DNLM: 1. Pain—nursing. 2. Pain—prevention & control. WL 704 P146596]
RT87.P35P36 1992
616'.472'024613—dc20
DNLM/DLC
for Library of Congress 92-1056
CIP

92 93 94 95 96 GW/DC/DC 9 8 7 6 5 4 3 2 1

Contributors

Judith E. Beyer, RN, PhD
Associate Professor
School of Nursing
University of Colorado
Health Sciences Center
Denver, Colorado

Marcia Sue DeWolf Bosek, RN, DNSc
Assistant Professor
Department of Medical Nursing and Section on Ethics and Department of Religion and Health
Rush-Presbyterian–St. Luke's Medical Center
Chicago, Illinois

Susan A. Clegg, RN, MS
Clinical Nurse Specialist, Neurosurgery
The Children's Hospital
Denver, Colorado

Joan M. Crook, RN, BS, MA, MSc, PhD candidate
Professor
Faculty of Health Sciences
McMaster University
Hamilton, Ontario

Linda Edgar, N, MSc(A)
Director of Nursing Research
Sir Mortimer B. Davis—Jewish General Hospital
Assistant Professor
School of Nursing
McGill University
Montreal, Quebec

Joann M. Eland, RN, PhD, FAAN
Associate Professor
College of Nursing
University of Iowa
Iowa City, Iowa

Betty R. Ferrell, RN, PhD, FAAN
Associate Research Scientist
Nursing Education and Research
City of Hope Medical Center
Duarte, California

Bruce Ferrell, MD
Assistant Professor of Medicine and Geriatrics
UCLA School of Medicine;
Clinical Director
Sepulveda VA Geriatric Research Education and Clinical Center
Sepulveda, California

Roxie L. Foster, RN, PhD
Assistant Research Professor
School of Nursing
University of Colorado
Health Sciences Center
Denver, Colorado

Nancy O. Hester, RN, BS, MN, PhD
Associate Professor and Assistant Director
Center for Nursing Research
School of Nursing
University of Colorado
Health Sciences Center
Denver, Colorado

Mary Ellen Jeans, N, PhD
Shaw Professor and Director
School of Nursing
McGill University
Montreal, Quebec

Celeste Johnston, RN, DEd
Associate Professor
McGill University;
Director of Nursing Research
Montreal Children's Hospital
Montreal, Quebec

Judith A. Knighton, RN, MScN
Clinical Nurse Specialist, Burns
The Wellesley Hospital;
Clinical Associate
Graduate School Division
Faculty of Nursing
University of Toronto
Toronto, Ontario

Sandra M. LeFort, RN, BA, BN, MN
Doctoral Student
School of Nursing
McGill University
Montreal, Quebec

Ronald Melzack, PhD
Professor
McGill University
Montreal, Quebec

Judith A. Paice, RN, MS
Assistant Professor
Rush-Presbyterian–St. Luke's Medical Center;
Doctoral Candidate
University of Illinois
Chicago, Illinois

Lori Palozzi, RN, BScN, MScN
Pediatric Clinical Nurse Specialist
The Hospital for Sick Children
Toronto, Ontario

Kathleen M. Rowat, N, PhD
Associate Director, Programs
School of Nursing
McGill University
Montreal, Quebec

Marybeth Singer, RN, BSN, OCN
Pain Consultant
Staff Nurse
Dana Farber Cancer Institute
Boston, Massachusetts

Caroline M. Smith-Hanrahan, BS, N, MSc, PhD
Assistant Professor
School of Nursing
McGill University
Montreal, Quebec

Judith A. Spross, RN, MS, OCN
Assistant Professor
MGH Institute of Health Professions
Boston, Massachusetts

Bonnie Stevens, RN, MScN, PhD Candidate
Assistant Professor
School of Nursing
McMaster University
Hamilton, Ontario

Tracy J. Wasylak, BN, MSc
Nursing Unit Director
Intensive Care Unit/Critical Care Unit
Holy Cross Hospital
Calgary, Alberta

Robin E. Weir, RN, BScN, MS, MEd, PhD
Associate Professor
School of Nursing
Faculty of Health Sciences
McMaster University;
Clinical Associate
Pain Clinic
Chedoke-McMaster Hospitals
Hamilton, Ontario

Susan M. Wright, RN, DNSc
Clinical Assistant Professor/Consultant in Pain Management
Department of Medical-Surgical Nursing
University of Illinois
Champaign/Urbana, Illinois

To those whose support was essential:
Peter and Mike, Simon, Emily, Stephen and Katie,
our parents,
colleagues, and friends.

PAIN

This eternal now
Which cannot remember
a time when it was not
nor a time when it shall not be
White-hot, incessant iron
inscrutable, beyond my knowing.
But I can see
the place where it dwells
how it has wrought
the tired agony of your face
branded every motion
of your body with invisible flames
forged the shape of the words
mouthed by a voice
from out of the fire.

—All I Feel
All
Pain

Carolyn Schmidt
BScN, Year 4
University of Toronto
with permission

Preface

Pain management presents many challenges for nurses working with patients in a variety of settings. Poor pain control for both adults and children has been well documented in practice and research.

Nurses have become more effective in managing pain through their increasing clinical expertise and their utilization of research. This book is a compilation of chapters written by nursing experts in both practice and research, who discuss practical approaches in working toward better pain control with their patients.

Each contributor has been asked to examine issues in his or her area of expertise; to discuss current research, literature, and experience as a rationale for practice; and to outline specific practical approaches to pain assessment and/or management in their area.

It is hoped that this book will contribute to more effective nursing practice in helping patients to manage their pain. To facilitate this, the fit between practice and research will be carefully analyzed. Our purpose is to clarify common areas of difficulty, present new knowledge, and stimulate the reader's own thinking toward possible solutions.

J.H.W.W.
M.I.D.

Contents

PART II
DEVELOPMENTAL DIFFERENCES IN PAIN MANAGEMENT

PART III
PAIN ISSUES FOR SELECTED PATIENTS

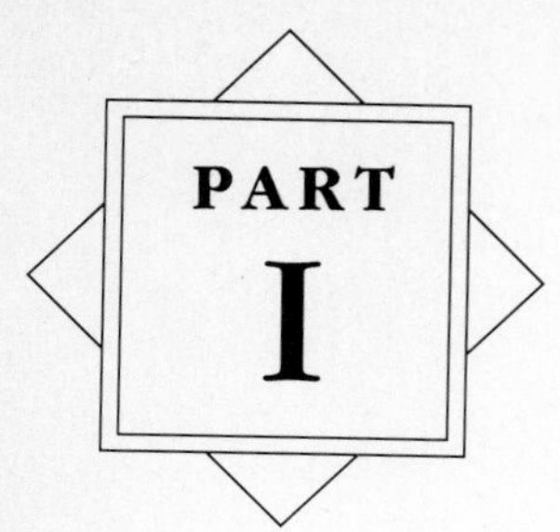

GENERAL UNDERSTANDING OF PAIN

1

Current Status of Pain Management

Marilee Ivers Donovan
Judith H. Watt-Watson

As we move through the last decade of this century, poor pain relief continues to be a problem for both patients and professional caregivers. Millions of people experience acute and chronic pain every year, yet effective pain management seems elusive. Consequently pain is the most frequent cause of suffering and disability for many people, significantly decreasing their quality of life.[5]

The approaches we use to manage pain represent a collage of reactions to a concept of pain that has evolved over thousands of years. Current practices in pain management seem to reflect outdated thinking rather than current knowledge and research. Aristotle, in the fourth century BC, believed that pain was an emotion. Today there are still those who practice, study, and publish in a manner that suggests they believe pain is primarily an emotional reaction that can be conquered by willpower. It is disconcerting to hear professional caregivers suggest that their patients with persistent pain "could get better if they really wanted to."

In the Middle Ages, pain was viewed as a possession by demons, punishment for sins, and the will of God. Kilwein[20] suggests that pain continues to be perceived as having some redeeming value and as synonymous with moral weakness. As a result, caregivers are unwilling to give adequate analgesic doses for pain relief, fears of addiction are exaggerated, and patients suffer needlessly. Research continues to demonstrate that professional caregivers do not have the goal of total relief for patients.[10,11,15,29,34]

In the nineteenth century, the role of the nervous system in the transmission of pain was discovered, and thus began our romance with neurosurgery and anesthesia. Removing the pain by severing or blocking a nerve became acceptable, but covering up the pain by using treatments, particularly medications, was a sign of weakness or a breach of morality. These beliefs are still evident among patients, family members, and caregivers. Their responses to pain management approaches, particularly analgesia, reflect some beliefs that do not encourage pain relief. These misbeliefs suggest that covering up pain is dangerous and that suffering has merit.

Melzack and Wall's gate control theory,[24] which proposed that the dorsal horn, the brain stem, and the cortex played essential roles in enhancing, modulating, and integrating the pain experience, brought a more holistic view of pain than earlier pain theories had allowed. The most significant contributions of Melzack and Wall to the understanding of pain were their identifications of the gating mechanism by which painful impulses are modulated in the dorsal horn of the spinal cord before ascending to the thalamus and cortex, where they are recognized as pain; and the interacting effects of cognitive and emotional processes within the cerebral cortex and midbrain on the transmission of painful impulses. The gate control theory acknowledged that emotional states, learning, knowledge, and thought processes help to determine whether the gating mechanism in the spinal cord allows or stops the transmission of pain impulses.

This suggestion of a link between cortical processes and pain transmission reactivated interest in the relationships between psychological states and pain perception. Indeed, gate control theory stimulated the development of a new field in psychology, and soon a variety of new techniques for pain management emerged. Many of these are discussed in the chapters that follow. Imagery, distraction, music therapy, laughter, and sensory information can be broadly classified as behavioral or cognitive approaches to the management of pain. The rationale for their use comes from the gate control theory, which links cognitive and emotional functioning with the transmission and perception of pain.

Cutaneous stimulation techniques interfere with the transmission of pain impulses, decreasing the perception of pain.

Cutaneous stimulation, such as the application of heat or cold, massage, acupuncture, transcutaneous electrical nerve stimulation (TENS), and implanted electrical stimulation of the dorsal columns and thalamus have also become increasingly common in practice. Biofeedback is both a distraction technique that modulates incoming painful stimuli and a method of reducing the muscle activity that may be contributing to the pain.

In the early 1970s, the discovery of endogenous opiates[26] suggested that spinal opioid analgesia might be useful in pain management. Nonnarcotic analgesics, particularly nonsteroidal antiinflammatory drugs, gained more prominence in the early 1980s. However, to date, the ideal therapy that would be simple, universally effective, nonaddicting, without side effects, inexpensive, able to meet every patient's needs, and requiring little nursing time has been elusive. Interventions that require large expenditures of nursing time have become less acceptable as a result of prospective reimbursement and nursing clinical pressures. Even the intervention that seems to be most effective, patient-controlled analgesia (PCA), is not embraced by all patients. Thus there is still no panacea for acute or chronic pain.

Unfortunately, the well-documented information from hospice programs in England and the United States has done little to correct the misbeliefs and practices of caregivers. The prevalence of misbeliefs is discussed in Chapter 3. It is still commonly but erroneously believed that tolerance inevitably develops if a patient is given a narcotic on a regular basis. The fear of addiction remains common among patients, family members, nurses, and physicians, despite large studies indicating a risk of less than 1%.[27] The erroneous belief that morphine commonly produces life-threatening respiratory depression has been reinforced most effectively by the notorious *Journal of the American Medical Association* article, "It's over Debbie."[16] The result of this misbelief is that patients are undermedicated.

We now have the ability to modulate or reduce pain at four points:

1. At peripheral sites of pain, nonopioid analgesics, heat and cold application, and local anesthetics can alter the release of nociceptive substances and decrease accompanying muscle spasm response.
2. In the spinal cord, stimulation of large nerve fibers (by

direct electrical stimulation, massage, heat and cold application, and therapeutic touch), epidural analgesics, tricyclic antidepressants, and neurosurgical procedures can interfere with the transmission of nerve impulses.
3. In the brain stem, electrical stimulation, tricyclic antidepressants, opioid analgesics, and neurosurgical procedures can effectively reduce or eliminate the transmission of pain impulses.
4. In the cortex, cognitive techniques (hypnosis, imagery, music therapy, relaxation), behavioral training, and opioid analgesics provide additional methods to control the pain experience.

With all of these interventions available, one would expect that pain would usually be adequately controlled; however, that is not the case.

In 1986, the NIH-sponsored consensus conference on pain concluded that despite all the resources and therapies available, acute pain and cancer pain are significantly undertreated, and chronic pain is often overmedicated. The pain management of children is significantly worse than that of adults.[25]

The current prevalence of ineffective pain management has been clearly documented with both adults and children. With adults, a significant lack of knowledge about pain assessment and management has been documented in both nurses and physicians.[6,7,34] Inadequate analgesic knowledge has been clearly evident for many years, with surgical patients,[8,19] medical patients,[21] and terminal cancer patients.[28,29] It is not surprising then, that pain relief has been frequently described as inadequate for a variety of patients.

In Donovan, Dillon, and McGuire's[11] sample of 465 medical and surgical patients, 58% had experienced excruciating or horrible pain in the previous 72 hours. Of these patients with pain, 55% could not recall having a nurse even ask about their pain, and only 31% had pain noted on their chart. It is interesting that a poor relationship was evident between the patient's self-reports of pain and the amount of analgesic given ($r = 0.27$). Camp's study[6] with 30 nurse-patient pairs in an oncology setting showed that nurses charted less than 18.5% of the patients' pain information and were less than 14% in agreement with what the patients described. Teske, Daut, and Cleeland[33] also showed a minimal relationship between patients' self-reports of pain and nurses' judgments of pain based on nonverbal behavior (r = 0.32 for acute pain, r = 0.28 for chronic pain). In Rankin and Snider's[29] sample of 52 nurses in an oncology setting, 82% of nurses believed their patients received adequate medications for pain control, but 67% stated their patients had moderate pain.

Pain complaints with older patients are often related to diseases associated with aging, such as postherpetic neuralgia, degenerative disc or joint disease, arthritis, diabetic neuropathy, or cancer. Some of these problems cause excruciating pain. Although assumptions are commonly made about pain in the elderly, there is minimal examination of this phenomenon in the literature. The effect of aging on the physiology of the pain experience is not well understood. Therefore the lack of substantive information encourages assumptions and misconceptions about the pain experience in the elderly population.[1]

With infants and children, pain measurement can be difficult, and there is a tendency for health providers to rely on personal belief systems and assumptions in assessing and managing their pain.[3,17] The discrepancy in the fewer analgesics given to children compared with the greater doses given to adults with the same diagnoses is a serious concern.

The inadequacy of analgesic administration with children experiencing postoperative pain has been clearly established in research over a considerable time period.[4,12,22,30-32] Beyer et al[4] compared the narcotics ordered for 50 adults and 50 children after open-heart surgery. Children were prescribed fewer narcotics than the adults, and the doses were often inaccurate and inadequate. The adults received almost two and a half times the analgesics given to the children, and 25% of the children received no analgesics. In a sample of adults and children with burns and abdominal and orthopedic surgery,[30] the adults received twice as many doses of narcotics per day compared with the children. Infants and young children were less likely to have narcotics ordered for them, and greater discrepancies between adults and children were evident with longer hospital stays.

The extent to which preterm and newborn infants feel pain is controversial. It has historically been suggested that infants do not feel pain and therefore do not need analgesics or anesthetics when undergoing procedures or surgeries. However, in spite of the fact that infants are unable to verbalize their experience,[9,23] recent work shows that full-term neonates do respond to painful stimuli.[2,13,18] Neonates and preterm infants undergoing surgery with deep anesthetics are more clinically stable during surgery, have a marked decrease in the physiological stress response, and have fewer postoperative complications than those receiving minimal or no anesthetics.[2] One hopes with the recent advances in neonatal research, practices will change.

The assessment and treatment of pain seems to be as problematic today as the ineffective pain management documented by Marks and Sachar[21] more than 18 years ago. It is important to acknowledge that for some patients, complete pain relief may not be possible. Although some pain involving peripheral or central pain pathway pathology is very difficult to manage, the patients with these problems are in the minority. Pain in the majority of individuals can be successfully assessed and managed, which brings us to the purpose of this book.

A serious gap exists in the fit between research findings and changes in pain management practices. Researchers tend to write for each other, in language not easily understood, and with minimal discussion of implications for day-to-day nursing practice.[14] Research findings need to be shared with nurses working daily with pain patients in order to generate new ways of looking at pain and new approaches to practice. This book is an attempt to communicate current research findings in a meaningful way to clinicians.

The following chapters describe pain management from a nursing perspective. The contributors are experienced clinicians as well as researchers. A general understanding of pain management is explored in the first section. This encompasses the conceptual basis for pain management, misbeliefs that obstruct effective practice, ethical issues complicating care, and specific assessment and management approaches with implications for families. Developmental differences in the pain management of infants, children, and elders are examined in the middle section. Finally, assessment and management of patients with specific pain problems related to surgery, cancer, arthritis, burns, and chronic pain are discussed with unique suggestions for each. The integration of the authors' theoretical and research knowledge with expertise in pain management provides rich, diverse content relevant to all nurses in clinical practice working with pain patients.

REFERENCES

1. Amadio P, Cummings D, and Amadio P. (Nov 1987). Pain in the elderly: management techniques. *Pain Manage,* 33-41.
2. Anand KJS and Hickey P. (1987). Pain and its effects in the human neonate and fetus. *N Engl J Med, 317*(21), 1321-1329.
3. Beyer J and Byers M. (1985). Knowledge of pediatric pain: the state of the art. *Child Health Care, 13*(4), 150-159.
4. Beyer J, DeGood D, Ashley L, and Russell G. (1983). Pattern of postoperative analgesia with adults and children following cardiac surgery. *Pain, 17,* 71-81.
5. Bonica J. (1990). *The management of pain,* (ed 2), London: Lea & Febiger, vol 1.
6. Camp L. (1988). A comparison of nurses' recorded assessments of pain with perceptions of pain as described by cancer patients. *Cancer Nurs, 11*(4), 237-243.
7. Chapman P, Ganendran A, Scott R, and Basford K. (1987). Attitudes and knowledge of nursing staff in relation to management of postoperative pain. *Aust N Z J Surg, 57,* 447-450.
8. Cohen F. (1980). Postsurgical pain relief: patients' status and nurses' medication choices. *Pain, 9,* 265-274.
9. Davis D and Calhoon M. (1989). Do preterm infants show behavioral responses to painful procedures? In Funk S, Tornquist E, Champayne M, et al (eds), *Key aspects of comfort* (pp. 35-45). New York: Springer Publishing Company.
10. Donovan M and Dillon P. (1987). Incidence and characteristics of pain in a sample of hospitalized cancer patients. *Cancer Nurs, 10*(20), 85-92.
11. Donovan M, Dillon P, and McGuire L. (1987). Incidence and characteristics of pain in a sample of medical-surgical inpatients. *Pain, 30,* 69-78.
12. Eland J and Anderson J. (1977). The experience of pain in children. In Jacox A (ed), *Pain: a source book for nurses and other professionals* (pp. 453-473). Boston: Little, Brown & Company.
13. Fletcher A. (1987). Pain in the neonate. *N Engl J Med, 317*(21), 1347-1348.
14. Funk S and Tornquist E. (1989). Patient comfort: from research to practice. In Funk S, Tornquist E, Champagne M, et al (eds), *Key aspects of comfort: management of pain, fatigue, and nausea* (pp. 3-21). New York: Springer Publishing Company.
15. Halvorson M and Page G. (1988). *The assessment and control of pain in preverbal infants.* Paper presented at a national conference on key aspects of comfort: management of pain, fatigue, and nausea, Chapel Hill, NC.
16. It's over Debbie. (1988). Letter to the editor. *JAMA, 259,* 272.
17. Jeans M. (1983). Pain in children: a neglected area. In Firestone P, McGrath P, Feldman W (eds), *Advances in behavioral medicine for children and adolescents.* Hillsdale, NJ: Lawrence Erlbaum Associates.
18. Johnston C and Strada M. (1986). Acute pain response in infants: a multidimensional description. *Pain, 24,* 373-382.
19. Keeri-Szanto M and Heaman S. (1972). Postoperative demand analgesia. *Surg Gynecol Obstet, 134,* 647-651.
20. Kilwein J. (1983). Valium and values. *Am Pharm, NS23*(12), 5-7.

21. Marks R and Sachar M. (1973). Undertreatment of medical inpatients with narcotic analgesics. *Ann Intern Med, 78,* 173-181.
22. Mather L and Mackie J. (1983). The incidence of postoperative pain in children. *Pain, 15,* 271-282.
23. McGrath P and Unruh A. (1987). *Pain in children and adolescents.* New York: Elsevier.
24. Melzack R and Wall P. (1965). Pain mechanisms: a new theory. *Science, 150,* 971-979.
25. National Institutes of Health. (1986). *Consensus development conference statement: the integrated approach to the management of pain.* USHHS, *6*(3), (document number 491-292:41148).
26. Pert C and Snyder S. (1973). Opiate receptor: demonstration in nervous tissue. *Science, 179,* 1001-1004.
27. Porter J and Jick H. (1980). Addiction rare in patients treated with narcotics. *N Engl J Med, 303*(2), 123.
28. Rankin M. (1982). Use of drugs for pain with cancer patients. *Cancer Nurs, 5,* 181-190.
29. Rankin M and Snider B. (1984). Nurses' perceptions of cancer patients' pain. *Cancer Nurs, 1,* 149-155.
30. Schecter N, Allen D, and Hanson K. (1986). Status of pediatric pain control: a comparison of hospital analgesic usage in children and adults. *Pediatrics, 77,* 11-15.
31. Strauss A, Fagerhaugh S, and Glaser B. (1974). Pain: an organizational-work-interactive perspective. *Nurs Outlook, 22,* 560-566.
32. Swafford L and Allen D. (1968). Pain relief in the pediatric patient. *Med Clin North Am, 52*(1), 131-135.
33. Teske K, Daut R, and Cleeland C. (1983). Relationships between nurses' observations and patients' self-reports of pain. *Pain, 16,* 289-296.
34. Watt-Watson J. (1987). Nurses' knowledge of pain issues: a survey. *J Pain Sympt Manage, 2*(4), 207-211.

2

Conceptual Basis of Nursing Practice: Theoretical Foundations of Pain

Mary Ellen Jeans
Ronald Melzack

◆ OVERVIEW

There is substantial evidence that current nursing practice often fails to meet patients' needs for adequate pain relief. Marks and Sachar,[30] Mather and Mackie,[32] and Donovan, Dillon, and McGuire,[13] have shown that there may also be a lack of accountability for pain relief. Although nurses have long been carrying out important research on many aspects of pain management, it is clear that there is a need for the development of a conceptual basis for the management of pain by nurses.

To strengthen the link between theory and practice, this chapter will describe a theoretical foundation for the understanding of pain and pain relief. The aim of the chapter is to provide a basis for understanding the possible mechanisms of action of the physical and psychological interventions used by nurses and described throughout this text. Clinical decisions as to which pain management approaches to select for an individual patient require a thorough understanding of the physiological and psychological aspects of pain and the many variables that influence pain and pain relief.

Pain is a highly personal and variable subjective experience that is influenced by cultural learning, the meaning of the situation in which it occurs, attention, anxiety, and a host of other cognitive and psychological variables. It is generally acknowledged that pain is a signal that body tissues are being or have been injured. However, it is important to remember that pain processes do not begin with the stimulation of receptors. Rather, injury or disease produces neural signals that enter an already active nervous system that represents the substrate of past experience, culture, anxiety, and other ongoing and current neural processes. These brain processes actively influence the selection, abstraction, and synthesis of information from the total sensory input at any given time. Pain, then, is not simply the end product of a linear sensory transmission system, but is a dynamic process involving continuous interactions among complex ascending and descending neural systems.[41]

◆ PSYCHOLOGICAL ASPECTS OF PAIN

When compared with vision or hearing, the perception of pain seems simple, urgent, and primitive. We expect the nerve signals evoked by injury or disease to be perceived, unless we are unconscious or anesthetized. But experiments and clinical observations show that pain is much more variable and modifiable than many people have believed in the past. Pain differs from person to person and from culture to culture. Stimuli that produce intolerable pain in one person may be well tolerated by another. Pain perception, then, cannot be defined simply in terms of particular kinds of stimuli. Rather, it is a highly personal experience that depends in part on psychological factors that are unique to each individual.[39]

Cultural Determinants

It is often asserted that variations in pain experience from person to person are due to different "pain thresholds"; however, there are several thresholds related to pain, and it is important to distinguish among them. Typically, thresholds are measured by applying a stimulus such as electric shock or radiant heat to a small area of skin and gradually increasing the intensity. Four thresholds can be measured by this technique:

1. Sensation threshold—the lowest stimulus value at which a sensation such as tingling or warmth is first reported;

2. Pain perception threshold—the lowest stimulus value at which the person reports that the stimulation feels painful;
3. Pain tolerance (or upper threshold)—the lowest stimulus level at which the subject withdraws or asks to have the stimulation stopped; and
4. Encouraged pain tolerance—the highest level the subject will tolerate after being encouraged to tolerate higher levels of stimulation than identified in 3.

There is now evidence that all people, regardless of cultural background, have a uniform sensation threshold. Sternbach and Tursky[52] made careful measurements of sensation threshold, using electric shock as the stimulus, in American-born women belonging to four different ethnic groups: Italian, Jewish, Irish, and Old American. They found no differences among the groups in the level of shock that was first reported as producing a detectable sensation. The sensory conducting apparatus, in other words, appears to be essentially similar in all people so that a given level of input always elicits a sensation.

Cultural background, however, does have a powerful effect on the *pain perception threshold.* For example, levels of radiant heat that are reported as painful by people of Mediterranean origin are described only as warmth by Northern Europeans.[20] Similarly, Nepalese porters on a climbing expedition are much more stoical than the Occidental visitors for whom they work. Even though both groups are equally sensitive to changes in electric shock, the Nepalese porters require much higher intensities before they report pain.[18] The most notable effect of cultural background, however, is on pain tolerance levels. Sternbach and Tursky[52] report that the levels at which subjects refuse to tolerate electric shock, even when they are encouraged by the experimenters, depend in part on the ethnic origin of the subject. Women of Italian descent tolerate less shock than women of Old American or Jewish origin. In another experiment, in which Jewish and Protestant women served as subjects, the Jewish, but not the Protestant, women increased their tolerance level after they were told that their religious group tolerated pain more poorly than others.[27]

These differences in pain tolerance reflect different ethnic attitudes toward pain. Zborowski[59] found that Old Americans have an accepting, matter-of-fact attitude toward pain and pain expression. They tend to withdraw when the pain is intense, and cry out or moan only when they are alone. Jews and Italians, on the other hand, tend to be vociferous in their complaints and openly seek support and sympathy. The underlying attitudes of the two groups, however, appear to be different. Jews tend to be concerned about the meaning and implications of the pain, whereas Italians usually express a desire for immediate pain relief.

Past Experience

The knowledge that pain is influenced by cultural factors leads one to examine the effect of early experience on adult behavior related to pain. It is commonly accepted that children are influenced by the attitudes of their parents toward pain. In some families, a great fuss is made about ordinary cuts and bruises, whereas in others there seems to be little sympathy expressed about even fairly serious injuries. There is reason to believe, on the basis of everyday observations, that attitudes toward pain acquired early in life are carried into adulthood. These observations have been confirmed experimentally in dogs[34] and monkeys.[29] In these studies, young animals were raised in cages that protected them from the usual injuries encountered in normal development. When mature, these animals exhibited little or no response to injurious stimuli. The monkeys, for example, when released into a normal environment, often engaged in dangerous attacks against older and stronger monkeys. They also viciously bit their own limbs. These acts of self-destruction by the monkeys "have on occasion resulted in broken bones and torn skin and blood vessels. After being repaired, many of these animals fail to profit from their experiences, continuing to bite themselves and to attack larger animals who inflict new wounds . . .".[29]

Meaning of the Pain-Producing Situation

There is considerable evidence to show that people assign various meanings to pain-producing situations and that the meaning greatly influences the degree and quality of pain they report. Beecher[3] observed that, in battle, wounded soldiers rarely complained of pain, whereas civilians with similar surgical wounds usually reported severe pain. Beecher concluded the following from his study[3]:

The common belief that wounds are inevitably associated with pain, and that the more extensive the wound the worse the pain, was not supported by observations made as carefully as possible in the combat zone . . . The data state in numerical terms what is known to all thoughtful clinical observers: there is no simple direct relationship between the wound per se and the pain experienced. The pain is in very large part determined by other factors, and of great importance here is the significance of the wound . . . In the wounded soldier (the response to injury) was relief, thankfulness at his escape alive from the battlefield, even euphoria; to the civilian, his major surgery was a depressing, calamitous event.

Another study of Israeli soldiers with traumatic amputations after the Yom Kippur War provided similar observations.[5] Most of the wounded men described their initial injury as painless and used neutral terms such as "bang," "thump," or "blow" to describe their first sensation. They often seemed surprised that the injury did not hurt.

Melzack, Wall, and Ty[40] studied features of acute pain in patients at an emergency clinic. Patients who had severe, life-threatening injuries or who were agitated, drunk, or "in shock" were not included in the study. Of the 138 patients who were assessed, 51 (37%) reported no pain at the time of injury. The majority of these patients stated that pain began within an hour of injury, although some patients reported onset of pain as long as 9 hours or more after injury. Delays in pain onset were related to the type of injury sustained. Of 46 patients whose injuries were limited to skin (lacerations, cuts, abrasions, burns), 53% had a pain-free period. Of 86 patients with deep-tissue injuries (fractures, sprains, bruises, amputation of a finger, stabs, and crushes), 28% reported a pain-free period. The findings suggest that the relationship between injury and pain is highly variable and complex.

Attention, Anxiety, and Distraction

When a person's attention is focused on a potentially painful experience, he tends to perceive more intense pain than he would normally. Hall and Stride[19] noted that the simple appearance of the word "pain" in a set of instructions made subjects more likely to report a given level of electric shock as painful. When the word was absent from the instructions, the same level of shock was seldom reported to be painful. Thus the mere anticipation of pain is sufficient to raise the level of anxiety and thereby the intensity of perceived pain. Similarly, Hill, Kornetsky, Flanary, and Wikler[21,22] have shown that if anxiety is relieved (by reassuring the subject that he has control over the pain-producing stimulus), a given level of electric shock or burning heat is perceived as significantly less painful than the same stimulus under conditions of high anxiety.

It is also well known that distraction of attention away from pain can diminish or abolish the pain. Distraction of attention may partly explain why athletes sometimes sustain severe injuries during the excitement of competition without being aware that they have been hurt. Distraction of attention may be most effective when the pain is steady or rises slowly in intensity.[36] When radiant heat is focused on the skin, for example, the pain intensity may increase so quickly and sharply that subjects are unable to control it by distraction. But when the pain intensity increases slowly, people may use various techniques to distract their attention from it. Distraction strategies are used effectively by some people to control pain produced by dental drilling and extraction.[18]

Feelings of Control Over Pain

The severity of postsurgical pain may be significantly reduced when patients are taught how to cope with their pain. Patients who were scheduled to undergo major surgery to remove the gall bladder, uterus, or portions of the digestive tract were given detailed information about the pain they would feel after the operation and how they could best cope with it. They were told where they would feel pain, how severe it could be, how long it might last, and that such pain is normal after an operation. They were also shown how to relax by using breathing and relaxation strategies. They were also told that they should request medication for pain whenever they were uncomfortable. The patients who received these instructions reported significantly less pain, requested much less medication after surgery, and spent less time in hospital than a similar group of patients who received no specific preoperative teaching.[14]

Originally, it was thought that information alone was sufficient preparation to reduce the uncertainty and anxiety associated with major surgery. It is now apparent that information alone may actually increase anxiety because of the expectation of pain and other discomforts. Recent studies have shown that simply giving patients information about their pain tends to make them focus on the discomforting aspects of the experience, and their pain is magnified rather than reduced; however, when the patients are taught skills to cope with their pain, such as relaxation or distraction strategies, the pain is less severe.[28] The positive effect of preoperative preparation, therefore, is more likely related to providing the patient with strategies to cope with the pain and anxiety and to provide him or her with a sense of control.[25,26,43] Other studies have shown that the amount of postsurgical pain is directly related to the level of anxiety experienced by the patient.[31] Feelings of control, then, appear to diminish both anxiety and pain.

Suggestion and Placebos

Studies of the effectiveness of placebos clearly demonstrate the effect of suggestion on the intensity of perceived pain. Clinical research shows that severe pain, such as postoperative pain, can be relieved in many patients by giving them a placebo (usually a nonanalgesic substance such as a sugar or salt solution) in place of morphine or other analgesics.[3] About 35% of patients reported a significant relief of pain after being given a placebo. This is a particularly high proportion because morphine, even in large doses, relieves severe pain in only about 75% of patients.

A surprising discovery about placebos is that their effectiveness is always about 50% of the potency of the drug for which they are being substituted, even in double-blind experiments;[15] that is, if the drug is a mild analgesic such as aspirin, then the pain relief produced by the placebo is half that of the aspirin. If it is a powerful drug such as morphine, the placebo has greater pain-relieving properties, again about 50% of that of morphine.

There are large individual differences in susceptibility to placebos, and research has been done to describe some of the factors involved.[15] These studies reveal that placebo responses are more evident for severe pain than for mild pain and are more likely to be evident when the patient is experiencing high levels of stress and anxiety than when he or she is not. McGlashan et al[33] have shown that placebo-induced analgesia is not significantly related to suggestibility, hypnotic susceptibility, or anxiety induced specifically by pain or the therapeutic situation (which is known as state-anxiety); however, placebo effects are more likely to occur in people who have longstanding generalized anxiety (personality trait-anxiety).

There are other interesting findings related to the placebo response. For example, two placebo capsules are more effective than one capsule, and large capsules are better than small ones. A placebo is more effective when injected than when given by mouth and is more potent when accompanied by strong suggestion that a powerful analgesic has been given. That is, the greater the implicit and explicit suggestion that pain will be relieved, the greater is the relief obtained by the patient. Unfortunately, however, patients tend to get less and less relief from repeated administration of placebos.

Summary

In this section we have reviewed the powerful role that psychological factors play in pain perception; however, they are seldom the primary or sole cause of pain. Labeling a person as "neurotic" or a pain syndrome as "psychogenic" implies psychological causation. It suggests that a person is in pain because he or she needs or wants the pain. While we must recognize the psychological contribution to pain, we must also maintain a balanced view. The psychological factors contributing to pain may be treated using psychological approaches and may help relieve pain. But there are also physical contributions.

Even when psychological factors are predominant, there is often associated tissue damage. In many cases, the physical and psychological symptoms both require treatment. Indeed, using various approaches to pain relief is required in the majority of patient situations. Using psychological labels to ascribe causation often reveals our profound ignorance of the complexity of pain mechanisms.

◆ THEORETICAL CONCEPTS OF PAIN

The traditional specificity theory of pain, which is still widely taught, proposes that pain is a specific sensation and that the intensity of pain is proportional to the extent of tissue damage. The theory implies a fixed, straight-through transmission system from pain receptors in the skin to a pain center in the brain. Today, we know that pain is not simply a function of the amount of bodily damage, but is influenced by attention, anxiety, suggestion, experience, and other psychological variables described earlier.[39] One outcome of the specificity concept of pain was the development of neurosurgical techniques to cut the so-called pain pathway. When failures occurred, they were attributed to an escape of "pain fibers," so that operations were carried out at successively higher levels of the nervous system. Generally, the results have been disappointing, particularly for low back pain, the neuralgias, and other chronic pain syndromes. Not only does the pain tend to return in a substantial number of patients, but other iatrogenic complications, such as dysesthesias, girdle pains, and various sensory-motor losses, have been described.[45]

More recent psychological and neurological data refute the concept of a single straight-through sensory transmission system. The evidence suggests that the central nervous system is characterized by plasticity and is capable of modifying inputs resulting from injury or pathology. The psychological data lend strong support to the concept of pain as a complex perceptual and affective experience determined by the unique history of the individual, by the meaning of the stimulus to him, by his "state of mind" at the moment, and by the sensory nerve patterns evoked by physical stimulation.

The Gate Control Theory of Pain

It was in the light of this understanding of pain processes that Melzack and Wall[37] proposed the gate control theory of pain. Basically, the theory states that neural mechanisms in the dorsal horns of the spinal cord act like a gate that can enhance or diminish the flow of nerve impulses from peripheral fibers to the spinal cord cells that project to the brain. Somatic input is therefore subjected to the modulating influence of the gate **before** it evokes pain perception and response. The theory suggests that large-fiber inputs tend to close the gate, small-fiber inputs generally open it, and the gate is also influenced by descending controls from the brain. It further suggests that sensory input is modulated at successive synapses throughout its projection from the spinal cord to the brain areas responsible for pain experience and response. Pain occurs when the number of nerve impulses that arrive at these areas exceeds a critical level.

Melzack and Wall[39] recently assessed the current status of the gate control theory in the light of new physiological research. It is clear that the theory has continued to thrive and evolve despite considerable controversy. The concept of gating, or input modulation, has gained increasing strength (Figure 2-1).

Spinal Cord Mechanisms

The dorsal horns, which receive fibers from the body or project impulses toward the brain, contribute to our understanding of information processing at the spinal cord level. The dorsal horns comprise several layers or laminae, each of which is now known to have specialized functions, although the inputs and outputs of each lamina are not entirely understood. But it now appears that input is modulated in the dorsal horns before it is transmitted to the brain.[23]

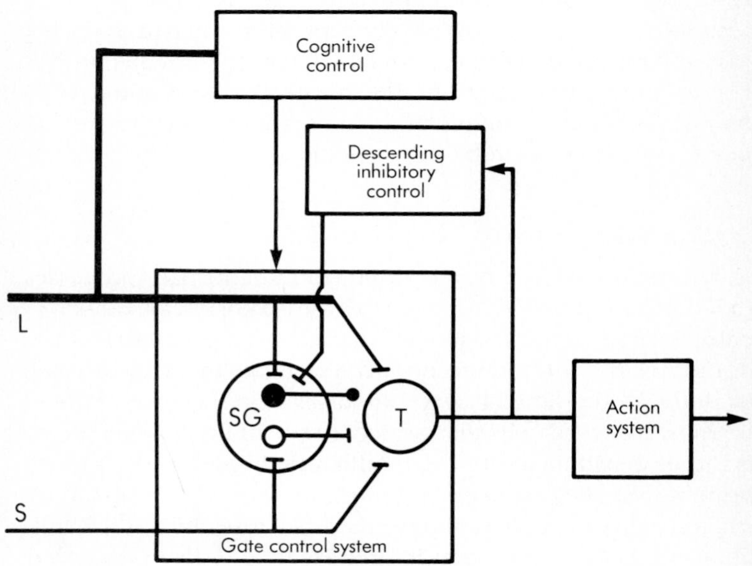

FIGURE 2-1. The gate control theory. The new model includes excitatory *(white circle)* and inhibitory *(black circle)* links from the substantia gelatinosa *(SG)* to the transmission *(T)* cells, as well as descending inhibitory control from brain-stem systems. The round knob at the end of the inhibitory link implies that its action may be presynaptic, postsynaptic, or both. All connections are excitatory, except the inhibitory link from the SG to the T cell.

The substantia gelatinosa, laminae 1 and 2, is of particular interest here because it represents a unique system on each side of the spinal cord where this modulating effect occurs.[56] Many afferent fibers from the skin terminate in the substantia gelatinosa, and the dendrites of many cells in lower laminae, whose axons project to the brain, lie within the substantia gelatinosa. This region, then, is situated between a major portion of the peripheral nerve fiber terminals and the spinal cord cells that project to the brain. There is convincing physiological evidence that the substantia gelatinosa has a modulating effect on transmission from peripheral fibers to spinal cells.[39]

Although cells in all laminae undoubtedly play a role in pain processes, lamina 5 cells are particularly responsive when noxious stimuli are applied within their receptive fields.[23] Their fields have a remarkably complex organization, and they respond with characteristic firing patterns to stimulation over a wide range of intensities. Moreover, lamina 5 cells receive multiple inputs. There is reason to believe that they receive inputs from the lamina 4 cells, which respond readily to light touch. In addition, they receive inputs from the small myelinated and unmyelinated fibers from the skin, from deeper tissues, such as blood vessels and muscles, and from the viscera.[47]

It is now also established that virtually all dorsal horn cells are under the control of fibers that descend from the brain. These cells, moreover, with the exception of the substantia gelatinosa, have extensive projections to the brain. In primates, the majority project through the spinothalamic tract, while some appear to project through the dorsalateral and dorsal column systems.

The mechanism of the inhibition produced by the large fibers and the facilitation produced by the small fibers is unknown, but Hillman and Wall[47] suggest that it may be due to presynaptic and postsynaptic effects produced by the small cells of laminae 1 and 2. A similar effect has been observed by Mendell and Wall.[42] They found that a single electrical pulse delivered to small fibers produces a burst of nerve impulses followed by repetitive discharges in spinal cord cells. Successive pulses, if delivered at sufficiently high frequency, produce a "wind-up" effect—a burst followed by a discharge of increasing duration after each stimulation. In contrast, successive pulses delivered to large fibers produce a burst of impulses followed by a "turn-off" or period of silence after each pulse. These opposing effects of facilitation and inhibition after small and large fiber stimulation are believed to be mediated by the substantia gelatinosa, and provide the physiological basis of the gate-control theory.[56]

The Gate Control Concept

The conceptual model (Figure 2-1) that underlies the gate control theory of pain is based on the following propositions:

1. The transmission of nerve impulses from afferent fibers to spinal cord transmission (T) cells is modulated by a spinal gating (SG) mechanism in the dorsal horns.
2. The spinal gating mechanism is influenced by the relative amount of activity in large-diameter (L) and small-diameter (S) fibers: Activity in large fibers tends to inhibit transmission (close the gate), and small-fiber activity tends to facilitate transmission (open the gate).
3. The spinal gating mechanism is also influenced by nerve impulses that descend from the brain.
4. A specialized system of large-diameter, rapidly conducting fibers (the central control trigger) activates higher cognitive processes that then influence, by way of descending fibers, the modulating properties of the spinal gating mechanism.
5. When the output of the spinal cord transmission (T) cells exceeds a critical level, it activates the action system—those neural areas that underlie the complex, sequential patterns of behavior and experience characteristic of pain.

The small (A-delta and C) fibers, in this conceptual framework, play a highly specialized and important role in pain processes in that they activate the T cells directly and contribute to their output. The activity of high-threshold small fibers, during intense stimulation, may be especially important in raising the T cell output above the critical level necessary for pain. But the small fibers are believed to do much more than this.[39] They facilitate transmission ("open the gate") and thereby provide the basis for summation, prolonged activity, and spread of pain to other body areas. This facilitative influence provides the small fibers with greater power than was envisaged in the concept of "pain fibers." Yet at the same time, the small-fiber impulses are susceptible to modulation by activities in the entire nervous system. This multifaceted role of the small fibers is consistent with the psychological, clinical, and physiological evidence.The substantia gelatinosa, laminae 1 and 2, appears to be the most likely site of the spinal gating mechanism.[39,56] It receives axon terminals from many of the large- and small-diameter fibers, and the dendrites of cells in deeper laminae project into it. The substantia gelatinosa, moreover, forms a functional unit that extends the length of the spinal cord on each side. Furthermore, its rostral extension is continuous with the substantia gelatinosa of the trigeminal system. Its cells connect with one another by short fibers and influence each other at distant sites on the same side by means of Lissauer's tract and on the opposite side by means of commissural fibres that cross the cord.[54] The substantia gelatinosa, then, consists of a highly specialized, closed system of cells throughout the length of the spinal cord on both sides; it receives afferent input from large and small fibers, and is able to influence the activity of cells that project to the brain.

We have already noted that cognitive or higher central nervous system processes exert a powerful influence on pain. It is also firmly established that stimulation of several different brain regions activates descending efferent fibers that can influence afferent conduction at the earliest synaptic levels of the somesthetic system. Thus it is possible for brain activities subserving attention, emotion, and memories of previous experience to exert control over the sensory input. This control of spinal cord transmission by the brain may be exerted through several systems.

Brain stem projections. Specialized areas in the brain stem, particularly, the midbrain, exert a powerful inhibitory control over information projected by the spinal transmission cells. The inhibition of activity in dorsal horn cells by descending fibers from the brain is at least partly due to brain stem influences on the dorsal horn gating system. This descending inhibitory projection is itself controlled by multiple influences, including somatic, visual, and auditory projections to the midbrain reticular formation.[48] Higher brain stem areas are also involved in descending control.[1,2] Injection of morphine into a lateral ventricle produces analgesia of only the ipsilateral side of the body, thus implicating an adjacent thalamic region.[9] Moreover, electrical stimulation of the habenula and adjacent thalamic areas produces a striking analgesia bilaterally.[10] Stimulation of hypothalamic areas also produces analgesia.[6] There is a rapidly growing body of evidence that several neuropharmacological systems are also involved in descending control.

Cortical projections. Fibers from the whole cortex, particularly the frontal cortex, project to the reticular formation. Cognitive processes such as previous experience and attention, which are subserved at least in part by cortical neural activity, are therefore able to influence spinal activities by way of the reticulospinal projection system. Cognitive processes can also influence spinal gating mechanisms by means of pyramidal (or corticospinal) fibers, which are known to project to the dorsal horns as well as to other spinal areas. These are large, fast-conducting fibers so that cognitive processes can rapidly and directly modulate neural transmission in the dorsal horns.

Concept of a central control trigger. It is apparent that the influence of cognitive "central control" processes on spinal transmission is mediated, in part at least, through the gate control system. Although some central activities, such as anxiety or excitement, may open or close the gate for all inputs from any part of the body, others are obviously more selective and localized in their influence on gate activity. Melzack and Wall[37] have therefore proposed that there exists in the nervous system a mechanism, which they have called the **central control trigger,** that activates the particular, selective brain processes. These brain activities, they suggest, do not give rise to sensory experience, but instead act, by way of central-control efferent fibers, on the gate control system. Part, at least, of their functions, then, could be to activate selective brain processes, such as memories of previous experience and preset response strategies that influence information that is still arriving over slowly conducting fibers or is being transmitted up more slowly conducting pathways. These functions will be discussed in more detail in the next section.

The Dimensions of Pain Experience

The concept of pain, since the beginning of this century, has been dominated by the notion that pain is purely a sensory experience. Yet pain also has a distinctly unpleasant, affective quality. It becomes overwhelming, demands immediate attention, and disrupts ongoing behavior and thought. It motivates or drives the organism into activity aimed at stopping the pain as quickly as possible. To consider only the sensory features of pain and ignore its motivational-affective properties is to look at only part of the problem. Even the concept of pain as a perception, with full recognition of previous experience, attention, and other cognitive influences, still neglects the crucial motivational dimension.

The motivational-affective dimension of pain is brought clearly into focus by clinical studies on frontal lobotomy, congenital insensitivity to pain, and pain asymbolia. Patients who have undergone a frontal lobotomy (which severs the connections between the prefrontal lobes and the thalamus) rarely complain about severe clinical pain or ask for medication.[17] Typically, these patients report that they still have pain but it does not bother them. When they are questioned more closely, they frequently say that they still have the "little" pain, but the "big" pain, the suffering, and the anguish are gone. It is certain that the sensory component of pain is still present because these patients may complain vociferously about pin prick and mild burn. The predominant effect of lobotomy, in relation to pain, appears to be on the motivational-affective dimension. The aversive quality of the pain and the drive to seek pain relief both appear to be diminished.

People who are congenitally insensitive to pain are still able to feel pricking, warmth, cold, and pressure. They give accurate reports of increasing intensity of stimulation, but the input, even at intense, noxious levels, never gives rise to reports of pain. The evidence[53] suggests that it is not the sensory properties of the input but rather the motivational-affective properties that are absent. Similarly, patients who have lesions of portions of the parietal lobe or the frontal cortex and exhibit "pain asymbolia" are able to appreciate the spatial and temporal properties of noxious stimuli but fail to withdraw or complain about them.[49]

These considerations suggest that there are three major psychological dimensions of pain: sensory-discriminative, motivational-affective, and cognitive-evaluative. Melzack and Casey[38] have proposed that they are subserved by physiologically specialized systems in the brain (Figure 2-2).

Physiological Mechanisms

The sensory-discriminative dimension. Physiological and behavioral data suggest that several rapidly conducting systems—the neospinothalamic tract, the spinocervical tract,

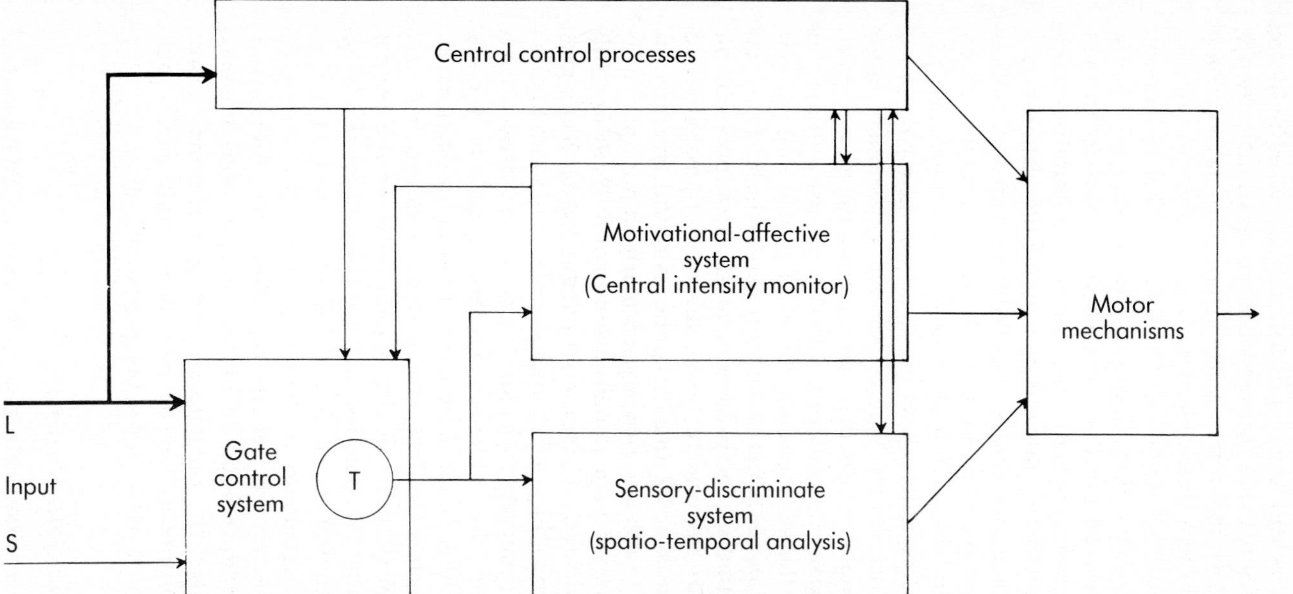

FIGURE 2-2. Conceptual model of the sensory, motivational, and central control determinants of pain. The output of the T cells of the gate control system projects to the sensory-discriminative system (via neospinothalamic fibers) and the motivational-affective system (via the paramedial ascending system). The central control trigger is represented by a line running from the larger fiber system to central control processes; these, in turn, project back to the gate control system and to the sensory-discriminative and motivational-affective system. All three systems interact with one another and project to the motor system.

and possibly the postsynaptic neurons in the dorsal column system—contribute to the sensory-discriminative dimension of pain. Neurons in the ventrobasal thalamus, which receive a large portion of their afferent input from these systems, have a discrete somatotropic organization. Studies in human patients and in animals have shown that surgical section of the dorsal columns, long presumed to subserve virtually all of the discriminative capacity of the skin sensory system, produces little or no loss in fine tactile discrimination and localization.[55] Furthermore, Semmes and Mishkin[51] found marked deficits in tactile discrimination that are attributable to injury of the cortical projection of the neospinothalamic system: Taken together, these data suggest that the rapidly conducting projection systems have the capacity to transmit precise information about the spatial, temporal, and magnitudinal properties of input that characterizes the sensory-discriminative dimension of pain.

The motivational-affective dimension. There is convincing evidence that the brain stem reticular formation and the limbic system, which receive projections from the spinoreticular and paleospinothalamic components of the anterolateral somatosensory pathway, play a particularly important role in the motivational-affective dimension of pain.[38] These medially coursing fibers, which comprise a "paramedial ascending system", tend to be short and connect diffusely with one another during their ascent from the spinal cord to the brain.[38] They are not organized to carry discrete spatial and temporal information. Their target cells in the brain usually have wide receptive fields, sometimes covering half or more of the body surface. In addition to the convergence of somatosensory fibers, inputs from other sensory systems, such as vision and audition, also arrive at many of these cells.

Reticular formation. It is well established that the reticular formation is involved in aversive drive and similar pain-related behavior. Stimulation of nucleus gigantocellularis in the medulla[7] and the central gray and adjacent areas in the midbrain[11] produces strong aversive drive and behavior typical of responses to naturally occurring painful stimuli. In contrast, lesions of the central gray or spinothalamic tract produce marked decreases in responsiveness to noxious stimuli.[35] In humans, lesions in the medial thalamus (parafascicular and centromedian complex) and intralaminar nuclei have provided relief from intractable pain.[58]

Limbic system. The reciprocal interconnections between the reticular formation and the limbic system is of particular importance in pain processes.[38] The midbrain central gray, which is traditionally part of the reticular formation, is also a major gateway to the limbic system. It is part of the "limbic midbrain area" that projects to the medial thalamus and hypothalamus, which in turn project to limbic forebrain structures.[44] Many of these areas also interact with portions of the frontal cortex that are sometimes functionally designated as part of the limbic system.

It is now firmly established that the limbic system plays an important role in pain processes.[38] Electrical stimulation of the hippocampus, amygdala, or other limbic structures may evoke escape or other attempts to stop stimulation.[12] After ablation of the amygdala and overlying cortex, cats showed marked changes in affective behavior, including decreased responsiveness to noxious stimuli.[50] Surgical section of the cingulum bundle, which connects the frontal cortex to the hippocampus, also produces a loss of negative affect associated with intractable pain in human subjects.[16] This evidence indicates that limbic structures, although playing a role in many other functions, provide a neural basis for the aversive drive and affect that make up the motivational dimension of pain. These data clearly demonstrate that the neural areas comprising the paramedial, reticular, and limbic systems are involved in the motivational and affective features of pain. The manner in which these areas are brought into play will be discussed shortly.

The cognitive-evaluative dimension. We have already noted that cognitive activities such as cultural values, anxiety, attention, and suggestion all have a profound effect on pain experience. These activities, which are subserved in part at least by cortical processes, may affect the sensory-discriminative dimension or the motivational-affective dimension. Thus excitement in games or war appears to block both of these dimensions of pain, but suggestion and placebos may modulate the motivational-affective dimension and leave the sensory-discriminative dimension relatively undisturbed.

Cognitive functions, then, are able to act selectively on sensory processing or motivational mechanisms. In addition, there is evidence that the sensory input is localized, identified in terms of its physical properties, evaluated in terms of past experience, and modified **before** it activates the discriminative or motivational systems. Men wounded in battle may feel little or no pain from the wound but may complain bitterly about an inept vein puncture.[3] Dogs that repeatedly receive food immediately after the skin is shocked, burned, or cut soon respond to these stimuli as signals for food and salivate, without showing any signs of pain, yet howl as normal dogs would when the stimuli are applied to other sites on the body.[46]

The neural system that performs these complex functions of identification, evaluation, and selective input modulation must conduct rapidly to the cortex so that somatosensory information has the opportunity to undergo further analysis, interact with other sensory inputs, and activate memory stores and preset response strategies. It must then be able to act selectively on the sensory and motivational systems to influence their response to the information being transmitted over more slowly conducting pathways. Melzack and Wall[37] have proposed that the dorsal column and dorsolateral projection pathways act as the "feed-forward" limb of this loop. The dorsal column pathway, in particular, has grown apace with the cerebral cortex, carries precise information about the nature and location of the stimulus, adapts quickly to give precedence to phasic stimulus changes rather than prolonged tonic activity, and conducts rapidly to the cortex so that its impulses may begin activation of central control processes.[4]

Influences that descend from the cortex are known to act, via pyramidal and other central-control fibers, on portions of the sensory-discriminative system such as the ventrobasal thalamus.[38] Moreover, the powerful descending inhibitory influences exerted on dorsal-horn cells in the spinal cord can modulate the input before it is transmitted to the discriminative and motivational systems (Figure 2-1).[23] These rapidly conducting ascending and descending systems can thus account for the fact that psychological processes play a powerful role in determining the quality and intensity of pain.

The Conceptual Model

The physiological and behavioral evidence described above led Melzack and Casey[38] to extend the gate control theory to include the motivational dimension of pain (Figure 2-2). They proposed the following:

1. The sensory-discriminative dimension of pain is influenced primarily by the rapidly conducting spinal systems.
2. The powerful motivational drive and unpleasant affect characteristic of pain are subserved by activities in reticular and limbic structures that are influenced primarily by the slowly conducting spinal systems.
3. Neocortical or higher central nervous system processes, such as evaluation of the input in terms of past experience, exert control over activity in both the discriminative and motivational systems.

It is assumed that these three categories of activity interact with one another to provide **perceptual information** regarding the location, magnitude, and spatiotemporal properties of the noxious stimulus, **motivational tendency** toward escape or attack, and **cognitive information** based on analysis of multimodal information, past experience, and probability of outcome of different response strategies. All three forms of activity could then influence motor mechanisms responsible for the complex pattern of overt responses that characterize pain.

A crucial question remains. The somatic input has access to reticular and limbic areas involved in both approach and avoidance, and stimulation of some areas can produce either kind of response. On what basis, then, are aversive rather than approach mechanisms triggered by the input?

Melzack and Casey propose that portions of the reticular and limbic systems function as a **central intensity monitor:** that their activities are determined, in part at least, by the intensity of the T cell output (the total number of active fibers and their rate of firing) after it has undergone modulation by the gate control system in the dorsal horns. The cells in the midbrain reticular formation are capable of summation of input from spatially separate body sites; furthermore, the poststimulus discharge activity of some of these cells lasts for many seconds, so that their activity may provide a measure of the intensity of the total T cell output over relatively long periods of time. Essentially, both kinds of summation transform discrete spatial and temporal information into intensity information. Melzack and Casey propose that the output of these cells, up to a critical intensity level, activates those brain areas that subserve positive affect and approach tendency. Beyond that level, the output activates areas that underlie negative affect and aversive drive. They suggest, therefore, that the drive mechanisms associated with pain are activated when the somatosensory input into the motivational-affective system exceeds the critical level. This notion fits well with observations that animals seek low-intensity electrical stimulation of some limbic system structures, but avoid or actively try to stop high-intensity stimulation of the same areas.[38] Signals from these limbic structures to motor mechanisms, together with the informationn derived from sensory and cognitive processes, could selectively activate neural networks that subserve adaptive response patterns.

The complex sequences of behavior that characterize pain are determined by sensory, motivational, and cognitive processes that act on motor mechanisms. By motor mechanisms, (Figure 2-2), Melzack and Casey[38] mean all of the brain areas that contribute to overt behavioral response patterns. These areas extend throughout the whole of the central nervous system, and their organization must be at least as complex as that of the input systems we have described here.

◆ CONCLUSION

The complexity of the neural substrates of pain, characterized by plasticity, interaction, and modulation, help to explain the highly variable and individual nature of pain perception and response. This theoretical position provides a basis for an expanded view of pain assessment and treatment. It unlocks some of the mystery posed by individual differences and enhances the role of nursing in pain management by providing the rationale to broaden our approaches to pain relief. It also confirms the fact that, because of the subjective and individual nature of pain, the patient is the primary source of information about his or her pain.

The topics of assessment and intervention will be dealt with in more detail in subsequent chapters. However, it is appropriate here to underscore the link between the theoretical perspective presented and these clinical skills. Pain assessment, in our view, must encompass the three major aspects of pain: sensory, affective, and cognitive/evaluative. As well, the physical and psychological factors that are known to influence pain must be assessed and considered within the total patient situation.

With the plastic and interactive nature of the neural substrates of pain established, there is now sound justification for the preparation of patients undergoing potentially painful procedures, such as diagnostic tests and surgery. Providing patients with accurate information, strategies to cope with pain, and a sense of control represents the first important step in preventing unnecessary and uncontrolled acute pain. It is also evident that pain relief may be approached in a large variety of ways ranging from peripheral—such as heat, cold, TENS, and massage—to cognitive/psychological—such as information, relaxation, and distraction. Neurochemical methods primarily involve the use of analgesic medications to modulate the nerve-impulse patterns that subserve pain.

All of these approaches are explored in later chapters of this text. The point here is that the theoretical perspective suggests that a simple, single approach to pain relief is unlikely to be successful, given the complexity of the nervous system processes that give rise to pain. In any specific patient situation, one may well require several methods of intervention to achieve adequate pain relief.

The perspective we have described is a broad and general framework for the understanding of pain. It is not specific to any syndrome but is capable of explaining a variety of pain conditions. The research and clinical examples used throughout refer primarily to adults, but the theory itself is applicable to all age groups. One may translate the theory within a developmental perspective to address the unique challenge of understanding pain in young children and the elderly. Indeed, people with sensory, cognitive, and physical deficits require special consideration in the clinical application of pain assessment and treatment.

We have not addressed the differences between acute and chronic pain in this chapter. However, the neural processes that may give rise to chronic pain are an integral part of the theory.[39] There is growing evidence that poorly controlled acute pain may contribute to prolonged hospitalization[57] and to the development of chronic pain.[24] Since the majority of nurses practice in acute care settings, their role in acute pain relief is enormous. To strive toward meeting this responsibility, practice based on current scientific theory is necessary.

REFERENCES

1. Abbott FV and Melzack R. (1982). Brainstem lesions dissociate neural mechanisms of morphine analgesia in different kinds of pain. *Brain Res, 25,* 149-155.

2. Abbott FV and Melzack R. (1983). Dissociation of the mechanisms of stimulation-produced analgesia in tests of tonic and phasic pain. In Bonica JJ, Lindblom U, and Iggo A (eds), *Advances in pain research and therapy: vol 5* (pp. 401-409). New York: Raven Press.
3. Beecher HK. (1959). *Measurement of subjective responses.* New York: Oxford University Press.
4. Bishop GH. (1959). The relation between nerve fiber size and sensory modality: phylogenetic implications of the afferent innervation of the cortex. *J Nerv Ment Dis, 128,* 89-114.
5. Carlen PL, Wall PD, Nadvorna H, and Steinbach T. (1978). Phantom limbs and related phenomena in recent traumatic amputations. *Neurology, 28,* 211.
6. Carstens E. (1982). Inhibition of spinal dorsal horn neuronal responses to noxious skin heating by medical hypothalamic stimulation in the cat. *J Neurophysiol, 48,* 808-822.
7. Casey KL. (1970). Somatosensory responses of bulboreticular units in awake cat: relation to escape-producing stimuli. *Science, 173,* 77-80.
8. Clark WC and Clark SB. (1980). Pain responses in Nepalese porters. *Science, 209,* 410.
9. Cohen SR, Abbott FV, and Melzack R. (1984). Unilateral analgesia produced by intraventricular morphine. *Brain Res, 303,* 277-287.
10. Cohen SR and Melzack R. (1985), Morphine injected into the habenula and dorsal posteromedial thalamus produces analgesia in the formalin test. *Brain Res, 359,* 131-139.
11. Delgado JMR. (1955). Cerebral structures involved in transmission and elaboration of noxious stimulation. *J Neurophysiol, 18,* 261-275.
12. Delgado JMR, Rosvold HE, and Looney E. (1956). Evoking conditioned fear by electrical stimulation of subcortical structures in the monkey brain. *J Comp Physiol Psychol, 49,* 373-380.
13. Donovan M, Dillon P, and McGuire L. (1987). Incidence and characteristics of pain in a sample of medical-surgical inpatients. *Pain, 30,* 69-78.
14. Egbert LD, Battit GE, Welch CD, and Bartlett MK. (1964). Reduction of postoperative pain by encouragement and instruction of patients. *N Engl J Med, 270,* 825.
15. Evans FJ. (1974). The placebo response in pain reduction. In Bonica JJ (ed), *Advances in neurology: vol 4.* New York: Raven Press.
16. Foltz EL and White LE. (1962). Pain "relief" by frontal cingulotomy. *J Neurosurg, 19,* 89-100.
17. Freeman W and Watts JW. (1950). *Psychosurgery in the treatment of mental disorders and intractable pain.* Springfield: CC Thomas.
18. Gardner WJ and Licklider JCR. (1959). Auditory analgesia in dental operations. *J Am Dent Assoc, 59,* 1144.
19. Hall KRL and Stride E. (1954). The varying response to pain in psychiatric disorders: a study in abnormal psychology. *Br J Med Psychol, 27,* 48.
20. Hardy JD, Wolff HG, and Goodell H. (1952). *Pain sensations and reactions.* Baltimore: Williams & Wilkins.
21. Hill HE, Kornetsky CH, Flanary HG, and Wikler A. (1952a). Effects of anxiety and morphine on discrimination of intensities of painful stimuli. *J Clin Invest, 31,* 473.
22. Hill HE, Kornetsky CH, Flanary HG, and Wikler A. (1952b). Studies of anxiety associated with anticipation of pain. I. Effects of morphine. *Arch Neurol Psychiatr, 67,* 612.

23. Hillman P and Wall PD. (1969). Inhibitory and excitatory factors influencing the receptive fields of lamina 5 spinal cord cells. *Exper Brain Res, 9,* 284-306.
24. Jeans ME, Gray-Donald K, Abbott FV, et al. (October 1989). Resolution of pain after hospitalization. Abstract. (Canadian Pain Society Annual Meeting, Banff, Alberta.)
25. Johnson J and Rice V. (1974). Sensory and distress components of pain implications for the study of clinical pain. *Nurs Res, 23,* 203-229.
26. Johnson J, Rice V, Fuller S, and Endress P. (1978). Sensory information, instruction in a coping strategy and recovery from surgery. *Res Nurs Health, 1,* 4-17.
27. Lambert WE, Libman E, and Poser EG. (1960). Effect of increased salience of membership group on pain tolerance. *J Pers, 28,* 350.
28. Langer E, Janis IL, and Wolfer JA. (1975). Reduction of psychological stress in surgical patients. *J Exp Soc Psychol, 11,* 155.
29. Lichstein L and Sackett GP. (1971). Reactions by differentially raised Rhesus monkeys to noxious stimulation. *Dev Psychobiol, 4,* 339.
30. Marks RM and Sachar EJ, (1973). Undertreatment of medical inpatients with narcotic analgesics. *Ann Intern Med, 78,* 173-181.
31. Martinez-Urrutia A. (1975). Anxiety and pain in surgical patients. *J Consult Clin Psychol, 43,* 437.
32. Mather L and Mackie J. (1983). The incidence of postoperative pain in children. *Pain, 15,* 271-282.
33. McGlashan TH, Evans FJ, and Orne MT. (1969). The nature of hypnotic analgesia and placebo response to experimental pain. *Psychosom Med, 31,* 227.
34. Melzack R and Scott TH. (1957). The effects of early experience on the response to pain. *J Comp Physiol Psychol, 50,* 155.
35. Melzack R, Stotler WA, and Livingston WK. (1958). Effects of discrete brainstem lesions in cats on perception of noxious stimulation. *J Neurophysiol, 21,* 353-367.
36. Melzack R, Weisz AZ, and Sprague LT. (1963). Stratagems for controlling pain: contributions of auditory stimulation and suggestion. *Exp Neurol, 8,* 239.
37. Melzack R and Wall PD. (1965). Pain mechanisms: a new theory. *Science, 150,* 971-979.
38. Melzack R and Casey KL. (1968). Sensory, motivational, and central control determinants of pain: a new conceptual model. In Kenshalo D (ed), *The skin senses* (pp. 423-443). Springfield: CC Thomas.
39. Melzack R and Wall PD. (1982). *The challenge of pain.* New York: Basic Books.
40. Melzack R, Wall PD, and Ty TC. (1982). Acute pain in an emergency clinic: latency of onset and descriptor patterns. *Pain, 14,* 33.
41. Melzack R. (1988). Psychological aspects of pain: implications for neural blockade. In Cousins MJ and Bridenbaugh PO (eds), *Neural blockade,* ed 2, (pp. 845-860). Philadelphia: Lippincott.
42. Mendell LM and Wall PD. (1965). Presynaptic hyperpolarization: a role for five afferent fibers. *J Physiol* (London), *172,* 274-294.
43. Mogan J, Wells N, and Robertson E. (1986). Effects of pre-operative teaching on post-operative pain: a replication and expansion. *Pain, 26*(1), 124.
44. Nauta WJH. (1958). Hippocampal projections and related neural pathways to the midbrain in the cat. *Brain, 81,* 319-340.

45. Noordenbos W. (1959). *Pain*. Amsterdam: Elsevier.
46. Pavlov IP. (1928). *Lectures on conditional reflexes*. New York: International Publishers.
47. Pomeranz B, Wall PD, and Weber WV. (1968). Cord cells responding to five myelinated afferents from viscera, muscle and skin. *J Physiol* (London), *199,* 511-532.
48. Rossi GF and Zanchetti A. (1957). The brainstem reticular formation. *Arch Ital Biol, 95,* 199-435.
49. Rubins JL and Friedman ED. (1948). Asymbolia for pain. *Arch Neurol* (Chicago), *60,* 554-573.
50. Schreiner L and Kling A. (1953). Behavioral changes following rhinencephalic injury in cat. *J Neurophysiol, 15,* 643-659.
51. Semmes J and Mishkin M. (1965). Somatosensory loss in monkeys after ipsilateral cortical ablation. *J Neurophysiol, 28,* 473-486.
52. Sternbach RA and Tursky B. (1965). Ethnic differences among housewives in psychophysical and skin potential responses to electric shock. *Psychophysiol, 1,* 73.
53. Sternbach RA. (1968). *Pain: a psychophysiological analysis*. New York: Academic Press.
54. Szentagothia J. (1964). Neuronal and synaptic arrangement in the substantia gelatinosa rolandi. *J Comp Neurol, 122,* 219-239.
55. Wall PD. (1970). The sensory and motor role of impulses travelling in the dorsal columns toward cerebral cortex. *Brain, 93,* 505-524.
56. Wall PD. (1978). The gate-control theory of pain: a re-examination and a re-statement. *Brain, 101,* 1-18.
57. Wasylak TJ, Abbott FV, English MJM and Jeans ME. (1990). Reduction of post-operative morbidity following patient-controlled morphine. *Can J Anaesth,* 37:7, 726-731.
58. White JC and Sweet WH. (1969). *Pain and the neurosurgeon*. Springfield: Charles C Thomas.
59. Zborowski M. (1952). Cultural components in responses to pain. *J Soc Issues, 8,* 16.

3

Misbeliefs About Pain

Judith H. Watt-Watson

◆ INTRODUCTION

Beliefs that are accepted as truths often guide the choice of approaches for pain assessment and management. Difficulties arise when decisions are based on erroneous beliefs or faulty assumptions that come from an incomplete or incorrect knowledge base. Professional caregivers involved in acute care seem to guess rather than assess the extent of pain or its relief,[18] and chronic pain management can be even more of a challenge. Perry and Heidrich[43a] suggest that when nurses do not know how to assess pain, they rely on their own judgment of how much pain they *think* patients are experiencing. The basis on which these judgments are made needs to be carefully examined.

Assumptions, personal experiences, and outdated or incorrect beliefs that are implemented as rationales for practice lead to inadequate pain relief for patients. This chapter will examine erroneous beliefs or *misbeliefs* frequently held by both nurses and patients that lead to inadequate pain control. Misbeliefs held by nurses will focus on pain assessment, pain management, particularly opioid administration, and pain in specific age groups, including children, infants, and elders. Patients have misbeliefs about the roles of professionals in treating pain, patients' role in management, and the modalities involved. Only by examining what we hold to be true and then using current scientific data to correct misbeliefs will we be effective in changing the inadequacy of pain management.

◆ NURSES' MISBELIEFS ABOUT THE PAIN EXPERIENCE

McCaffery and Beebe[38] have stated that "pain is whatever the person experiencing it says it is." Although it is frequently stated that the patient is the one with the pain, not the caregiver, patient self-reports of pain are not valued by nurses.[10,17,58] It is crucial both to ask patients about their pain experiences and to believe their responses, but actual practices do not reflect this. In reality, patients frequently do not receive effective pain management because of some commonly held misbeliefs that are used as a basis for practice (see box). These erroneous beliefs have no basis in fact and make solutions to pain management more difficult than is necessary.

Misbelief 1. Patients should expect to have pain in hospital.

Studies have shown that nurses identified no problem with patients experiencing moderate pain and thought their pain management for these patients was satisfactory. In fact, significant percentages thought that patients should increase their tolerance to pain.[49,64] Of the nurses interviewed by Chapman et al, 25% would wait for their postoperative patients to be in severe pain before offering analgesics, and 32% would wait for the patient to request pain medication before giving it. People do have varying ways of responding to, reporting, and dealing with pain. A belief that everyone must tolerate pain or respond to an illness experience in the same way, including reporting it, is unfair.

If moderate pain is considered to be an acceptable part of the hospital experience, then relief of pain will not be a management goal. This premise needs to be challenged! Although

◆ NURSES' MISBELIEFS ABOUT THE PAIN EXPERIENCE

1. Patients should expect to have pain in hospital.
2. Obvious pathology, test results, and/or the type of surgery determine the existence and intensity of pain.
3. Patients who are in pain always have observable signs.
4. Chronic pain is not as serious a problem for patients as acute pain.
5. Patients are not the experts about their pain, health professionals are.
6. Patients will report that they are in pain and will use the term "pain."

not all pain can be removed, it can usually be significantly decreased with the multiple modalities now available for pain management (see Chapters 7, 8).

Misbelief 2: Obvious pathology is necessary for pain to be real; test results and the type of surgery determine the existence and intensity of pain.

Diagnostic tests are thought to be infallible and conclusive; therefore negative results are interpreted to mean that the pain is not real and that the patient is "malingering" or "psychogenic." Donovan[16] suggests, however, that with bone metastases in cancer patients, 60% of the bone density must be destroyed before the lesion will show on the standard x-ray. Thus the patient will have pain long before objective signs of pathology become available. Health professionals seem to be afraid of patients "putting one over on us," and as a result waste energy trying to decide whether the person *really* has pain. Malingerers are people who lie and say they have pain when they do not and comprise only 1% to 2% of the population. One has the choice of suspecting all patients of malingering and being wrong 98% of the time, or believing all patients who report pain and being wrong 1% to 2% of the time.[16]

Either the diagnosis or the type of surgery may be the primary basis used by nurses to determine the degree of patients' pain and the dose of analgesics required to alleviate it. For example, why are hysterectomy patients postoperatively given Demerol 75 to 100 mg every 3 to 4 hours for 48 hours, but cesarean section patients receive Demerol for 24 hours and then are given Tylenol #3? Although having a baby is usually a happier context than losing a uterus, both women have abdominal incisions that may necessitate significant analgesia for 48 to 72 hours. In reality, opioids are minimally secreted through breast milk,[26] and few women in considerable pain will be successful in breast feeding.

Patterns of pain in response to selected diagnoses, tests, or surgeries have been clinically described, but people's responses vary. Individual endorphin levels may differ and directly effect the amount of analgesia required.[56] The amount of preoperative opioid analgesia and the type of anesthetic given, i.e., general or regional, may greatly influence the level of postoperative pain.[62]

Misbelief 3: Patients who are in pain always have observable signs.

Health professionals tend to be most familiar with the

acute pain model, which is frequently the only pain model taught in educational programs. Pain is consistently assessed as acute pain, with the clinician looking for signs of sympathetic overactivity. Using only this model impedes the assessment of people with chronic pain who have learned a variety of coping styles to reduce the visibility of their pain. As well, the physiological adaptation that occurs with chronic pain (and sometimes with acute pain), results in the absence of evidence of sympathetic overactivity, such as increases in pulse, blood pressure, and respirations. Response indicators, such as changes in mood, sleeping, eating, and sex patterns may be more sensitive gauges of pain with these patients.

Where acute pain is superimposed on chronic pain, such as a patient with lupus undergoing a hysterectomy, chronic pain is rarely treated as a separate entity. Cancer patients may experience acute recurrent pain with both the "fight or flight" signs of acute pain and the response indicators of chronic pain. Therefore acute and chronic pain are separate entities that need to be assessed differently. In a population of patients with growing numbers of chronic illnesses, both phenomena are commonly experienced concurrently by the same individual (see Chapters 14 and 17).

Misbelief 4: Chronic pain is not as serious a problem for patients as acute pain.

Chronic pain patients are challenging, and their repeated hospitalizations or clinic visits can be frustrating when approaches to pain treatment are unsuccessful. Because these patients may have few objective signs to support their pain complaints, and because their use of coping strategies, such as socializing, negates the "pain image," the seriousness of this problem may not be recognized. Chronic pain patients are given less attention than acute pain patients, particularly if they are younger, have negative signs of pathology, and are depressed.[57] However, chronic pain patients can have tremendous disruptions in all aspects of their life because of the pain, including sleep, social interaction, emotional behavior, home management, work, and recreation.[65] Therefore it is important to assess not only the pain symptom but the related changes in their everyday lived experience.[65a]

One has to question whether covertly these patients are held responsible for their pain and lack of relief. Chronic pain may be considered the fault of the individual because projecting blame is less threatening to health professionals. Some clinicians state overtly that many chronic pain sufferers could get better if they wanted to get better. Using this misbelief as a rationale for practice can lead only to failure. The ongoing search for creative multimodal approaches and the belief in the seriousness of this challenging problem will lead to increased pain management success for the chronic pain patient (see Chapters 7 and 8).

Misbelief 5: Patients are not the experts about their pain, health professionals are.

In Donovan, Dillon, and McGuire's study,[17] fewer than 50% of patients in pain were asked about their pain or had anything charted about their pain. McCaffery's definition that pain is whatever and whenever the person says it is, is frequently not evident in the assessment and documentation for people experiencing pain.[38] One should not assume there is no pain just because pain isn't obvious. Alternatively, when patients with guarding, pallor, and/or general malaise refuse analgesics, it is important to explore this refusal further including the meaning of the pain and their understanding of analgesics. It is difficult to quantify pain and the pain experience, but good tools for pain assessment are available to make this easier (see Chapters 4, 9, and 10). Pain assessment must go beyond location, intensity, and duration to include the meaning of pain for patients and their families, and how they are coping with it.[13]

Donovan et al[17] stress that to accurately quantify the pain experience, one must systematically use assessment tools such as scales. One practical, easy approach would be to teach patients the 0 (no pain) to 10 (worst pain) scale beginning at the intake assessment history. Nurses need to assure patients that their input is very necessary in assessing the pain level and that their help will be expected. Health professionals then need to make sure to implement their part of this contract by regularly asking patients to rate their pain.

Misbelief 6: Patients will report that they are in pain and will use the term "pain."

We cannot assume that every patient's vocabulary includes *pain* or that pain will be described as such. Some cancer and postoperative patients may talk about "pressure," "soreness," or "discomfort." These words can be used similarly to "pain" in a pain rating scale (see Chapter 4). Even if English is their first language and the term "pain" is used, patients for various reasons may not ask for something to relieve it (see the following box). The majority of the postoperative patients (n = 259) in Owen, McMillan, and Rogowski's [42] sample wanted effective pain control but would not ask for an analgesic until their pain was severe.

Health professionals tend to ask patients to rate their pain when they are sitting or lying absolutely still, and therefore they may answer "no pain." Questions about pain must be related to activities, such as "How much do you hurt when you turn over, get up to walk, go to the bathroom, or swallow?" Too many patients, because of erroneous beliefs discussed later in this chapter, do not ask for help with their pain until it is almost unbearable. The more intense the pain, the greater the analgesic dose needed to control it. Patients cannot maintain their maximum activity level or usual lifestyle patterns if pain relief is not available or adequate.

◆ NURSES' MISBELIEFS ABOUT PAIN MANAGEMENT

Many misbeliefs about pain management relate to the administration of analgesics. Some of the nurses' erroneous beliefs (see box) are similar to those misbeliefs of patients discussed later in this chapter. When both patients and health professionals hold similar but incorrect beliefs about pain and treatment, pain relief is unlikely. Resistance to trying alternatives will obstruct potential successes.

Misbelief 1: One pain treatment or strategy is all that is needed.

Pain is a complex experience having sensory, affective, and

◆ NURSES' MISBELIEFS ABOUT PAIN MANAGEMENT

1. One pain treatment or strategy is all that is needed.
2. Addiction is a major problem with patients taking opioids.
3. The nurse is the best person to give out opioids.
4. Patients must demonstrate pain before receiving medication.
5. Placebo responders do not have real pain.
6. Injectable opioids are the most effective.
7. Respiratory depression is a common side effect of opioids in all patients.

behavioral components and therefore may require a multimodal treatment approach. Pain such as muscle spasms in the lower back may be relieved more effectively by heat and ultrasound than by medications. Strategies such as breathing exercises, muscle relaxation, imagery, and distraction do not replace analgesia for patients who need pharmacological management. However, they can be very useful adjuncts in reducing the dose required and in decreasing the pain while waiting for titration to work. Because pain is multidimensional, encouraging patients to use a broad range of methods will result in more effective pain management.

Misbelief 2: Addiction is a major problem with patients taking opioids.

A nursing colleague called me in tears. Her father was dying in hospital of bowel cancer and was constantly in pain. His oncologist refused to increase his morphine dose because he "might get addicted and the medication wouldn't work at the end when he needed it." My advice was to change physicians, for this irrational fear could only result in an agonizing experience for the patient and the family. It is important to clearly understand the terms confused or associated with addiction (see box).

Fear of patient addiction is well documented and has been identified as a key contributor to undermedication of patients.[6,9,12,16,36,38] The majority of nurses in the author's survey[64] believed that over 10% of hospitalized patients in pain became addicted, whereas in reality the incidence is less than 1%.[39,46] What the health professional sees as asking for anal-

◆ CLARIFICATION OF TERMS USED IN REFERRING TO OPIOIDS

ADDICTION	A behavioral response demonstrating a compulsion to take drugs for their psychic effect; a psychological dependence
TOLERANCE	An involuntary physiological response of the body to repeated opioid use, resulting in the need for larger doses to obtain the same analgesic use
DEPENDENCE	A physiological response when an opioid is withdrawn abruptly after continued use

gesia "by the clock" may be the vigilant behavior of an astute patient who knows the medication may not come on time. There are no guarantees for patients that pain medications will be given before pain escalates to an unbearable level, particularly if the regular dosing does not give adequate relief. Even with a conscientious nurse, the difficulty of finding the narcotic keys or the necessity of meeting an emergency need of another patient can mean significant delays in administering analgesics. Clock watching behavior reflects inadequate dosing and poor pain control for the patient.

Problems arise for patients with a history of long-term opiod use or drug abuse. Fears of increasing or reestablishing a habit seem to take precedence over pain control. For example, I have been told that nothing stronger than codeine can be given to a terminal head-neck cancer patient because "he's a dependent personality and will probably get addicted." We should not be concerned about the long-term use of opioids with terminal cancer patients. Although it is important to recognize that drug abusers do exist in our society, pain control plans can be discussed preoperatively in consultation with the patient, nurse, anesthetist, and surgeon. Patients who need increasing doses of opioids for pain control, including drug abusers, are not becoming addicted or increasing their habit, but demonstrating drug tolerance (see box on p. 42). This tolerance slows with more chronic opioid use, particularly if the oral route and round-the-clock scheduling are used.[59]

Misbelief 3: The nurse is the best person to give out analgesics.

Some nurses believe addiction can be prevented by carefully giving out opioids on demand,[64] and then only if the pain is thought to justify analgesics. However, patients who receive round-the-clock analgesia, particularly if it is self-regulated, may require lower total daily doses and have fewer side effects.[30,33,35] Anxiety about whether the pain will return before the analgesic arrives increases one's distress and probably the perceived pain. The misbelief that control should lie with health professionals is obstructing the implementation of self-dosing, although research has documented the effectiveness of this approach.

Misbelief 4: Patients must demonstrate pain before receiving analgesic.

Clinicians erroneously treat pain rather than prevent it. The misbelief that pain must return before analgesia can be given is still prevalent. In explaining the need to prevent peaks and valleys of pain intensity, as indicated by a postoperative patient's 0 to 10 ratings, a nurse asked me, "Why are we giving him morphine if his pain is only 3?" Unfortunately, nurses still expect patients to justify their need for pain medication, with the result that analgesics, particularly opioids, are frequently given only if pain ratings are high. Regular dosing (see Chapter 7) is one of the keys to pain relief. For acute-pain patients who feel their need for analgesia decreasing as they recover from surgery or treatments, the strength of the analgesic can be reduced or another analgesic given.

Misbelief 5: Placebo responders do not have real pain.

One third of all patients, when given a pseudotreatment with implied therapeutic effects, will turn on their own morphine-like substances called endorphins, resulting in pain relief. This is a physiological response to decreased anxiety and the belief in the person and/or the treatment.[28] Patients supply their own endogenous opioid to relieve the pain. These responses tend not to last, and patients become aware of the deception. The result is a lack of trust in the health professionals. Deliberately giving placebos may be helpful in detoxification programs and in research situations where the patient has given consent, but they have no role in clinical pain management.

Misbelief 6: Injectable opioids are the most effective.

If the patient is able to swallow, is not vomiting, and is not in acute pain, the oral route is more comfortable than injections. Oral doses of opioids at equianalgesic doses (see Chapter 7) are as potent as intramuscular opioids, and morphine pills including slow release are small and easily swallowed. The intravenous and epidural routes are being considered more frequently with postoperative patients, and suppositories are available for some drugs and may be very helpful when the oral route is not possible (see Chapter 7). Patients with chronic or persistent pain should not be receiving routine injections. Injections add to patients' discomfort and the potential for skin breakdown. Continuous subcutaneous infusions of opioids can be helpful for pain control, with the small needle being changed every three to seven days. A stopcock in the catheter equipment allows for painless subcutaneous injection of analgesics for breakthrough pain. Regular dosing shows a decrease in dose requirements as a steady state is maintained and acute episodes decrease (see Chapter 7).

Misbelief 7: Respiratory depression is a common side effect of opioids in all patients.

Although respiratory depression is a possible problem with opiate-naive patients, it usually does not happen because of standard doses and careful titration (see Chapters 6 and 7). The one group where caution in dosing is required is the group over 75 years old. Dosages must be titrated with consideration given to the elongated detoxification time in this age group. This caution is particularly relevant if liver disease is present. If respiratory depression does occur, it can be easily reversed by the antagonist naloxone (Narcan) (see Chapter 7). It is interesting to find that first-year nursing students, even before taking formal pharmacological lectures, always express fears of opioids related to respiratory depression. Perhaps our national nursing organizations should be correcting the scripts of common television soaps that may perpetuate these myths with the public.

◆ NURSES' MISBELIEFS RELATED TO PATIENT AGE

Age is a significant factor influencing pain assessment and management. Two particular groups of patients are treated differently because of their ages: children including infants, and the older person. Misbeliefs are used to justify these practices.

Children, Including Infants

The general belief that children do not experience pain is still prevalent.[21] Eland[20] has stated that health professionals tend either to assume their knowledge of adults is relevant to children in pain or to deny that pain exists. Karen Eng, a fourth-year nursing baccalaureate student, graphically describes treatment given without analgesia to a 20-month-old girl with 30% body burns: "Jane's piercing screams as flaps of cheesy eschar were scraped from her wound were met with disgusted looks and the comment, 'I hate doing this kid.' Questions arise as to why pain relief for children is so inadequate: Do health professionals, including nurses, still believe the old myth that children, including infants, do not experience pain? Are analgesics not being ordered in sufficient dosages? Are children refusing analgesics? Erroneous beliefs that confound effective pain relief for infants and children (see

◆ NURSES' MISBELIEFS ABOUT PAIN AND AGE

CHILDREN, INCLUDING INFANTS

1. Children do not experience pain.
2. Children cannot accurately describe their pain.
3. Children should not be given opioids for pain.
4. Opioids are best given by the intramuscular route.
5. Children forget painful experiences.
6. Children who are playing, or, conversely, sleeping do not have pain.
7. Parents should not stay with children during painful procedures.

THE OLDER PERSON

1. Pain is a normal part of getting older and can never be very intense; pain sensation decreases with age.
2. Opioids are too potent for elderly patients.
3. Pain cannot be assessed with elderly patients who are cognitively impaired.

box) need to be recognized and clarified in order to change practices.

Misbelief 1: Children do not experience pain.

Although authors have suggested that children don't respond to painful experiences as adults do, there is no evidence that this is true.[29,37,41] Infants, children, and neonates are subject to a stress response similar to that of adults when exposed to pain.[66] Infants have demonstrated behavioral changes, such as increased crying for up to 72 hours, after procedures such as circumcision.[50] Frequently children are taken off intravenous opioids when they leave the recovery room and given no analgesics in the unit setting. Too many heart-breaking stories are heard about children experiencing burns and related treatments with no or minimal analgesics. Knighton and Palozzi's discussion of the pain experienced by children after burns is found in Chapter 19, and the importance of careful assessment is underlined in Chapters 9 and 10.

The prevalent myth that infants don't feel or respond to pain is based on incorrect data that infants lack pain receptors and have an underdeveloped nervous system. It is now known that myelination begins in utero and includes the sensory roots at birth.[60] Pain impulses are transmitted by unmyelinated as well as myelinated fibers (see Chapter 2).[48] Behavioral and physiological responses to painful stimuli, such as circumcision and blood work, have been shown with full-term neonates.* An increased incidence of physiological stress response and more severe postoperative complications have been found in preterm babies undergoing cardiac surgery with anesthetic but no fentanyl.[4] Unfortunately, because neonates are thought to have no pain, analgesics and/or anesthesia are frequently not given during invasive procedures, including surgery.[3,52,54]

Misbelief 2: Children cannot accurately describe their pain.

The assumption that children are unable to communicate their pain experience has been challenged in the literature.[54] The recent development of instruments such as Hester's Poker Chip Tool[31] and Beyer's Oucher[6a] are designed to assist the child in describing pain and are described in more detail in Chapter 10. The reliability and validity of these tools continue to be developed, and these approaches are very useful along with other modes of subjective and behavioral data to confirm or reevaluate assumptions about children's pain.[53] Infants and preverbal children are the most difficult to assess, and increasingly research is being done in this area (see Chapter 9).

Misbelief 3: Children should not be given opioids for pain.

Foster and Hester,[23] in their study of 120 children experiencing either postoperative pain or pain related to their medical diagnosis, found only a moderate relationship between high pain ratings of the nurse or the child and analgesic administration. Of the medications ordered, nurses more readily gave Tylenol plain or Tylenol #3 than morphine. The cues that this sample of nurses used to determine the child's pain intensity often provided little rationale for their interventions. Foster and Hester refer to the statement from the National Institute of Health Consensus Development Conference that "even when pain is reported and assessed, it may not necessarily be attended, monitored, treated, and satisfactorily managed" (p. 6). This may relate to the considerable emphasis on potential side effects of opioids rather than on the studies of their therapeutic use, which are rarely discussed.[66]

* References 5, 14, 22, 24, 43, 47, 61.

Eland[20,21] (see Chapter 12) has been one of the first to encourage nurses to examine erroneous beliefs guiding their practices, particularly related to analgesic administration. Fears of addiction need to be clarified, and physiological and psychological dependency need to be clearly differentiated. With the current emphasis in both the schools and the media on "saying no to drugs," both parents and children may need help to distinguish between drug abuse on the street and therapeutic use to decrease pain and facilitate recovery. With appropriate use of opiates and careful monitoring, pain in infants and children can be effectively managed.

Misbelief 4: Opioids are best given by the intramuscular route.

Injections, particularly intramuscular injections, are not the treatment preferred by any patient, and children are no different. A child may deny absolutely the presence of pain to avoid being pricked. If a child can be persuaded to have the injection, the resulting pain relief may promote less resistance the next time. However, similarly for adults, one has to ask why this route is used so frequently when it is not necessary (see Chapter 12).

Misbelief 5: Children forget painful experiences.

It has been suggested that children do not remember painful experiences to the same degree as adults do.[66] There is no evidence that this is true, and the long-term effects of pain on infants and children are not known. One only has to see children after hospital discharge giving a needle to a doll, repeating the coping strategy suggested to them: "Don't cry. It will only hurt for a minute and then you can play," to realize how much they do remember. To what degree these pain experiences affect future pain trajectories and coping patterns is not known.

Specific behavioral changes in neonates after circumcision imply the presence of memory[3] and may disrupt adaptation to the postnatal environment.[15,36a,50] Therefore health professionals need to be encouraged to administer analgesics in appropriate doses and intervals to children undergoing painful procedures.

Misbelief 6: Children who are playing or, conversely, sleeping do not have pain.

A commonly held misbelief is that children's increased activities, loud verbalizations, and more aggressive body movements indicate the absence of pain.[8] The more quiet, restrained behaviors, such as sleeping, are also taken as indicators of the absence of pain. In fact, children may use both approaches in coping with their pain. Hester[31] has suggested that increased verbalizations and behaviors may be used by children to reduce stress and tension. Play, sleeping, and aggressive activities can all be distractors rather than indicators of the absence of pain. Labels can be misleading and result in incorrect pain assessment. McCaffery and Beebe[38] suggest that the expected behavioral manifestations of pain may decrease because of parental and/or nurse expectations, children's own coping strategies, cultural strategies, fatigue, and distractibility.

Misbelief 7: Parents should not stay with children during painful procedures.

Nurses and parents do not always agree on the parents' role when the child is undergoing painful procedures. Nurses have expressed confidence in working with families of children but also anxiety about the presence of parents during difficult and painful procedures.[27] Many parents are now asking to stay with their children when they are hurting even when procedures are involved.[1,63] In preparation for this, possible roles for the parents in comforting their child could be discussed. Parents could be quickly taught basic relaxation and distraction techniques, and breathing exercises to help the child. Stoddard[55] has suggested that the most effective analgesic very often is the presence of a well-prepared parent who can increase the child's feeling of security.

In summary, pain assessment in children is complex, particularly if the child seems anxious and/or does not express discomfort because of fear of potential interventions. Nurses need to systematically assess pain and to act on these judgments knowledgeably. Effective treatments exist for children experiencing pain. However, common misbeliefs about children's pain experiences as well as the difficulties assessing pain in children and infants interfere with effective pain management for this population.

The Older Person

Physiological changes do occur as one grows older, but the clinical implications of these changes are not clear. The response of elders to the analgesic effect of opioids is known to be more sensitive than that of the younger population. Therefore any analgesic treatment for pain has the potential to alter the already compromised physiological status of these patients.[2] Pharmacokinetic changes resulting from alterations in the absorption, distribution, metabolism, and excretion of drugs may result in higher blood levels of analgesic drugs. Therefore older patients need to be assessed differently than younger patients with the same diagnosis, and the treatments of the older patients need to be carefully monitored. The previously discussed misbeliefs that influence pain assessment and management relate to this age group as well. To deal with pain in the older age group, health professionals have to recognize the legitimacy of this symptom and the need for treatment with this group. Several beliefs that obstruct this process are listed (see box on p. 46) and need to be challenged.

Misbelief 1: Pain is a normal part of getting older and can never be very intense; pain sensation decreases with age.

Pain is thought to be not only normal but irreversible for the older person. However, pain and suffering are not necessarily consequences of normal aging.[34] The incorrect belief that pain sensitivity and perception decrease with age has resulted in patients being treated minimally if at all for pain. Although superficial sensitivity to pain may decrease with age, no documentation has been found that age affects visceral or bony pain. Older patients do have altered body responses to processes such as inflammation, and although the effect of physiological changes is unclear, older patients do experience pain. No age differences in density or morphology of nociceptor endings have been found, suggesting that basic processes of nociception are influenced only minimally by age.[11]

Misbelief 2: Opioids are too potent for elderly patients.

Although it is unclear how age affects the presentation of clinical pain, the elderly are significantly more sensitive to the pain-relieving effect of opioids because of alteration of receptors, changes in plasma protein binding, and prolonged clearance.[34] However, this does not mean that opiate use is contraindicated, only that opioids should be used in smaller doses. Careful titration is imperative, with the dose being gradually increased until the patient obtains maximum relief for at least 4 hours or the appropriate drug duration. This will result in a therapeutic rather than a toxic dose, as older patients show enhanced pain relief from opiates as compared with younger patients.[32]

◆ NURSING OBSERVATIONS OF PAIN IN THE OLDER PERSON*

The older person in pain may:

1. Not be mobilizing
2. Have changes in continence
3. Not be eating
4. Be restless
5. Have poor chest expansion postoperatively
6. Push the examining hand away
7. Pull at tubes, even those distant from the operative site

*Galloway, S., Clinical Nurse Specialist in Surgery, Sunnybrook Health Science Centre, Toronto, Canada, 1990. Printed with permission.

Misbelief 3: Pain cannot be assessed with elderly patients who have cognitive impairment.

It is difficult to assess a patient's pain if the patient is unable to describe it, such as with infants and cognitively impaired elders. Assessment is possible, however, and requires careful observation of responses both at rest and during movement. Flinching, guarding, grimacing, whimpering, and aggression may all indicate some degree of discomfort for the patient if these behaviors are present. Galloway[25] suggests some concrete observations to use in assessing whether cognitively impaired adults are in pain (see box). The same patient assignment for several days helps to establish a baseline for judging pain in the elderly. Using a variety of modalities, such as massage and analgesics, may increase the effectiveness of pain management, and one has to be attuned to positive behavioral responses where they occur.

◆ PATIENT MISBELIEFS ABOUT PAIN

Patients who are experiencing pain utilize their own beliefs about pain and treatments that reflect past experiences, family mores, and/or advice from friends. The beliefs that describe effective past treatments and individual responses to pain are crucial to effective planning. However, not all beliefs that an individual brings to the pain context are therapeutic, and some may prove detrimental to pain management. Unfortunately, some health professionals may contribute to these er-

◆ PATIENT MISBELIEFS ABOUT PAIN

1. Pain is to be expected with treatments and diagnoses such as cancer.
2. I have no control over my pain.
3. Surgery or a pill will fix me up.
4. I should not ask for anything for pain unless I'm desperate.
5. Opioids cause too many problems, such as addiction.

roneous beliefs by implying that pain mechanisms are unidimensional and simplistic. If the designated treatment doesn't work, the patient is expected to cope anyway, without guidance from health professionals. The most common patient misbeliefs that may interfere with an individual's ability to control pain are outlined in the accompanying box.

Misbelief 1: Pain is to be expected with treatments and diagnoses such as cancer.

Many people going into hospital for tests and/or treatment expect to have pain and to have no choice but to tolerate it. The inevitability of pain may also be associated with certain diagnoses such as cancer. This misbelief could be dispelled by nurses in the admission history, where patients could be reassured that good pain relief is expected and that to do this we need to work together. The expectation that patients will be involved in their pain management needs to be stressed along with the methods to do this. Patients can be taught a rating scale, as described in Chapter 4, and asked to communicate their pain to their health professional. Patients with cancer don't necessarily have pain, and clarifying concerns about the incidence of pain from the point of diagnosis would decrease some of the anxiety associated with these diseases.

Misbelief 2: I have no control over my pain.

Patients, particularly those with chronic pain, frequently deny that anything has helped their pain. Patients often do not recognize the methods they have developed and use routinely to alleviate pain. Because these approaches may involve common everyday practices such as massage, application of heat, or exercise, patients do not consider them to be as legitimate as medical treatments. Some patients therefore may need help to recognize the strategies they are using to control their pain;

they may also need encouragement to continue using them.[51,65]

Misbelief 3: Surgery or a pill will fix me up.

Some patients may see the physician as the only member of the health team capable of treating their pain. They believe that a single modality prescribed by a physician is all that is needed to treat the pain. Immediate medical solutions are expected, such as surgery "to cut out the pain" or pills to take the problem away. If surgery or pills are not available or are not successful, some patients are unwilling to try other approaches. This resistance creates a significant problem for people with chronic or recurrent pain. The availability and benefits of multiple approaches for pain management should be discussed with patients from the beginning assessment.

Misbelief 4: I should not ask for anything for pain unless I'm desperate.

Clinically it has been noted that some patients who report severe pain have not asked for the prescribed analgesia. Often they have made this choice for reasons such as, "I stood lots of pain in the war, and I can tough this out," "You'll think I'm not coping if I keep asking for drugs," and "Nurses are too busy to ask them for help." It is important to clarify with patients, especially those who seem to be in pain, their reasons for refusing analgesics. Patients often need encouragement to seek help when they are hurting. They need to understand that pain is restrictive and may prevent mobilization, resulting in complications. Unfortunately, with the current staffing crises and the time needed to find the narcotic keys and prepare the dose for an individual patient, delays in analgesic administration are too frequent. Some patients respond to these system problems with a reluctance to ask for analgesics, and others demand analgesia "on the dot." Patient-controlled analgesia is proving to be a very effective way of solving this problem with patients (see Chapter 7).

Misbelief 5: Opioids cause too many problems, such as addiction.

Fears about taking analgesics, particularly opioids, focus on addiction, symbolic meanings that opioids imply dying, and the possibility that strong drugs won't be effective at the end when they are really needed. A group of nurses from Montreal, Canada,[19] outlined seven common erroneous beliefs about pain medications commonly reported from the patients' perspective (see box). It is important to validate with patients

◆ PATIENT MISBELIEFS ABOUT ANALGESICS

1. I should wait as long as possible before taking a pain medication.
2. If I need a higher dose of narcotic, I am addicted.
3. Medications are best given by injection.
4. Larger pills or greater volume of medication means better relief.
5. I need my pain medication only when I'm awake.
6. Only opioids are strong enough to control pain.
7. Morphine is the last resort.

Modified from *Managing your pain effectively*, Dupont, 1987.[19] Reprinted with permission.

whether these misbeliefs are interfering with effective pain relief.

Patients need clarification and reassurance about how to appropriately use opioids. Deliberate delays in asking for medications only increase the amount of drug needed to bring the pain under control. The need to increase doses of an analgesic does not indicate addiction; this may indicate that the pain is increasing or the patient is developing tolerance (see Chapter 7). Larger pill size or liquid volume have nothing to do with analgesic strength. Moreover, the injection route is not necessarily the most potent or effective one. In fact, slow release pills, such as MS Contin, are often preferable to parenteral routes because they permit independence and less frequent dosing with equivalent stable blood levels. Pain medication should not be limited to the times when the person is awake. Although dosages for chronic pain may permit a prenight loading of analgesic to allow uninterrupted sleep, acute pain sufferers need analgesics around the clock during the first 48 to 72 hours to prevent pain.

Morphine may symbolize dying, and reassurance needs to be given that this drug can be taken for years for good pain control. Some physicians are now proposing long-term treatment of chronic pain with morphine.[44,45] Patients frequently do not understand that nonopioids such as nonsteroidal anti-inflammatory drugs (NSAIDs) may be the drug of choice (superior to opioids) for some pain, such as bone pain. In some situations, nondrug methods, such as relaxation exercises, may be the most effective treatment. As no single method of pain relief works for everyone or even consistently for the same person, *multiple approaches are likely to be the most effective.*

In summary, patients bring their own beliefs that influence the way they perceive pain and respond to related treatments. Nurses have the most consistent involvement with patients in working toward pain relief. The nurse, therefore, has a major role in assessing the meaning of the situation for the patient and how the patient is dealing with it. In addition to identifying the patient's misbeliefs, we must recognize our own erroneous beliefs about pain management as well. Erroneous beliefs held by patients and/or professional caregivers can restrict effective pain management.

◆ CONCLUSION

Difficulties in understanding and recognizing another's pain are well known. Pain cannot be quantified like the symptom of diarrhea, and responses to painful contexts can vary for each individual as well as between individuals. It is crucial to gain as much information from the patient about his or her pain and pain relief as possible and to avoid making assumptions about what is or is not happening. Recognizing erroneous beliefs or misbeliefs that obstruct effective pain relief is a necessary step in effecting change in pain management. The following chapters in this book will help to dispel these misbeliefs.

REFERENCES

1. Algren C. (1985). Role perception of mothers who have hospitalized children. *Child Health Care, 15*(1), 6-9.
2. Amadio P, Cummings D, and Amadio P. (Nov 1987). Pain in the elderly: management techniques. *Pain Manage,* 33-41.
3. Anand KJS and Hickey P. (1987). Pain and its effects in the human neonate and fetus. *N Engl J Med, 317*(21), 1321-1329.
4. Anand KJS, Sippell W, and Aynsley-Green A. (1987). Randomized trial of fentanyl anesthesia in preterm babies undergoing surgery: effects on the stress response. *Lancet, 1,* 243-248.
5. Anders T and Chalemian R. (1974). Effect of circumcision on sleep-wake states in human neonates. *Psychosom Med, 36,* 174-179.
6. Angell M. (1982). The quality of mercy. *N Engl J Med, 306*(92), 98-99.

6a. Beyer J and Aradine C. (1986). Content validity of an instrument to measure young children's perceptions of the intensity of their pain. *J Pediatr Nurs, 1,* 386-395.

7. Beyer J, DeGood D, Ashley L, and Russell G. (1983). Pattern of postoperative analgesia with adults and children following cardiac surgery. *Pain, 17,* 71-81.
8. Broome M, Lillis P, and Smith M. (1989). Pain interventions with children: A meta-analysis of research. *Nurs Res, 38*(3), 154-158.
9. Charap A. (1978). The knowledge, attitudes, and experience of medical personnel treating pain in the terminally ill. *Mt Sinai J Med, 45,* 561-580.
10. Camp L. (1988). A comparison of nurses' recorded assessments of pain with perceptions of pain as described by cancer patients. *Cancer Nurs, 11*(4), 237-243.
11. Cauna N. (1965). The effects of aging on the receptor organs of the human dermis. In Montagna W (ed), *Advances in biology of the skin.* vol 6, (pp. 63-96). New York: Pergamon Press.
12. Cohen F. (1980). Postsurgical pain relief: patients' status and nurses' medication choices. *Pain, 9,* 265-274.
13. Copp L. (1985). Pain coping model and typology. *Image, 17*(3), 69-71.
14. Davis D and Calhoon M. (1989). Do preterm infants show behavioral responses to painful procedures? In Funk S, Tornquist S, Champayne M, et al (eds), *Key aspects of comfort* (pp. 35-45). New York: Springer Publishing Company.
15. Dixon S, Snyder J, Holve R, and Bromberger P. (1984). Behavioral effects of circumcision with and without anesthetics. *J Dev Behav Pediatr, 5,* 246-250.
16. Donovan M. (1982). Cancer pain: you can help. *Nurs Clin North Am, 17*(4), 713-728.
17. Donovan M, Dillon P, and McGuire L. (1987). Incidence and characteristics of pain in a sample of medical-surgical inpatients. *Pain, 30,* 69-78.
18. Donovan M, Slack J, Faut M, and Wright S. (1989). Factors associated with inadequate management of acute pain. American Pain Society Scientific Meeting, Poster Presentation.
19. Dupont Pharmaceuticals. (1987). *Managing your pain effectively.* Montreal, Canada Nursing Group.
20. Eland J. (1985). The role of the nurse in children's pain. In Copp L (ed), *Perspective on pain* (pp. 29-45). Edinburgh: Churchill Livingstone.
21. Eland J and Anderson J. (1977). The experience of pain in children. In Jacox A (ed), *Pain: a source book for nurses and other professionals* (pp. 453-473). Boston: Little, Brown & Company.
22. Emde R, Harmon R, Metcalf D, et al. (1971). Stress and neonatal sleep. *Psychosom Med, 33,* 491-496.
23. Foster R and Hester N. (1989). The relationship between assessment and pharmacologic intervention for children in pain. In Funk S, Tornquist E, Champayne M, et al (eds), *Key aspects of comfort* (pp. 72-79). New York: Springer Publishing Company.
24. Franck L. (1986). A new method to quantitatively describe pain behavior in infants. *Nurs Res, 35*(1), 28-31.
25. Galloway S. (1990). Clinical nurse specialist in surgery, Sunnybrook Health Science Centre, Toronto, Canada (personal communication).
26. Gilman A, Goodman L, and Gilman A. (1980). *The pharmacological basis of therapeutics.* New York: MacMillan Publishing Company.
27. Goodhall A. (1979). Perceptions of nurses toward parents' participation on pediatric oncology units. *Cancer Nurs, 2*(1), 38-46.
28. Goodwin J, Goodwin J, and Vogel A. (1979). Knowledge and use of placebos by house officers and nurses. *Ann Intern Med, 91,* 106-110.

29. Gross S and Gardner G. (1980). Child pain: treatment approaches. In Smith W, Merskey H, and Gross S (eds), *Pain meaning and management.* New York: SP Medical & Scientific Books.
30. Hecker B and Albert L. (1988). Patient-controlled analgesia: a randomized, prospective comparison between two commercially available PCA pumps and conventional analgesic therapy for postoperative pain. *Pain, 35,* 115-120.
31. Hester N. (1979). The preoperational child's reaction to immunization. *Nurs Res, 28*(4), 250-254.
32. Kaiko R, Wallenstein S, Rogers A, et al. (1982). Narcotics in the elderly. *Med Clin North Am, 66,* 1079-1089.
33. Keeri-Szanto M and Heaman S. (1972). Postoperative demand analgesia. *Surg Gynecol Obstet, 134,* 647-651.
34. Kwentus J, Harkins S, Lignon N, and Silverman J. (1985). Current concepts of geriatric pain and its treatment. *Geriatrics, 40*(4), 48-57.
35. Lange M, Dahn M, and Jacobs L. (1988). Patient-controlled analgesia versus intermittent analgesia dosing. *Heart Lung, 17,* 495-498.
36. Marks R and Sachar M. (1973). Undertreatment of medical inpatients with narcotic analgesics. *Ann Intern Med, 78,* 173-181.
36a. Marshall R, Stratton W, Moore J, and Boxerman S. (1980). Circumcision: effects upon newborn behaviour. *Infant Behav Dev, 3,* 1-14.
37. Mather L and Mackie J. (1983). The incidence of postoperative pain in children. *Pain, 15,* 271-282.
38. McCaffery M and Beebe A. (1989). *Pain: clinical manual for nursing practice* (p. 7). St. Louis: Mosby–Year Book, Inc.
39. Miller R and Jick H. (1978). Clinical effects of meperidine in hospitalized medical patients. *J Clin Pharmacol, 18*(4), 180-189.
40. National Institutes of Health. (1986). *Consensus development conference statement: the integrated approach to the management of pain.* USHHS, *6*(3), (document number 491-292:41148).
41. Owens M. (1984). Pain in infancy: conceptual and methodological issues. *Pain, 20,* 213-230.
42. Owen H, McMillan V, and Rogowski D. (1990). Post-operative pain therapy: a survey of patients' expectations and their experiences. *Pain, 41,* 303-307.
43. Owens M and Todd E. (1984). Pain in infancy: neonatal reaction to a heel lance. *Pain, 20,* 77-86.
43a. Perry S and Heidrich G. (1982). Management of pain during debridement: survey of US burn units. *Pain, 13,* 267-280.
44. Portenoy R. (1990). Chronic opioid therapy in nonmalignant pain. *J Pain Sympt Manage, 5*(1), 546-562.
45. Portenoy R and Foley K. (1986) Chronic use of opioid analgesics in non-malignant pain: report on 38 cases. *Pain, 25,* 171-186.
46. Porter J and Jick H. (1980). Addiction rare in patients treated with narcotics. *N Engl J Med, 303*(2), 123.
47. Porter F, Miller R, and Marshall R. (1986). Neonatal pain cries: effect of circumcision on acoustic features and perceived urgency. *Child Devel, 57*(3), 790-802.
48. Price D and Dubner R. (1977). Neurons that subserve, the sensory-discriminative aspects of pain. *Pain, 3,* 57-68.
49. Rankin M and Snider B. (1984). Nurses' perceptions of cancer patients' pain. *Cancer Nurs, 1,* 149-155.

50. Richards M, Bernal J, and Brackbill Y. (1976). Early behavioral differences: gender or circumcision? *Dev Psychobiol, 9,* 89-95.
51. Rowat K. (1983). The meaning and management of chronic pain: the family's perspective. (Doctoral dissertation, University of Illinois, 1983). *Dissertation Abstracts International, 44*(4-B), 1239-1240.
52. Shearer M. (1986). Editorial: surgery on the paralyzed unanesthetized newborn. *Birth, 13,* 79.
53. Stevens B. (1989). Nursing management of pain in children. In Foster R, Husberger M and Anderson J (eds), *Family-centered nursing care of children* (pp. 864-893). Toronto: WB Saunders.
54. Stevens B, Hunsberger M, and Browne G. (1987). Pain in children: theoretical, research and practice dilemmas. *J Pediatr Nurs, 3,* 154-166.
55. Stoddard F. (1982). Coping with pain: a developmental approach to treatment of burned children. *Am J Psychiatry, 139,* 736-740.
56. Tamsen A, Sakurada T, Wahlstrom A, et al. (1982). Postoperative demand for analgesics in relation to individual levels of endorphins and substance P in cerebrospinal fluid. *Pain, 13,* 171-183.
57. Taylor A, Skelton J, and Butcher J. (1984). Duration of pain condition and physical pathology as determinants of nurses' assessments of patients in pain. *Nurs Res, 33*(1), 4-8.
58. Teske K, Daut R, and Cleeland C. (1983). Relationships between nurses' observations and patients' self-reports of pain. *Pain, 16,* 289-296.
59. Twycross R and Lack S. (1983). *Symptom control in far advanced cancer: pain relief.* London: Pitman.
60. Volpe J. (1981). *Neurology of the newborn.* Philadelphia: WB Saunders.
61. Wachter-Shikora N. (1981). Pain theories and their relevance to the pediatric population. *Iss Comp Pediatr, 5,* 321-326.
62. Wall P. (1988). The prevention of post-operative pain. *Pain, 33,* 289-290.
63. Watt-Watson J, Evernden C, and Lawson C. (1990). Parents' perceptions of their child's acute pain experience. *J Pediatr Nurs, 5*(5), 344-349.
64. Watt-Watson J. (1987). Nurses' knowledge of pain issues: a survey. *J Pain Sympt Manage, 2*(4), 207-211.
65. Watt-Watson J, Evans R, and Watson P. (1988). Relationships among coping responses and perceptions of pain intensity, depression, and family functioning. *Clin J Pain, 4,* 101-106.
65a. Watt-Watson J. (In press). Neurological patient with chronic pain. In Baumann A and Dewis M (eds), *Decision making in neuroscience nursing,* St. Louis: Mosby–Year Book, Inc.
66. Yaster M and Deshpande J. (1988). Management of pediatric pain with opioid analgesics. *J Pediatr, 113*(3), 421-429.

4

A Practical Approach to Pain Assessment

Marilee Ivers Donovan

◆ ASSESSMENT VS. MEASUREMENT

The terms *pain measurement* and *pain assessment* are often used interchangeably by clinicians. However, these terms differ significantly in their goals and methods. The primary goal of pain measurement is the precise assignment of numbers to variables to represent quantities of these attributes according to rules required for research. The primary goal of pain assessment is to aid in the selection of alternative treatments and then evaluate the efficacy of the selected treatment(s) in clinical practice. For research purposes, one might want to know the exact site of each pain; for clinical therapy, knowing the general area(s) is usually adequate. In clinical practice, for instance, if the pain is localized to one discrete site, interventions that reduce the release of nociceptive substances are likely to be effective. If the patient reports multiple pain sites, the same interventions are inappropriate. Because these goals are different, the characteristics of the ideal process and/or tools for research measurement are different from those for clinical assessment. The primary characteristics of ideal research measurements and clinical assessments are outlined in Table 4-1. Their similarities and differences are evident.

Many methods of estimating and describing pain have been developed. The spectrum of these varies from the most subjective self-reports to the use of physiological correlates such as electromyographic readings, autonomic indices, and central nervous system indicators (Figure 4-1). Within the literature

◆ **Table 4-1**
Desired characteristics of pain measurement/pain assessment tools

Measurement for research	Assessment for clinical practice
Precise/standardized method	A method that will suggest the intervention to be used
High reliability/validity	Moderate reliability/validity
Able to assign numbers	Able to rank lowest to highest
Objective	Subjective
Comprehensive	Focused/individualized
Complex/multidimensional	Multidimensional/brief/easy
Independent factors	All factors are assumed to be interrelated
Uncontrolled variables are omitted, controlled, limited	Uncontrolled variables are accepted as inevitable
Computer compatible	Able to be clearly and consistently shared among colleagues

on pain measurement—and sadly in many practice settings—there are those who believe that pain measurement should be completely objective, i.e., free from the biases of the patient. Since the issues of subjectivity, reliability, and validity are crucial to the subject of clinical pain assessment, these topics will be addressed before the process of clinical assessment is described.

◆ VALIDITY AND RELIABILITY IN CLINICAL ASSESSMENT

Validity is the extent to which an instrument/tool/method measures the phenomenon under study. Reliability is the extent to which the method can be expected to give similar results when used again. The validity and reliability of self-reports (subjective) are frequently challenged in the clinical setting. Yet clinicians often accept without question the reports of objective tests known to have problems of reliability and validity, e.g., a test for cholesterol. The reliability of many of the objective measures listed in Figure 4-1 is high, and their validity for the physiological processes they measure is also very high. However, their validity as a measure of pain is

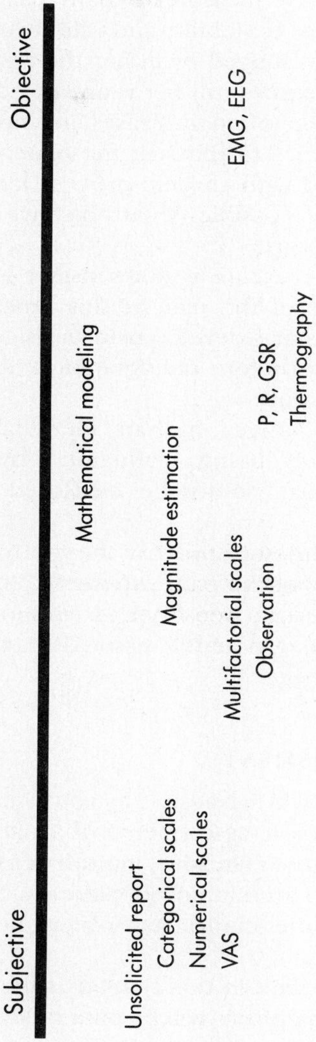

Subjective — Objective

Mathematical modeling

Unsolicited report

Categorical scales

Magnitude estimation

Numerical scales

VAS

Multifactorial scales

EMG, EEG

Observation

P, R, GSR

Thermography

FIGURE 4-1. Variety of measures of pain.

questionable. On the other hand, most subjective measures of pain (e.g., unsolicited complaints of pain, categorical, numerical, or visual analogue scale [VAS] estimates of intensity) have a reliability and validity thought to be moderate.[7,57,63] When subjective and objective measures of pain disagree, the reality of the pain experience (reliability and validity of the subjective measure) is often challenged by either the researchers or clinicians. The lack of agreement between subjective and objective measures of pain often increases in chronic pain and, therefore, the tendency to mistrust the patient is even more frequently associated with chronic pain. At least two alternative explanations are possible when objective and subjective measures of pain disagree:

1. The objective measure is not sensitive enough to indicate the cause of the pain at this time. For example, cancer patients may develop pain as a sign of recurrence days to months before radiographic evidence can confirm the recurrence.
2. The pain no longer has an identifiable peripheral stimulus but is being maintained by central pain mechanisms that cannot be measured using present technology.

The International Association for the Study of Pain recognizes the subjectivity of the pain experience in its definition: pain is ". . . an unpleasant sensory and emotional experience associated with actual or potential tissue damage, or described in terms of such damage."[44]

◆ CLINICAL ASSESSMENT

The clinical research literature has consistently confirmed that even the most basic assessments of a patient's pain are not being done.* Before extensive, multidimensional methods of pain measurement are employed clinically, the results of a regular, systematic, brief clinical assessment need to be used and evaluated.

The process described in this chapter is that of a practical clinical assessment. Emphasis will be on a process that is brief, intervention-focused, and individualized. The total clinical assessment consists of four phases:

---

* References 5, 10, 15, 28, 33, 58.

1. Basic
2. Personalized
3. Functional
4. Comprehensive

The data from each phase are used to develop and implement a plan of care. The outcomes of this plan are evaluated. If the evaluation indicates the need for additional information, the next phase of assessment is initiated. Evaluation information that clearly indicates the need for additional assessment may include: limited relief, dissatisfaction with the therapy or its effects, chronic pain, and observed dysfunctional interactions between patient and family or patient/family and caregivers.

Phase I, the basic assessment, will usually be adequate to manage uncomplicated acute pain, such as postoperative pain. Completion of all phases, best done in a multidisciplinary pain clinic, will usually be necessary to plan an effective program for a patient who has been housebound with chronic pain for months or years. Assessment of pain in children poses unique challenges and is addressed in detail in Chapters 9 and 10.

Phase I: The Basic Assessment

Even the most straightforward acute pain is a complex, multidimensional, neurophysiological, and psychosocial process fully known only to the person experiencing it. Therefore any assessment must be multidimensional. Since part of the complexity of pain is its variability over time, all pain assessment must also be longitudinal (repeated assessments at specified intervals).

Location

Failure to consistently confirm the location of pain can lead to treatment of the wrong pain or to selection of a method of treatment that is unlikely to be effective, e.g., choice of a localized therapy for a multisite pain. Patients tend to report only the most intense pain even when they have multiple sites of pain. In a recent study of 254 hospitalized medical, surgical, and pediatric patients, 34% reported multiple sites of pain.[16] For most patients, it is equally effective to ask the patient to point with one finger to each site of pain as it is to ask him or her to fill in the human figure (Figure 4-2). The effects of

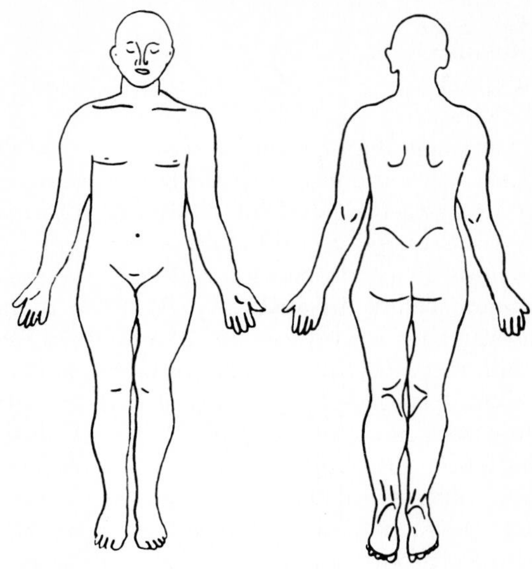

FIGURE 4-2. Pain figure.

mental status changes on the patient's ability to complete these tasks are unpredictable. For some patients whose mental status is deteriorating, it is easier to complete the human figure, and for others it is easier to point to each area of pain. The clinician needs to be prepared to try both methods and to search for secondary sites of pain. Repeated measures of location are the only effective method of determining whether and how pain moves over time.

Intensity

Categorical scales, numerical scales, and visual analogue scales (VAS) are commonly used to quantify the intensity of the pain experience (Figure 4-3). The horizontal VAS is considered by some to be the best scale for research purposes, but elderly patients and patients who are critically ill have difficulty understanding these scales. The correlations among categorical, numerical, and visual analogue scales are generally high ($r > .80$).[17,34,35,46,49] Therefore, for clinical assessment, any of these scales is adequate and appropriate. This author now routinely uses a 0 to 10 numerical scale for both clinical and research purposes. In addition to current pain intensity, it is useful to determine the intensity of the pain

Categorical scale

0 - No pain
1 - Mild pain
2 - Discomforting pain
3 - Distressing pain
4 - Horrible pain
5 - Excruciating pain

Numerical scale

0 - 1 - 2 - 3 - 4 - 5 - 6 - 7 - 8 - 9 - 10

No pain — Worst pain imaginable

VAS

No pain — Worst pain

FIGURE 4-3. Intensity scales.

when it "was at its worst in the past 24 hours" *(worst pain).* Some experts also assess *average pain* within the past 24 hours. Both *worst pain* and *average pain* are quantified using the same scale used for *current pain.* Specific methods of assessing childhood pain are described in Chapters 9 and 10.

Influencing Factors

Factors that precipitate or intensify the pain are often overlooked. Certain activities, positions, weather changes, times of day, moods, and cognitive appraisals are commonly associated with variations in pain. Obviously it isn't possible to eliminate everything that intensifies or causes pain, but it is essential to identify those factors that can be eliminated or treated as part of the pain relief plan.

All human experiences, including pain, have psychological as well as physiological components. It is often assumed that patients experiencing acute pain are anxious and patients experiencing chronic pain are depressed. However, either anxiety or depression may accompany either acute or chronic pain.[8,39] It is imperative that all assumptions about a patient's mood state or cognitive appraisal of the pain experience be verified using a validated clinical assessment tool.

The limited research available on factors that impede adequate pain control suggests that attitudes of patients, families, and caregivers are a primary impediment to rational and effective control of pain.[36,38,45] Identification of the counterproductive attitudes operating in a patient-setting interaction is prerequisite to the implementation of a satisfactory pain management program. Some of the common misconceptions leading to poor treatment of pain include:

1. Suspicion that the patient is a malingerer if a pathological reason for the pain cannot be found
2. Belief that health care professionals know more about pain than the patient
3. Assumption that the physiological changes associated with acute pain are valid indicators of pain
4. Fear that patients in pain are at significant risk of addiction and tolerance
5. Belief that waiting as long as possible between doses of an analgesic will prevent addiction.[9,20,36,39,45]

Where possible these erroneous beliefs need to be identified and corrected (see Chapter 3).

The pattern of *use* of therapy (analgesic or nonpharmacological method) must be analyzed. One cannot assume that what is ordered is actually used. In the author's research to date (n = 706 patients), only a quarter of the analgesic ordered was actually taken by the patients.[15,16]

Effects of Therapy

The effectiveness of pharmacological and nonpharmacological treatments in the past is a good predictor of what will be acceptable to the patient and what is likely to be effective during a current pain episode. Patients may be hesitant to report that distraction, heat, therapeutic touch, or massage effectively relieve their pain because they fear that the caregivers will not believe that they are "really having pain." Dr. Susan Wright (Chapter 17) proposes that pain relief measures that do not have an obvious clear physiological action are discounted as universally as is pain that is not accompanied by measurable pathological changes (x-ray, biochemical, etc.). This process of devaluing nontraditional approaches occurs

Relief

0% - 10% - 20% - 30% - 40% - 50% - 60% - 70% - 80% - 90% - 100%

No pain relief — Complete pain relief

Satisfaction

How satisfied are you with the pain relief you are receiving?

0 - 1 - 2 - 3 - 4 - 5 - 6 - 7 - 8 - 9 - 10

Not at all satisfied — Completely satisfied

How do you rate the side effects which accompany your pain treatment?

0 - 1 - 2 - 3 - 4 - 5 - 6 - 7 - 8 - 9 - 10

No problems — Very distressing

FIGURE 4-4. Measures of relief and satisfaction.

even though many of these nonanalgesic techniques have been demonstrated empirically to be effective, can be explained biochemically, and have been reported to be effective in relieving pain by patients in unrelated studies.*

Many pain assessments do not have a measure of relief included. The brief pain inventory (BPI) was one of the first to include a relief scale.[12] This relief scale (Figure 4-4) is brief, easy to use, valid, and easily understood by patients. In addition, patients should be asked to rank their satisfaction with the degree of pain relief and with the effects/side effects of the treatment being used.

Phase II: Personalizing the Assessment

Goal Identification

If patients are to be active members of the pain management team, they must be involved in the process early. One of the most significant roles for the patient is in goal setting.

* References 2, 8, 11, 15, 37, 43, 61.

Goals set *for* the patient are often inappropriate, misleading, and destined for failure. Even patients with acute postoperative pain differ in their goals. For example:

1. Some patients want "the nurse to take care of me." For a patient with this goal, PCA (patient-controlled analgesia) is not the preferred therapy even though current research supports the effectiveness of PCA.[3,52]
2. Patients with severe pain (acute or chronic in origin) differ in the degree of pain relief that is satisfactory and the magnitude of side effects they are willing to experience.

Psychosocial Modifiers

It is important to understand the person who is in pain if a truly personalized treatment plan is to be implemented. Zbrowski and others demonstrated that individuals raised in different cultures reacted to and expressed pain very differently.[13,55,64] However, an understanding of pain in various cultures and subcultures is almost nonexistent among health care providers. If the caregiver asks the patient to describe what they do in common situations involving pain (visit to a dentist, stubbing a toe, birth of a child, headache), even acutely ill patients are generally able to describe when and how they express pain, and the cultural and family rules that govern this expression.

Throughout the process of assessment, the clinician needs to be aware of cues the patient gives about personal ways of perceiving and coping with pain. The patient who answers every question in detail will probably be able to remember, when he returns home, to take his medications according to the schedule developed. The patient who gives brief, vague responses may need to be taught how to set up a schedule and a reminder system. The patient who says that "my doctor will handle it" is likely to accept a different range of approaches to pain control than the person who makes it clear, "I want to get control of this thing."

The emotions most commonly associated with pain have been anxiety and depression. Extensive evaluation of the psychological status of *every* patient is not warranted. In fact, some investigators have demonstrated that negative mood states are less common in patients experiencing pain than is generally assumed.[60] An estimate of the extent to which anxi-

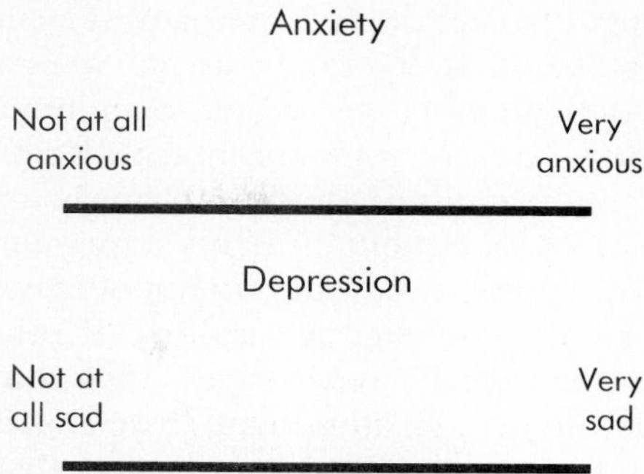

FIGURE 4-5. Assessing emotional state.

ety or depression may be altering the patient's perception of pain can be produced by a simple 10 cm VAS for depression and for anxiety[6] (Figure 4-5). Patients who have been living with pain for a long time may not recognize their own depression or anxiety and may not accurately respond to a simple screening tool such as a VAS. If the caregiver has reason to suspect that the patient is depressed or anxious even though his response to a VAS or numerical scale doesn't indicate such a state, the patient should be asked to complete brief, valid measures of depression or anxiety to determine the extent to which these mood states are contributing to the suffering of pain and whether a psychological referral is warranted.*

The way in which patients describe past successes and failures of treatment is also beneficial in planning current and future therapy. Patients who ascribe success only to medications are unlikely to be receptive to behavioral approaches, massage, or therapeutic touch. Patients who make it clear that they do not want to take "drugs" may be more receptive to nonpharmacological interventions.

Observations

Careful observation of the patient's behavior is part of any assessment.[32] The most important observations include facial expression, grimacing, movement, posture, and interactions with others. Measuring vital signs is also a form of observation. Since many of these observations are signs of autonomic stim-

* References 4, 7, 8, 25, 26, 54, 57.

ulation, occurring mainly with acute pain, the clinician needs to be aware of the duration of the pain and the possibility that autonomic stimulation is no longer operational. Although changes in vital signs are common in acute pain, the specific changes and the magnitude of these changes are unpredictable from patient to patient. Patients experiencing chronic pain may look depressed, but they do not necessarily look like they are in pain. Observing the actions of others, such as family, friends, and other caregivers, and their interaction with the patient is often more important than observing the patient. These interactions yield clues to factors that are intensifying, compounding, or reducing the pain. For instance, a husband who is urging his wife to wait a little longer before she asks for her postoperative analgesic is reducing the effectiveness of the pain relief plan. Such behavior requires family/patient education, stressing the benefits of preventing pain rather than treating pain. However, this same observation would be more serious if the patient was suffering from an advanced stage of a slow-growing sarcoma. To allow the husband's behavior to persist would be to subject his wife to much needless pain in the final months of her life. The families of those living with chronic pain have often developed behaviors that reinforce or intensify the pain. Treatment of these interpersonal factors may be essential to adequate pain relief. Early intervention by a knowledgeable and sensitive caregiver could alter family beliefs and behaviors, spare patients and family members a great deal of agony, and minimize the risk of developing countertherapeutic behavior patterns.

Phase III: Functional Assessment

Demographic Factors

Factors such as age (young), sex (male), education (less), socioeconomic status (lower), ethnicity, and religion have been suggested as risk factors for the development of pain or predictors of response to treatment. However, one could ask whether the high risk *young* man with *less education* who *earns less money* is not actually at risk because he is working in a job where he does the kinds of tasks that more often lead to injury. A description of the tasks one must perform at work may be more useful in planning therapy than a job title or a comprehensive list of demographic variables.

Functional Ability

If the above information is insufficient to determine an appropriate plan of therapy, the next most frequently explored areas are the effects the pain has on the patient's life in general and ability to function in particular. The interference scores on the brief pain inventory (BPI) are a simple indication of the effect the pain has had on the patient's mood and ability to work, sleep, walk, relate to significant others, and enjoy life.[12] Williams, in his review of the literature on measures for chronic pain assessment, suggested the following additional methods: a daily record or log of the exact amount of time the patient spends mobile and the exact amount of time the patient spends in bed; measures of disability and self-care ability; and evaluation of ambulation.[63]

Qualitative data (gathered by structured or unstructured interview) may include: living arrangements (size of dwelling, one story or two, placement of key rooms, who else lives in home, other help available); degree of independence expressed by patient; and relations with significant others.

Phase IV: Comprehensive Assessment

Economic Effect

The costs of medical care, surgery, hospitalization, medications, nonpharmacological interventions, missed income, and visiting (hotel, travel, parking, meals, babysitting, etc.) by significant others should be estimated for all patients with a chronic pain problem. In addition, an inventory of the available financial resources (salary, disability payments, settlements) must also be computed.

Psychological/Behavioral/Cognitive Measures

The instruments most commonly employed to assess psychological aspects of pain are listed in Table 4-2. The ability to replicate findings that suggest certain risk factors or predictors of success with pain therapy in other populations has consistently been a problem.[63] It is difficult to decipher the meanings of these contradictory findings. Are they:

1. The result of other unknown uncontrolled variables
2. An artifact of the treatment setting
3. Evidence of a relationship between psychosocial variables and pain/pain relief

◆ **Table 4-2**
Standardized measures of pain modifiers

Factor	Examples of instruments	Reference
Psychological		
Depression	YAS-D	Cella and Perry, 1986
	BDI	Beck et al, 1961
	CES-D	Radloff, 1977
Anxiety	VAS-A	Cella and Perry, 1986
	STAI	Speilberger et al, 1970
Multifactor	IBQ	Pilowsky and Spence, 1983
	MMPI	Fordyce et al, 1978
Cognitive errors	CEQ	Smith et al, 1986
Coping	?	Tunks and Bellissimo, 1988
Functional abilities	ADL	Katz, 1983
	AIMS	Heenan, 1982
	BPI	Daut et al, 1983
	SIP	Follick et al, 1984
	Up-time	Sanders, 1983
Multidimensional	MPQ	Melzack, 1975
	Memorial pain assessment card	Fishman et al, 1986
Physical	Algometer	Jensen et al, 1986
	EMG activity	
Quality of life	FLIC	Schipper et al, 1984
	Quality of life index	Padilla et al, 1983
	Quality of life index	Ferrans and Powers, 1985

4. Evidence that psychosocial factors are intervening variables in the pain experience
5. Evidence that the pain is causing the factor observed

Williams[63] cautions that it is premature to interpret even such commonly used measures as the MMPI, BDI, and coping scales in a diagnostic manner. They provide information that may help the clinician understand the pain experience from the patient's perspective; they do not diagnose pain (Table 4-3).

◆ **Table 4-3**
Standardized tests and alternative meanings

Conclusion of report	Alternative meanings
Patient has fewer than normal emotional supports	1) The result of pain-related depression, causing the patient to withdraw from social contact 2) The result of withdrawal secondary to severe pain even without depression 3) The result of perceptual distortions that lead the patient to answer the questions in a way that suggests social isolation but that cannot be objectively confirmed (i.e., the patient feels isolated but the social supports are available and not used)

All standardized tests need to be cautiously interpreted.

Other behavioral measures frequently suggested include a count of the number of visits to a physician/year, number of hospitalizations, number of hospitalizations for pain, and number of surgeries. Although some investigators suggest that these variables are predictors of response to therapy, replication of these studies has been inconsistent.[63]

Recently, interest in the interaction between family dynamics and pain has begun to be explored. Observation of family interaction was suggested in phase II. As part of a comprehensive psychosocial evaluation, assessment of family interaction should include some standardized tests and interviews of family members to explore the degree of positive feelings among family members, the support available, the beliefs and agreement regarding the pain, cause of pain and goals, and identification of reinforcing behaviors that exist within the family to maintain the pain and pain behaviors.

Physical Measures

These measures are usually the most invasive and most costly. They are used when clearly indicated or when other measures have been inconclusive. They measure physiological states that have at times been associated with pain; they do not measure pain. Tests such as EMG, EEG, algometry (and other measures of pressure sensitivity), and thermography have been suggested as measures of chronic pain. In some patients and to round out a comprehensive assessment, they can be appropriate. However, their validity and reliability for the assessment of clinical pain have not been well established.[7,57,63]

◆ SUMMARY

The four-phase clinical assessment described is based on reliable and valid components of clinical assessment and was developed to provide a practical framework within which clinicians in a variety of settings could work. It is not meant to be applied as a single process to all patients. Clinical judgment is required in the selection of the factors to assess and in the breadth and depth of the assessment. Because clinical judgment is critical to the implementation of this assessment, novice practitioners, including expert practitioners who are new to the field of pain assessment and pain control will need guidance and supervision in its use.

The goals of the clinical assessment process are to characterize the pain experience, to direct the selection of appropriate intervention strategies, and to verify the effectiveness of the pain therapy employed. A consistently applied measure of relief and a measure of satisfaction with the relief and the therapy are essential to any clinical assessment process.

The educational deficits, cultural biases, and system obstacles that lead to poor pain assessment and poor pain treatment affect all caregivers. No one is naturally better prepared to care for the patient in pain. Therefore effective pain management is more likely if a variety of professional perspectives are focused on the assessment and treatment planning for patients with pain. This team must include at least the patient, the nurse, and the physician. In addition, for patients with more complex pain problems, it may include many of the following: psychologist, pharmacist, social worker, clergy, and occupational, physical, and vocational therapists. In support of this interprofessional approach, throughout this chapter, reference has been to the clinician or the caregiver rather than to the nurse.

McCaffery[38] and Strauss et al[56] suggest that lack of accountability for pain relief is one of the causes of poor pain control.

A single caregiver needs to undertake the leadership of this team and assume *responsibility* for the effective relief of pain. Data is beginning to accumulate that suggests that the nurse is the most crucial person in the link between pain, pain assessment, and pain relief in the hospital setting.[15,16] Therefore, it follows logically that in most situations, the nurse should function as the leader of the pain relief team.

Some of the behaviors described in this chapter may be beyond those regularly practiced by the reader. Not every nurse will be prepared, willing, or able to perform all phases of the assessment. However, every nurse who cares for a patient in pain must be proficient in the basic assessment, including the evaluation of relief and satisfaction. With these basic tools the nurse is an irreplaceable contributor to the ongoing process of patient assessment, pain therapy, and evaluation of relief.

REFERENCES

1. Ahles TA, Blanchard EB, and Ruckdeschel JC. (1983). The multidimensional nature of cancer-related pain. *Pain, 7,* 277-288.
2. Barbour LA, McGuire DB, and Kirchoff KT. (1986). Nonanalgesic methods of pain control used by cancer outpatients. *Oncol Nurs Forum, 13,* 56-60.
3. Barkas G and Duafala M. (Summer 1988). Advances in cancer pain management: a review of patient-controlled analgesia. *J Pain Sympt Manage, 3,* 150-160.
4. Beck AT, Ward CH, Mendelsohn M, et al. (1961). An inventory for measuring depression. *Arch Gen Psychiatry, 4,* 561-571.
5. Camp LD. (1988). A comparison of nurses' recorded assessment of pain with perceptions of pain as described by cancer patients. *Cancer Nurs, 11,* 237-243.
6. Cella D and Perry SW. (1986). Reliability and concurrent validity of three visual analogue mood scales. *Psychol Rep, 59,* 827-833.
7. Chapman CR, Casey KL, Dubner R, et al. (1985). Pain measurement: an overview. *Pain, 22,* 1-31.
8. Chapman CR and Turner JA. (1986). Psychological control of acute pain in medical settings. *J Pain Sympt Manage, 1,* 9-20.
9. Charap AD. (1978). The knowledge, attitudes and experience of medical personnel treating pain in the terminally ill. *Mt Sinai J Med, 45,* 561-580.
10. Cohen FL. (1980). Postsurgical pain relief: patients' status and nurses' medication choices. *Pain, 9,* 265-274.
11. Dalton JA. (1987). Education for pain management: a pilot study. *Patient Education Counsel, 9,* 155-165.
12. Daut RL, Cleeland CS, and Flanery RC. (1983). Development of the Wisconsin Brief Pain Questionnaire to assess pain in cancer and other diseases. *Pain, 17,* 197-210.
13. Davitz LJ, Davitz JR. (1981). *Inferences of patients' pain and psychological distress: studies of nursing behaviors.* New York: Springer.

14. Derogatis LR. (1975). *SCL-90R: administration, scoring and procedures manual II.* Towson, Md: Clinical Psychometrics Research.
15. Donovan M, Dillon P, and McGuire L. (1987). Incidence and characteristics of pain in a sample of medical-surgical inpatients. *Pain, 30,* 69-78.
16. Donovan M, Slack J, Wright S, and Faut M. (1989). Factors associated with inadequate pain control in hospitalized patients. American Pain Society Annual Scientific Meeting. Phoenix Ariz, October 26-29, 1989. (Abstract)
17. Ekblom A and Hansson P. (1988). Pain intensity measurements in patients with acute pain receiving afferent stimulation. *J Neurol Neurosurg Psychiatry, 51,* 481-486.
18. Ferrans C and Powers M. (1985). Quality of life index: development and psychometric properties. *Adv Nurs Res, 8,* 15.
19. Fishman B, Pasternak S, and Wallenstein RW, et al. (1986). The memorial pain assessment card: a valid instrument for evaluation of cancer pain. *Proc ASCO, 5,* 239. (abstract).
20. Foley KM. (1985). The treatment of cancer pain. *N Engl J Med, 313,* 84-95.
21. Foley KM. (1986). The treatment of pain in the patient with cancer. *CA, 36,* 194-215.
22. Follick MJ, Ahern DK, and Laser-Wolston N. (1984). Evaluation of a daily activity diary for chronic pain patients. *Pain, 19,* 373-382.
23. Follick MJ, Smith TW, and Ahern DK. (1984). The sickness impact profile: a global measure of disability in chronic low back pain. *Pain, 21,* 67-76.
24. Fordyce WE, Brena SF, Holcomb RJ, et al. (1978). Relationship of patient semantic pain descriptions to physician diagnostic judgements, activity level measures and MMPI. *Pain, 5,* 293-303.
25. Frank-Stromborg M (ed). (1988). *Instruments for clinical nursing research.* Norwalk, Conn: Appleton-Lange.
26. Gobel B and Donovan M. Depression and anxiety. (1986). *Semin Oncol Nurs, 3,* 267-276.
27. Gracely RH and Kwilosz DM. (1988). The descriptor differential scale: applying psychophysical principles to clinical pain assessment. *Pain, 35,* 279-288.
28. Graffam SR. (1981). Congruence of nurse-patient expectations regarding nursing in pain. *Nurs Leader, 4,* 12-15.
29. International Association for the Study of Pain. (1986). Pain terms: a current list with definitions and notes on usage. *Pain, 3,* S216-S221.
30. Jensen K, Andersen HO, Oleson J, and Lindblom U. (1986). Pressure-pain threshold in human temporal region. Evaluation of a new pressure algometer. *Pain, 25,* 313-325.
31. Katz S. (1983). Assessing self-maintenance: activities of daily living, mobility, and instrumental activities of daily living. *J Am Geriatr Soc, 31,* 721.
32. Keefe FJ and Block AR. (1982). Development of an observation method for assessing pain behavior in chronic low back pain. *Behav Ther, 13,* 363-375.
33. Ketovuori H. (1987). Nurses' and patients' conceptions of wound pain and the administration of analgesics. *J Pain Sympt Manag, 2,* 213-218.
34. Kremer E, Atkinson JH, and Ignelzi RJ. (1981). Measurement of pain: patient preference does not confound pain measurement. *Pain, 10,* 241-248.
35. Lee KA and Kreckhefer GM. (1989). Technical notes: measuring human responses using visual-analogue scales. *West J Nurs Res, 11,* 128-132.

36. Marks RM and Sachar EJ. (1973). Undertreatment of medical inpatients with narcotic analgesics. *Ann Intern Med, 78,* 172-181.
37. Mast DE. (1986). Effects of imagery. *Image, 18,* 118-120.
38. McCaffery M. (1979). *Nursing management of the patient with pain* (ed 2). Philadelphia: Lippincott.
39. McCaffery M and Beebe A. (1989). *Pain: clinical manual for nursing practice.* St Louis: Mosby.
40. McGuire DB. (1984). The measurement of clinical pain. *Nurs Res, 33,* 152-156.
41. Meenan RF. (1982). The AIMS approach to health status measurement: conceptual background and measurement properties. *J Rheumatol, 9,* 785.
42. Melzack R. (1975). The McGill pain questionnaire: major properties and scoring methods. *Pain, 1,* 277-299.
43. Melzack R. (1985). Hyperstimulation analgesia. In Brena SF and Chapman SL (editors). *Clin Anesthesiol, 3,* 81-92.
44. Merskey H (ed). (1986). Classification of chronic pain: description of chronic pain syndromes and definitions of pain terms. *Pain Suppl, 3,* S217.
45. Myers JS. (1985). Cancer pain: assessment of nurses' knowledge and attitudes. *Oncol Nurs Forum, 12,* 62-66.
46. Ohrhaus EE and Adler R. (1975). Methodological problems in the measurement of pain: a comparison between the verbal rating scale and the visual analogue scale. *Pain, 1,* 379-384.
47. Padilla G, Present C, Grant M, et al. (1983). Quality of life index for patients with cancer. *Res Nurs Health, 6,* 117.
48. Pilowsky I and Spence ND. (1983). *Manual for the illness behavior questionnaire* (IBQ). (ed 2). Adelaide, Australia, University of Adelaide.
49. Price DS, McGrath DA, and Rafil A. (1983). The validation of visual analogue scales as ratio scale measures for chronic experimental pain. *Pain, 17,* 45.
50. Radloff L. (1977). The CES-D scale: a self-report depression scale for research in the general population. *Appl Psychol Measur, 3,* 385-401.
51. Schipper H, Clinch J, McMurray A, and Levitt M. (1984). Measuring the quality of life of cancer patients: the functional living index-cancer: development and validation. *J Clin Oncol, 2,* 472.
52. Sheidler VR. (1989). Patient-controlled analgesia. *Curr Con Nurs, 1,* 13-16.
53. Smith TW, Aberger EW, Follick MJ, and Ahern DK. (1986). Cognitive distortion and psychological distress in chronic low back pain. *J Consult Clin Psychol, 54,* 573-575.
54. Spielberger CD, Gorsuch RL, and Luschene RE. (1970). *Manual for the state-trait anxiety inventory* (STAI). Palo Alto, Calif: Consulting Psychologist Press.
55. Sternbach RA. (1974). *Pain patients: traits and treatment.* Orlando, Fla: Academic Press.
56. Strauss A, Fagerhaugh SY, and Glaser B. (1974). Pain: an organization-work-interactional perspective. *Nurs Outlook, 22,* 560-566.
57. Syrjala KL, Chapman CR. (1984). Measurement of clinical pain: a review and integration of research findings. *Adv Pain Res Ther, 7,* 71-101.

58. Teske K, Daut RL, and Cleeland CS. (1983). Relationships between nurses' observations and patients' self reports of pain. *Pain, 16,* 289-296.
59. Tunks E and Bellissimo A. (1988). Coping with the coping concept: a brief comment. *Pain, 34,* 171-174.
60. Turk DC, Meichenbaum D, and Genest M. (1983). *Pain and behavioral medicine.* New York: Guilford Press.
61. Turner JA and Romano JM. (1984). Evaluating psychologic interventions for chronic pain: issues and recent developments. *Adv Pain Res Ther, 7,* 257-296.
62. Ventafridda V, Ripamonti C, Bianchi M, et al. (1986). A randomized study on oral administration of morphine and methadone in the treatment of cancer pain. *J Pain Sympt Manag, 1,* 203-207.
63. Williams RC. (1988). Review article: toward a set of reliable and valid measures for chronic pain assessment and outcome research. *Pain, 35,* 239-251.
64. Zborowski M. (1969). *People in pain.* San Francisco: Jossey-Bass.

5

Living with Chronic Pain: A Family Perspective

Kathleen M. Rowat

THE FAMILY OF the chronic pain sufferer faces a number of challenges as the family, like the patient, learns to live with the pain. Recent writings within the area of chronic pain and the family suggest four aspects of the pain experience that challenge the family:

1. Understanding the pain
2. Dealing with its effects on their lives
3. The uncertainty of management
4. Confronting the health care system

◆ UNDERSTANDING CHRONIC PAIN

The meaning given to any illness experience has been cited as an important feature of such an experience in both how the illness affects the individual and family, and their attempts at management.[60] Schwenk and Hughes,[55] in their review of several studies dealing with the effect of an illness on the family, concluded that "the way in which the family perceived (defined) the illness . . . was directly related to the eventual level of family stability and coping" (p. 9).

For the family experiencing chronic pain, issues of understanding and defining likewise are central. The meaning families ascribed to their situations was found to be associated both with family adjustment[7,53] and with treatment outcomes for the pain sufferer.[62,69] The family most often is the first group to whom the individual in pain turns for validation of his experience. However, comprehending chronic pain presents a particular challenge to families. Two factors may contribute to the family's difficulty in understanding the pain: the unique and distinctive characteristics of chronic pain, and the family's encounters with the health care system concerning the pain problem.

A number of authors have suggested that the uncertainties surrounding chronic pain are among its most troublesome features.[25,34,54,59] The absence, often, of identifiable organic etiology or pathology and the lack of usefulness of the pain as a signal or warning are two such characteristics. In their attempt to understand the pain, family members may compare the present chronic pain with other episodes of pain they have witnessed or experienced in the past.[49] The models used for comparison may be those of acute pain in which the pain is time-limited, has a clearly defined cause, evokes commonly understood and easily recognized behaviors or responses, and generally is responsive to treatment. With the present pain, however, the family now finds itself facing a perplexing and unfamiliar situation. Rather than showing signs of abating, this pain continues with no signs of relief and no clear endpoint. Furthermore, there may be little evidence of the predisposing cause or pathology, and those behaviors commonly associated with acute pain may be absent.

When the family is unable to find a fit between the present pain and that which is familiar, uncertainty and anxiety follow. To reduce such distress, family members may develop their own cognitive meanings to fill the void. They may conclude either that the pain is not real or that it is a manifestation of a far more severe, even life-threatening illness.[49] As attribution theory posits, when symptoms are unfamiliar or difficult to evaluate, highly speculative inferences and subsequently erroneous attributions may be made.[24] Adding to the complexity of the attribution or defining process is the likelihood that very disparate interpretations of the pain may exist within the family. The importance of obtaining both the pain sufferer's and family members' assessment of the pain was suggested in the findings of one study that looked at the pain ratings of spouses and their partners, using the McGill pain questionnaire.[49] In this study, spouses deemed to be highly stressed rated their mate's pain significantly higher than a group of low-stressed spouses even though the levels of pain as reported by the patients (partners) in each of these groups were almost identical. The author postulated that the spouse's pain rating might be more a reflection of the meaning and perception the spouses held concerning the pain than a rating of the pain per se.

In addition to the particular characteristics of chronic pain, the family's encounters with health professionals may be a second major factor contributing to its difficulty in understanding the pain. As family members, along with the patient, attempt to gain some insight into this health problem, they often find themselves embarking on an arduous and frustrating search for the answer. Indeed, ongoing and frequent contacts with a variety of health professionals may become an established way of life. When no answers are forthcoming and when the health care professional is unable to produce a definitive explanation as expected, feelings of anger, frustration, and distress are experienced by family members.[49,60] Family members may detect the health professional's own uncertainty concerning chronic pain, adding further to the anxieties the family is experiencing. A number of authors are critical of the slowness of those in the health field to recognize and deal with the differences between acute and chronic pain.[23]

◆ DEALING WITH THE EFFECTS OF THE PAIN

Not infrequently the family of the chronic pain patient is held suspect in terms of its possible influence on the pain behaviors of the sufferer and as possibly one of the predisposing factors in the development of the pain.*

Recent writings, however, have suggested that the family as well as the patient may be suffering the consequences of the pain and facing the challenge of dealing with its effects on their lives.[65] Unfortunately, there has been a delay in acknowledging that chronic pain is more than a symptom, that it is a chronic illness in its own right. This delay in recognition has resulted in a lack of awareness that chronic pain shares with other chronic illnesses many of the attendant disruptions.[8]

Severe chronic pain has been shown to have profound consequences for those in close contact with the patient, particularly those from whom the patient seeks understanding and assistance.† Furthermore, it has been suggested that the

---

* References 18, 20, 21, 28, 44, 58.

† References 9, 11, 13, 38, 39, 46, 49.

pain may evoke behaviors in others that in many respects resemble those of the patient.

The health of all family members may be at risk when chronic pain is present.* Of the spouses in one study, 83% reported experiencing some form of health problem that they attributed directly to the pain of their mate.[53] The most prevalent of such effects were emotional, such as feelings of depression, fear, and terror associated with a sense of uncertainty. Other authors likewise have noted the presence of depression in spouses of chronic pain patients.[1,19,57]

Increased physical and emotional illnesses in the children of chronic pain families also were linked in the minds of the respondents in Rowat's study[49] to the stress of having a parent with a long-term illness. Similar findings were reported by Dura and Beck,[15] who found that children who had mothers with chronic pain had significantly higher depression scores when compared with children whose parents had no illness.

Not only has chronic pain been shown to affect the health of individual family members, but like other long-term illnesses, chronic pain may affect family life as a whole by disrupting family roles and relationships.[6,15,53] Benoliel[4] notes that it is not the medical aspects of an illness that create the family's problems but rather it is the impingement of the disease and its treatment on family interactions and relationships and on normal activities and habits.

In their study of family functioning when mothers had chronic pain, Dura and Beck[15] found that members of these families perceived their family environments to have more problems than those of families in which the mother had a diagnosis of diabetes or no illness. More specifically, they noted that families with a mother experiencing chronic pain perceived the family environment as less cohesive and containing more conflict compared with families in which there was no illness in the parent. Respondents in Rowat's study[49] also spoke of the family environment as tense, conflictive, and unhappy.

Family activities may be dictated and/or altered by the pain. Pain becomes the pivotal point around which family life revolves, and those areas of family life normally within the control of the family are now to a greater or lesser extent within

* References 6, 13, 15, 27, 38, 46, 49.

the hold of the pain. Pain determines what the family is able to do and when it does it.[50] Terzian[63] refers to the individual with chronic pain as being without freedom and imprisoned by the pain. Those who share the patient's world, particularly the family, likewise feel the restrictive powers of pain.[50] Families describe themselves as "not free," with the selection and timing of activities and events subect to the vagaries of the pain.[49] Janis and Rodin[24] note that to be deprived of options is to lose one's freedom. Conversely, to be able to determine one's goals and the means by which these will be achieved implies freedom and choice, and consequently a sense of control.

The disruption of family relationships that has been observed to occur in families with chronic pain is another aspect of family life that presents a challenge. The direction of the relationship between chronic pain and marital disruption is controversial. Although writings on chronic pain and the marital relationship have tended to suggest that a disturbed relationship may lead to the development of a health problem such as chronic pain,[42,43,68] data from other studies support the conclusion that the stresses associated with a long-term illness contribute to strained relationships.[57]

In one study, over three quarters of spouses married to chronic pain sufferers believed that their marital relationship was affected by the chronic experience.[49] "Well" spouses spoke of the "binding" and "separating" force of the pain. Descriptions of feeling restricted and being unable to have a life of their own because of their mate's pain were given as evidence of the "binding force" of the pain. On the other hand, even more distressing and indeed prevalent in this same study were the reports of the "distancing" effects of the pain. The inability of spouses to comprehend and share with their mate "what it must feel like," coupled with the reality that physical closeness was not always possible because of the pain, led to statements by these spouses such as, "I didn't get married to be alone, now I am alone; I feel to a certain extent separated from my wife by this experience."

Evidence of the effect of chronic pain on the marital relationship also exists in the findings of a number of other studies.[1,19,27,37,42] Maruta and associates,[37] for example, found that 65% of the spouses in their study reported a negative change in marital satisfaction after the onset of pain. Similarly, Flor and associates[19] demonstrated substantial marital dissatisfaction in the spouses of chronic pain patients, dissatisfaction closely associated with that of the patients and with the spouses' mood.

Changes in the parent-child relationship also have been attributed to the presence of chronic pain in the parent.[49] Alterations in both the mood and the behavior of the parent as a result of the pain were seen as contributing to the child's fear and withdrawal from the parent. The erratic and often unpredictable behaviors of a once-predictable and certain parent were cited as one of the major factors leading to such strained relationships. Other authors have proposed that in those families in which the parent's illness may have affected the parent's ability to perform in the parental role, the children may feel resentful, "cheated," or burdened as a result of the additional responsibilities placed on them.[14]

◆ UNCERTAINTY OF MANAGEMENT

A third challenge facing the chronic pain family is that of managing the pain and its associated effects. The failure of the health care system to organize for the systematic care of the chronically ill has led to the individual and family becoming the prime managers of such health problems.[12,22,47,61] The challenge of managing chronic pain may be one for which the majority of families are ill prepared. The person with chronic pain and his family frequently are given the mandate, "You must learn to live with the pain." The question of how this is to be accomplished, however, rarely is addressed. Coping skills that the family may have used in the past to manage short-term crises now may be found ineffectual. Indeed, as the spouses in one study reported, the most distressing aspect of their experience as a family member was the sense of helplessness at being unable to effect any change in their mate's pain.[49] The sense of uncertainty about what to do was compounded by a sense of fear that if indeed they did intervene, their intervention might cause further harm. A striking finding in this study, however, was that over three quarters of the spouses could indeed identify factors that either augmented or reduced their mate's pain. However, spouses did not recognize these factors as potential control measures.

Much of the research on coping with the stresses of illness has focused on those conditions that for the most part present with well-defined stages or phases or that carry the expectation of recovery.[10] Little attention appears to have been directed toward those coping or management processes required for such long-term, unpredictable, and ill-defined health conditions as chronic pain.

The family faces not only the issue of coping with the pain itself but also questions concerning their own behavior. Management questions such as, "How do I act, sympathetic or firm? Do I ignore him? How will my behaviors affect his pain?" were some of the questions spouses posed in the study by Rowat.[49]

The uncertainty and anxiety surrounding issues of management are not surprising, perhaps, in light of the widespread uncertainty associated with the pain itself. As noted earlier, if an event such as chronic pain cannot be interpreted or understood, it may preclude the development of appropriate management strategies and lead to a sense of helplessness.[30] Studies in the area of coping point to the fact that the way in which individuals interpret or appraise a situation influences their coping as well as their emotional, physiological, and behavioral reactions to stressful events.[29,31,33]

◆ DEALING WITH THE HEALTH CARE SYSTEM

As families attempt to understand the world of pain within which they are living and as they struggle to manage not only the pain itself but also its effects on their health and family functioning, they, like the patient, look to the health care system for assistance. All too often, however, this presents still another challenge. The family frequently encounters a system that has not yet recognized the place of the family in such matters, leaving the family with a sense of being ignored, avoided, and abandoned by health professionals.[49] It appears evident that the place of the family within the present health care scene has not yet been established as legitimate, and the family finds itself confronting a system that is still geared to only the ill individual. As the family, like the patient, attempts to overcome feelings of helplessness and distress and to gain some sense of control, it may embark on an arduous search for answers. Frequently such behaviors are given the pejorative label of 'doctor-shopping.' This label may result in the eventual discounting of the pain problem by the health professional and an even wider gap between the health care provider and the family. Rowat[49] proposes that such labeling may obscure what is in fact a healthy and positive response by the family. The family's relentless pursuit of answers to its questions may be seen as a form of control. Availability of options, according to Averill,[3] is a form of control. Where options are lacking or perceived to be lacking, feelings of helplessness and hopelessness may follow. Seligman[56] argues that the inability to control events produces fear. However, such fear may be useful if it promotes the search for a response that will work to regain control.

◆ THE NURSE'S ROLE

As demonstrated in the previous sections, there is compelling evidence that the family as a whole, not only the individual in pain, must become the focus of the nurse's attention. The family shares with the individual in pain a number of challenges and concerns and, like the patient, must learn to live with the pain. Not only does the family play a possible role in shaping the patient's experience, but the family too may be affected by the experience. Nurses have an important role in helping patients and families to cope more effectively with this experience (see box).

The importance of viewing the family as the unit of care is receiving increased emphasis in the literature.[55] Livsey[35] notes, "It is essential to keep in mind the conceptual framework of the family as a whole when evaluating the family when one of its members is ill" (p. 248). Unfortunately, however, the difficulties that family members frequently encounter with the health system suggest that such a perspective has not yet been widely adopted. Although the patient's significant others

◆ NURSING THE FAMILY

1. Involve the total family in "learning to live with pain."
2. Create a positive and trusting relationship.
3. Assess the family's perceptions and understanding of the pain problem.
4. Augment the family's understanding of chronic pain and its manifestations.
5. Promote a sense of control.
6. Have a "staying" approach.

ideologically may not be forgotten by caretakers, designed or planned intervention with them often is overlooked, even in the face of acute family disruptions.[35]

Turk and Kerns[64] argue that chronic illness necessitates a general, long-term, supportive relationship among the patient, family, and health care system. One of the characteristics of the present system of health care, however, is that it is geared to short, intensive patient encounters. Chronically ill patients and their families, on the other hand, require longer encounters for effective dialogue to be established.[2] Waring[69] stresses that communication and collaboration with the health professional within a positive and trusting atmosphere are an essential aspect of the family's learning to live with chronic pain. Support is mounting for the necessity of incorporating the spouse, if not all family members, into a program of learning to live with the pain.*

Flor et al,[17] in their study of the effect of chronic pain on the spouse, concluded that it was not the chronic pain per se but the patients' and spouses' coping with it that determined the spouses' responses. Following from this, the authors went on to suggest that including the spouse in stress management and coping skills training might be one way of improving both the emotional and physical well-being of the spouse. However, as these same authors note, little attention appears to have been given in pain treatment programs to the possible effect of the patient on the spouse or on family interaction.[19]

A review of the challenges facing the chronic pain family would suggest that there are two major stressors that are central to the family's experience with chronic pain, namely feelings of uncertainty and helplessness. These stressors, it has been hypothesized, may contribute significantly to the distress of the family.[49] As proposed by Rowat,[49] the uncertain nature of the chronic pain itself may be at the heart of the uncertainties experienced by family members. Therefore assessing family members' perceptions and understanding of the pain problem may be an important first step in working with the chronic pain family.[51] Questions such as, "Can you describe for me what your husband/wife's pain is like?" "What do *you* think has caused the pain?" and "How serious do *you* think the problem is?" can yield valuable data on this key aspect of the pain experience. Obtaining such information not only will

* References 6, 7, 16, 27, 37, 41, 50, 53, 57, 66, 69.

enable the nurse to clarify, correct, or confirm where necessary, but also will provide the opportunity of comparing the family's understanding of the situation with that of the patient. Studies have shown that congruence or lack of congruence of family perceptions of a health problem with those of the patients not only was associated with treatment outcomes for the patient but also played a critical role in the family's overall experience with the problem.[26,36,49,62] Therefore decreasing the uncertainty regarding the pain and clarifying meanings through a total family involvement in learning about chronic pain may be one approach to assisting families to cope more effectively and ultimately to gain a sense of control.

With the experience of chronic pain, many uncertainties, such as those relating to etiology or prognosis, will remain. An important component of any intervention might be to develop those cognitive processes that would enable family members to tolerate a certain level of ambiguity. Pearlin and Schooler[45] note that some problems may be impervious to personal efforts to change, and therefore coping must be directed toward identifying strategies that enable the individual to endure that which cannot be avoided. Strategies such as reframing, which may control the meaning of the stressful experience and which functions to control the stress that arises out of such experiences, may be appropriate. LeShan[34] speaks of the universe of the person in chronic pain, a universe he likens to a nightmare in which outside forces are in control and the will is helpless. Family members, too, reside in such a universe. Altering the family's perception of helplessness may be as critical a feature of the nurse's intervention as providing the family with actual skills of management. Vachon et al[67] found wives of cancer patients to be more stressed than those whose husbands suffered from some form of cardiovascular disease. These authors attributed this difference to the differing perceptions of the control held by the two groups of spouses. The wives of cancer patients felt particularly impotent regarding the management of pain.

Miller[40] points out that most research on the response to aversive events has focused on the escape or avoidance response. However, many real-life situations only allow people to reduce the severity of the stressor. Little research has been carried out that investigates situations in which the controlling response is difficult or where the subject must learn the controlling response. As Roskies and Lazarus[48] observe, areas relating to severe chronic stress remain relatively untouched in coping-skills training programs.

Facilitating the deliberative and conscious assessment and planning by family members is an important aspect of the nurse's involvement with the family. Rowat[49] found that pain-augmenting or reducing factors often went unrecognized by family members as possible features of control. These findings suggest that assisting families to see this association and to identify ways in which such factors might be altered or enhanced by their own behaviors would promote feelings of control.

Assisting families to assume control of their own health, however, does not mean abandonment by the health care provider. Rather, evidence suggests that reliance on some "external power," such as that offered by the health care system, may be the enabling factor permitting families to assume control of their own welfare.[49] Benoliel and Crowley[5] refer to the concept of "staying," that is, of being open and available to the client, as being an important aspect of long-term care.

◆ CONCLUSION

To deal effectively with a long-term health problem, such as chronic pain, demands a partnership of the family and the nurse. As family members are incorporated into the team dealing with the chronic pain problem, and as recognition is given to the vital role they play in the total pain experience, not only may family distress be reduced, but the ultimate goal of enhanced quality of family life for all members may be realized.

REFERENCES

1. Ahern DC, Adams AE, and Follick MJ. (1985). Emotional and marital disturbance in spouses of chronic low back pain patients. *Clin J Pain, 1,* 69-74.
2. Aiken L. (1976). Chronic illness and responsive ambulatory care. In Mechanic D, (ed), *The growth of bureaucratic medicine* (pp. 239-251). New York: John Wiley & Sons.
3. Averill J. (1973). Personal control over aversive stimuli and its relationship to stress. *Psychol Bull, 80,* 286-303.
4. Benoliel JQ. (1979). Dying is a family affair. In Prichard E, (ed), *Home care: living with dying* (pp. 17-34). New York: Columbia University Press.
5. Benoliel JQ and Crowley D. (1977). The patient in pain: new concepts. *Nurs Digest,* Summer, 41-48.

6. Block A. (1981). An investigation of the response of the spouse to chronic pain behavior. *Psychosom Med, 43,* 415-422.
7. Block A and Boyer S. (1984). The spouse's adjustment to chronic pain: cognitive and emotional factors. *Soc Sci Med, 19,* 1313-1317.
8. Bonica J. (1973). Management of pain. *Postgrad Med, 53,* 56-57.
9. Bonica J. (1973). Introduction. In Brena S, (ed), *Chronic pain: America's hidden epidemic* (pp. v-ix). New York: Atheneum/SMI.
10. Cohen F and Lazarus R. (1980). Coping with the stresses of illness. In Stone G, Cohen F, and Adler F (eds), *Health Psychol* (pp. 217-254). San Francisco: Jossey-Bass.
11. Conlon P and Merskey H. (1988). The effect of chronic disability on a family. *Clin J Pain, 4,* 41-45.
12. Corbin J and Strauss A. (1988). *Unending work and care. Managing chronic illness at home.* San Francisco: Jossey-Bass.
13. Crowley D. (1975). Chronic pain: social aspects. In *A.N.A. clinical sessions, American Nurses Association* (pp. 257-266). New York: Appleton-Century-Crofts.
14. Davis M. (1973). *Living with multiple sclerosis.* Springfield, Ill: Charles C Thomas.
15. Dura J and Beck S. (1988). A comparison of family functioning when mothers have chronic pain. *Pain, 35,* 79-89.
16. Flor H and Turk D. (1985). Chronic illness in an adult family member: pain as a prototype. In Turk D and Kerns R (eds), *Health, illness and families* (pp. 255-278). New York: Wiley.
17. Flor H, Turk D, and Rudy T. (1987). Pain and families. II. Assessment and treatment. *Pain, 30,* 29-45.
18. Flor H, Turk DC, and Rudy TE. (1989). Relationship of pain impact and significant other reinforcement of pain behaviors: the mediating role of gender, marital status and marital satisfaction. *Pain, 38*(1), 45-50.
19. Flor H, Turk D, and Scholz O. (1987). Impact of chronic pain on the spouse: marital, emotional and physical consequences. *J Psychosom Res, 31*(1), 63-71.
20. Fordyce W. (1976). Behavioral concepts in chronic pain and illness. In Davidson P (ed), *The behavioral management of anxiety, depression, and pain* (pp. 147-188). New York: Brunner/Mazel.
21. Fordyce W. (1978). Learning processes in pain. In Sternbach R (ed), *The psychology of pain* (pp. 49-72). New York: Raven Press.
22. Gerson E and Strauss A. (1975). Time for living: problems in chronic illness care. *Soc Pol, 6,* 12-18.
23. Hendler N and Fenton J. (1979). *Coping with chronic pain.* New York: Clarkson N. Potter.
24. Janis I and Rodin J. (1980). Attribution, control, and decision making. In Stone G, Cohen F, and Adler N (eds), *Health psychology* (pp. 487-522). San Francisco: Jossey-Bass.
25. Jeans ME, Stratford J, Melzack R, and Monks R. (1979). Assessment of pain. *Can Fam Phys, 25,* 159-162.
26. Kaplan D, Grobstein R, and Smith A. (1976). Predicting the impact of severe illness in families. *Health Soc Work, 1*(3), 71-82.
27. Kerns R and Turk D. (1984). Depression and chronic pain: the mediating role of the spouse. *J Marr Fam, 46,* 845-852.

28. Khatami M and Rush J. (1978). A pilot study of the treatment of outpatients with chronic pain: symptom control, stimulus control and social system intervention. *Pain, 5,* 163-172.
29. Lazarus R. (1966). *Psychological stress and the coping process.* New York: McGraw-Hill.
30. Lazarus R and Averill J. (1972). Emotion and cognition: with special reference to anxiety. In Spielberger C (ed), *Anxiety: current trends in theory and research, vol II* (pp. 241-283). New York: Academic Press.
31. Lazarus R, Averill J, and Opton E. (1970). Towards a cognitive theory of emotion. In Arnold M (ed), *Feelings and emotions* (pp. 207-232). New York: Academic Press.
32. Lazarus R, Averill J, and Opton E. (1974). The psychology of coping: issues of research and assessment. In Coelho G, Hamburg D, and Adams J (eds), *Coping and adaptation* (pp. 249-315). New York: Basic Books.
33. Lazarus R and Launier R. (1978). Stress-related transactions between person and environment. In Pervin L and Lewis M (eds), *Perspectives in interactional psychology* (pp. 287-327). New York: Plenum Press.
34. LeShan L. (1964). The world of the patient in severe pain of long duration. *J Chron Dis, 17,* 119-126.
35. Livsey C. (1972). Physical illness and family dynamics. *Adv Psychosom Med, 8,* 237-251.
36. Llewellyn-Thomas H. (1982). Patient and spouse perceptions in malignant lymphoma. A research proposal. In Cahoon M (ed), *Recent advances in nursing 3. Cancer nursing* (pp. 101-119). Edinburgh: Churchill Livingstone.
37. Maruta T, Osborne D, Swanson D, and Halling J. (1981). Chronic pain patients and spouses: marital and sexual adjustment. *Mayo Clin Proc, 56,* 307-310.
38. Melzack R and Chapman C. (1973). Psychological aspects of pain. *Postgrad Med, 53,* 69-75.
39. Merskey H. (1965). Psychiatric patients with persistent pain. *J Psychosom Res, 9,* 291-309.
40. Miller S. (1979). Controllability and human stress: method evidence and theory. *Soc Res Ther, 17,* 287-304.
41. Mohamed S. (1982). The patient and his family. In Roy R and Trunks E (eds), *Chronic pain: psychosocial factors in rehabilitation* (pp. 145-150). Baltimore: Williams & Wilkins.
42. Mohamed SN, Weisz GM, and Waring EM. (1978). The relationship of chronic pain to depression, marital adjustment, and family dynamics. *Pain, 5,* 285-292.
43. Nichols E. (1978). *Chronic pain: a review of the intrapersonal and interpersonal factors and a study of marital interaction.* Doctoral dissertation, University of Tennessee, Knoxville.
44. Payne B and Norfleet M. (1986). Chronic pain and the family: a review. *Pain, 26,* 1-22.
45. Pearlin L and Schooler C. (1978). The structure of coping. *J Health Soc Behav, 9,* 2-21.
46. Pinsky J. (1979). Aspects of the psychology of pain. In Crue B (ed), *Chronic pain* (pp. 301-314). New York: Spectrum.
47. Pratt L. (1973). The significance of the family in medication. *J Compar Fam Studies, IV,* 13-35.

48. Roskies E and Lazarus R. (1980). Coping theory and the teaching of coping skills. In Davidson PD and Davidson S (eds), *Behavioral medicine: changing health lifestyles* (pp. 38-69). New York: Brunner/Mazel.
49. Rowat K. (1983). The meaning and management of chronic pain: the family's perspective. (Doctoral dissertation, University of Illinois at the Medical Center, 1983). *Dissertation Abstracts International, 44,* 1414B.
50. Rowat K. (1985a). Chronic pain: a family affair. In King K (ed), *Recent advances in nursing: long-term care* (pp. 137-149). Edinburgh: Churchill Livingstone.
51. Rowat K. (1985b). Assessing the chronic pain family. *Int J Fam Ther, 7*(4), 284-296.
52. Rowat K and Jeans ME. (1989). *A collaborative model of care: patient, family and health professionals.* In Wall P and Melzack R (eds), *Textbook of pain* (pp. 1010-1014). Edinburgh: Churchill Livingstone.
53. Rowat K and Knafl K. (1985). Living with chronic pain: the spouse's perspective. *Pain, 23,* 259-271.
54. Saunders C. (1967). *The management of terminal illness.* London: Hospital and Medicine Publications.
55. Schwenck T and Hughes C. (1983). The family as patient in family medicine. *Soc Sci Med, 17,* 1-16.
56. Seligman M. (1975). *Helplessness.* San Francisco: W.H. Freeman.
57. Shanfield S, Heiman E, Cope N, and Jones J. (1979). Pain and the marital relationship: psychiatric distress. *Pain, 7,* 343-351.
58. Shanfield S and Killingsworth R. (1977). The psychiatric aspect of pain. *Psych Ann, 7,* 24-35.
59. Sternbach R. (1974). *Pain patients: traits and treatment.* New York: Academic Press.
60. Stewart D and Sullivan T. (1982). Illness behavior and the sick role in chronic disease. The case of multiple sclerosis. *Soc Sci Med, 16,* 1397-1404.
61. Strauss A. (1975). *Chronic illness and the quality of life.* St. Louis: Mosby.
62. Swanson D and Maruta T. (1980). The family's viewpoint of chronic pain. *Pain, 8,* 163-166.
63. Terzian M. (1980). Neurosurgical interventions for the management of chronic intractable pain. *Top Clin Nurs, 2,* 75-88.
64. Turk D and Kerns R. (1985). *Health, illness and families.* New York: Wiley.
65. Turk D, Flor H, and Rudy T. (1987). Pain and families. I. Etiology, maintenance and psychosocial impact. *Pain, 30,* 3-27.
66. Turk D, Rudy T, and Flor H. (1985). Why a family perspective for pain? *Int J Fam Ther, 7,* 223-233.
67. Vachon ML, Freedman K, Formo A, et al. (1977). The final illness in cancer: the widow's perspective. *Can Med Assoc J, 117,* 1151-1154.
68. Waring EM. (1977). The role of the family in symptoms selection and perpetuation in psychosomatic illness. *Psychother Psychosom, 28,* 253-259.
69. Waring EM. (1982). Conjoint marital and family therapy. In Roy R and Tunks E (eds), *Chronic pain: psychosocial factors in rehabilitation* (pp. 151-165). Baltimore: Williams & Wilkins.

6

Ethical Decision-Making in Pain Management

Marcia Sue DeWolf Bosek

◆ INTRODUCTION

In every arena of health care, nurses are confronted with ethical situations that they must resolve to provide care for the patient. When asked to describe an ethical situation in which she had been involved, Nurse A describe the following scenario[7]:

Today, I cared for a terminal chronic obstructive pulmonary disease (COPD) patient, who had some unusual medical orders written. Several of the nurses on the unit thought that these orders were questionable. The orders stated: "This man is dying of emphysema be liberal with meds: Roxinal 2 mg PO every 4 hours, morphine IM PRN. The patient may request that the oxygen be increased to 5 liters per nasal cannula." The nurses knew the narcotics would make the patient unresponsive and the high oxygen levels would eventually kill him. But the patient was terminal. These orders were written based on the physician's and the family's joint decision about the patient's care. This was an ethical situation because if a nurse went in the room and turned the oxygen up, the patient would likely die. And that would be like euthanasia.

Nurse A's story (in which some details have been changed for confidentiality) is typical of stories elicited from female nurses in a recent study. These nurses worked in acute medical units and described ethical situations in which they had been involved. Such situations posed ethical problems that nurses had to solve, and the solutions were summarized by the means of a conceptual model called the Nurses' Clinical Descriptive Ethical Decision-Making Model (NCDEDMM) (see Figure 6-1).[7]

Before a nurse perceived a clinical situation as an ethical situation, five factors were found to be present. These factors were: emotional reaction, perceived time constraints, personalizing the situation, a communication failure, and a disagreement about the right thing to do.

When describing what made the clinical situation an ethical situation, the nurses discussed experiencing an emotional reaction or being uncomfortable. Second, the nurses experienced a sense of urgency created by perceived time constraints. Third, they personalized the situation by considering what they would want done if they or a loved one were the patient. Thus decision options or goals may often be determined by the nurse's value system rather than the patient's. Fourth, the nurses experienced a communication failure that created a lack of information necessary for the nurse to make a knowledgeable decision. Finally, a disagreement occurred about the right thing to do. This disagreement may be between the nurse and patient, or the nurse and another health care professional, or it may be a conflict between the nurse's personal and professional belief systems.

After the nurse encountered these five precipitating factors, the nurse perceived the ongoing situation to be an ethical situation. After perceiving an ethical situation, the nurse sought additional information that might help her determine the right thing to do. For example, the nurse may consult the institution's policy and procedure manual, the patient's chart, or another nurse. In addition, the nurse may receive unsolicitated information, such as a family member commenting that the patient has a living will.

Once the nurse perceived that an ethical situation was occurring, the nurse began to consider the possible options. But, rather than identifying the options herself, the nurse considered options that had been identified by the physician, patient, and/or family. Concurrently, the nurse often sought personal support from colleagues.

Although advice may have come from others, the nurse independently evaluated and chose an option. The nurse evaluated the identified options by considering her emotional comfort with the option and the option's anticipated consequences, especially those concerning the patient's physical

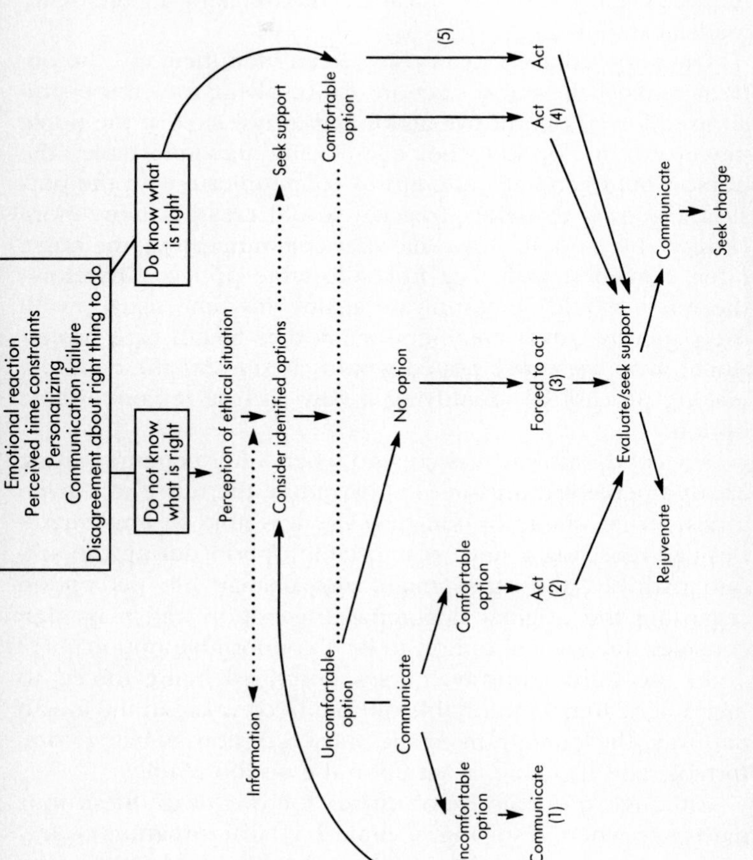

FIGURE 6-1. Nurses' clinical descriptive ethical decision-making model.

comfort. The nurse did not evaluate the appropriateness of the identified options by considering the cost, ease of implementation, or ethical principles. When choosing an option, the nurse ranked the identified options along a comfortable-uncomfortable continuum. Therefore comfort (the nurse's emotional and patient's physical) becomes the core variable influencing the nurse's ethical decision-making in the acute medical setting.

Once the ethical situation has been identified and the options ranked, the nurse's actions for resolving the ethical situation followed one of five action pathways. First, if the nurse perceived the option choice as being uncomfortable, the nurse would generally attempt to communicate with the physician, hoping that the physician would create a new, more comfortable option. However, after communicating, the nurse often remained with that uncomfortable option. Therefore, the nurse would communicate again, this time usually with the patient's family members or another health care professional, who the nurse hoped would circumvent the decision-making process by identifying a new and more comfortable option.

A second pathway was created when, after communicating about a perceived uncomfortable option, the nurse was given a new, comfortable option that she was able to implement. Besides receiving a new, comfortable option during the second pathway, the nurse might also change her perception regarding the original uncomfortable option and may then consider the original option to be a comfortable option.

In the third pathway, nurses described being forced to implement an uncomfortable option. In contrast, in the fourth pathway, the nurse ranked the chosen option as being comfortable and was able to act upon the option readily.

Although the majority of nurses follow one of these four pathways when resolving a clinical ethical situation, a few nurses reported that knowing the right thing to do can create a fifth pathway, which can eliminate the nurse's perception that an ethical situation is occurring. In this "right thing to do pathway," the nurse typically experienced an emotional reaction, perceived a time constraint, personalized the situation, and had a communication failure. However, even though the various individuals involved in the situation may have disagreed about the right thing to do, the nurse believed that she in fact did know the right thing to do. The nurse based this knowledge on her experiences and personal values. Since the nurse already knew the right thing to do and a comfortable option was available, the nurse did not need to seek information and support or to consider options. Thus the nurse implemented her perceived "right thing to do" option without evaluating or considering the moral implications of her "right thing to do" decision.

Regardless of which of the five pathways the nurse implemented when resolving a clinical ethical situation, the nurse would evaluate the resolved ethical situation and seek support from colleagues and significant others. In the majority of situations described, the nurses stopped their decision-making at this point and attempted to put the situation behind them. In other words, the nurses went home to rejuvenate so that they could return to work the next day with the stamina to withstand future ethical situations. Occasionally after evaluating the resolved ethical situation, however, the nurse would communicate to seek a change to prevent a similar ethical situation in the future.

In summary, the nurse experienced five factors before perceiving an ethical situation. The nurse evaluated the identified options by considering how comfortable she was with implementing the option. Comfortable options were acted on freely, but the nurse used communication techniques to change uncomfortable options to comfortable options. After the nurse acted, the situation was evaluated and support sought. Generally, the nurse gave up and rejuvenated. However, the nurse may again have communicated to facilitate change. Nurses may not have perceived that an ethical situation was occurring, much less considered options, when they believed they knew the right action for resolving the situation.

The purpose of this model was to describe the nurse's ethical decision-making process and not to make normative claims or advocate one particular ethical perspective. However, several obstacles to effective ethical decision-making by nurses can be identified from the Nurses' Clinical Descriptive Ethical Decision Making Model. These obstacles include: the inability to identify the ethical problem, identify the decision maker, and/or identify the goal; perceived time constraints; emotionalism; inadequate communication and negotiating skills; insufficient vocabulary; limited recognition of alternatives, ethical resources, and ethical perspectives; and ambiguous roles and accountability for the decision-making. In the remainder of this chapter, these obstacles to effective ethical decision-making will be discussed in relation to selected situations described by nurses that involve ethical questions concerning pain management.

◆ ETHICS

Ethics is the process of determining how one ought to act in a particular situation. Individuals have been considering what ought to be done since at least 500 BC, when Socrates contemplated what "good" meant. Typically, individuals base their ethics on moral customs. Morals are learned cultural beliefs that an individual affirms.[3,15] However, ethical decision-making skills based on traditional moral customs are being challenged by the rapid advancement of medical technology, changes in family structures, and increasing societal diversity. Because of this blurring of traditional moral customs, situations with new ethical questions are being experienced.

Relying on ethical theories and principles is another means by which ethical decisions can be justified. Two major ethical theories are used today, utilitarianism and deontology.

Utilitarianism was established on the Greatest Happiness Principle, which suggests that, "actions are right in proportion as they tend to promote happiness, wrong as they tend to produce the reverse of happiness."[4] Options are evaluated according to their expected consequences concerning happiness. Group happiness is emphasized rather than individual happiness when one is making a choice. A rule is considered a guide for conduct but may be broken if breaking the rule would result in better consequences. When justifying a choice retrospectively, the utilitarian considers the actual consequences and not the intent or adequacy of the decision-making process.[3,4,6,7,8]

In contrast to utilitarianism, deontologists proposed that actions may be supported as right or wrong regardless of their consequences. Deontology emphasizes the dignity of the individual rather than the importance of the group. Deontologists consider other criteria besides the consequences when determining the rightness of an action. These criteria include promise-keeping, fairness, duty, and the generalizability of the action to similar situations. Thus rules for deontologists are rarely broken.[3,4,6,7,8]

Nurses make ethical decisions daily in the clinical setting

utilizing a variety of rationales. Since no one true ethical decision-making process exists to ensure morally praiseworthy decision-making, nurses need to become knowledgeable about ethical issues. Therefore, rationales nurses have used to resolve clinical ethical situations involving pain management issues will be discussed in the following pages.

Euthanasia

Nurse A, in the original scenario, identified a patient pain management problem when she described an ethical situation. In this situation, Nurse A, the physician, and the patient's family acknowledged that the patient was dying. In addition, everyone seemed to agree that the treatment goal was to keep the patient comfortable. However, Nurse A identified an ethical question when attempting to incorporate the treatment goal into nursing care. The specific ethical question is, "Would Nurse A be committing euthanasia by implementing the physician's orders to liberally administer pain medications and increase the oxygen flow rate on the patient's request?"

Euthanasia is Greek for "good death." Euthanasia is an intentional act to painlessly end another person's life before that person can die from natural causes. To qualify for euthanasia, the person should have, or be dying from, an incurable, debilitating, and often painful disease. Four concepts are considered when evaluating euthanasia: active, passive, voluntary, and involuntary.[15,17,18]

In active euthanasia, the agent intends to relieve another's suffering by directly causing the other's death. Thus active euthanasia is sometimes called "mercy killing." In passive euthanasia, however, actions are taken that indirectly cause the person's death. For example, food and fluids may be withheld, and the person dies from dehydration. Voluntary euthanasia requires that the person initiate the request for his death to occur. In contrast, involuntary euthanasia occurs when the individual is not capable of making such a request or is not involved in the decision-making process by the party who will carry out the euthanasia decision.[17,18]

In this situation, Nurse A has incorrectly identified the ethical problem as euthanasia. Nurse A does not desire to end the patient's life, nor has the patient asked for his life to be terminated. Rather, the patient's death would be a side effect of the actions, administering pain medicine and oxygen, Nurse

A carries out to promote the patient's comfort. Therefore, Nurse A's questions about euthanasia are caused by the doctrine of double effects.

In the doctrine of double effects, a person acts to facilitate a certain goal. However, when acting to achieve this goal, a second outcome occurs that is not directly intended. In the situation described by Nurse A, the goal is to promote the patient's comfort. Thus, according to the doctrine of double effects, if the patient were to die after an injection administered for pain relief, the death would be considered an undesired side effect.[3] Therefore, since the intent of Nurse A's actions was to promote the patient's comfort, Nurse A should not be held morally responsible for the patient's death or accused of performing euthanasia.

Nonmaleficence/Beneficence

Instead of being a euthanasia question, the ethical question in this situation seems to be about how to justify the increase or lack of increase in the amount and frequency of pain medication. Nurse A may find the principles of nonmaleficence and beneficence helpful in resolving this moral quandary. To act nonmaleficently, Nurse A must always prevent harm from occurring. In addition to physical harm, Nurse A should also be concerned about preventing psychological and spiritual harm.

In contrast, the principle of beneficence requires that Nurse A not only do no harm, but also benefit the patient. Benefitting the patient encompasses helping, healing, or, in the more metaphysical sense, creating "happiness." Before the nonmaleficence/beneficence issues can be addressed further, Nurse A, along with the patient and his family, must determine whether the patient's death is to be perceived as a harm to be avoided or at least delayed or as a benefit to be accepted if not welcomed. Other questions Nurse A will need to consider include:

1. If I increase the oxygen and morphine, will I be harming the patient?
2. If I decrease the oxygen and morphine, will I be harming the patient?
3. If I increase the oxygen and morphine, will I be benefitting the patient?
4. If I decrease the oxygen and morphine, will I be benefitting the patient?

When considering these questions, Nurse A may realize that not giving or limiting the oxygen and pain medications could cause physical harm (pain), psychological harm (fear), and possibly spiritual distress related to suffering. However, Nurse A may not be as certain that increasing the oxygen and pain medication frequency and amounts would create further harm.

This scenario described by Nurse A illustrates how ethical decision-making can become complex when terminology, such as euthanasia and comfort, are poorly defined and/or poorly understood. Although the goal of comfort had been established, ambiguity existed regarding how comfort was to be evaluated and how to rank competing values, such as the right to life. Resources were needed to assist nurses in differentiating between euthanasia and actions that allowed patients to die.

Veracity

Another ethical situation involving a pain management question was described by Nurse B, who has 10 years of acute care medical nursing experience. During the past month, Nurse B had established a strong relationship with Mrs. M and her family while functioning as Mrs. M's primary nurse. Mrs. M was 45 years old and had breast cancer with metastases. Mrs. M's condition had been deteriorating rapidly. Mrs. M's husband or parents were at her bedside almost continuously and actively participated in Mrs. M's physical care. One evening, Nurse B described the following ethical situation.

> Mrs. M's pain is being treated with continuous morphine infusion. Despite the morphine, Mrs. M often experiences severe pain with movement. Everyone involved agrees that the primary goal is to keep Mrs. M as comfortable as possible. However, tonight Mrs. M is somnolent with respirations at 10 per minute. I think I should decrease the morphine rate, but I don't know whether I should decrease the rate without first telling Mr. M. What if Mrs. M wakes up later in pain and they discover that I've turned the morphine down?

In this situation, Nurse B was experiencing a moral quandary about how truthful she ought to be with Mrs. M and her family about nursing care decisions.

Beauchamp and Childress[3] claim that as a health care professional, Nurse B has a duty to be truthful and to follow the moral rule of veracity. Veracity requires individuals not only to be truthful, but also to avoid deceiving others. Are moral rules, such as veracity, absolutes that should always be followed regardless of the situation or the consequences? Rule deontologists would adamantly repond, "Yes, moral rules must always be followed." However, other ethical perspectives, such as act utilitarians, would suggest that veracity is only a prima facie duty since veracity may conflict with other higher moral rules or principles.

Beauchamp and Childress have proposed three arguments for not promoting veracity: respect for persons, fidelity, and trust. These arguments may prove helpful in resolving Nurse B's moral quandary.

Respect for Persons

First, Nurse B might be justified in not telling Mrs. and Mr. M that she is decreasing the morphine infusion rate if by not telling, Nurse B would be facilitating Mrs. M's autonomy. The principle of autonomy is concerned with self-will or governance. To act autonomously, one must be fully informed and be free from coercion while making the decision. When a person is allowed to act autonomously, the person is being respected as a person.

The opposite of autonomy is paternalism. When acting paternalistically, an individual makes decisions for another without the other's input or permission. Thus, to justify acting paternalistically, Nurse B must demonstrate that acting paternalistically prevented more harm and fostered more benefit than would have occurred if Mrs. M's autonomy had been respected.

Fidelity

Second, Nurse B may decide not to tell if he or she believes that not telling would support fidelity. Fidelity is concerned with promise-keeping. What promises has Nurse B made to Mrs. M and her family that might require Nurse B to not communicate the decision about the morphine rate? Has Nurse B promised that Mrs. M or her surrogate would always approve drug dosages? Has a promise been made that Mrs. M would be kept pain free regardless of side effects such as respiratory depression? Or has Nurse B promised not to overburden Mrs. M and her family with decisions that require experience and professional judgment? In addition, if multiple promises have been made, Nurse B may need to rank these promises to determine which has the greatest bearing on her decision to reveal to the family that she is decreasing the morphine.

Trust

Third, Nurse B needs to consider whether not telling would influence the trust established with Mrs. M and the family. A strong relationship that includes trust exists between Nurse B, and Mrs. M and the family. Undoubtedly, this trust was forged as Mrs. M and her family realized that Nurse B was competent, supported Mrs. M's wishes and decisions, and desired the best for Mrs. M. Again, Nurse B must consider whether Mrs. M and her family would perceive not telling as a form of incompetence or as not being supportive of Mrs. M's decisions.

In addition, Nurse B needs to examine whose needs are being supported by not telling that the morphine rate is being decreased. Is Nurse B becoming too personally involved in Mrs. M's care and, therefore, losing objectivity? By not telling, is Nurse B attempting to avoid a discussion about Mrs. M's deteriorating condition and imminent death? Similarly, does Nurse B feel responsible for Mrs. M's somnolent condition and thus feel guilt that affects the decision to decrease the morphine?

Advance Directives

Nurse B's moral quandary might have been eased if Mrs. M had provided an advance directive. An advance directive fosters a person's autonomy by allowing the individual to communicate in advance feelings about the use of certain treatment options, how aggressive treatment should be, and/or the goal by which any treatment option should be evaluated. A variety of advance directives exist: values history, living will, durable power of attorney for health care, and medical directives.

Values History

In a values history (see box), the health care professional asks open-ended questions about the patient's life, important decisions made in the past, support systems, and valuable

◆ **SAMPLE QUESTIONS FOR A VALUES HISTORY**

How do you feel about the use of life-sustaining treatments?

What are your wishes regarding the use of a respirator, kidney dialysis, organ donation, cardiopulmonary resuscitation, and tube feedings?

Do you believe that your doctor should make the final decision about your medical treatment?

What are your beliefs about death?

How do your religious beliefs influence your health care decisions?

Which person understands your beliefs, dreams, and fears the best?

Have you ever signed a document containing your wishes about health care or medical treatments if you are ever seriously ill or dying and cannot communicate your wishes?

What makes life meaningful for you?

Have you made any funeral arrangements? If so, please describe.

Would you like your obituary printed in the paper?

features of the patient's present life. Taking a values history is a means of initiating a discussion about quality of life issues and ascertaining which values have guided previous life decisions and may influence future decisions. A values history ought to be updated periodically, such as during annual checkups. In addition, mechanisms need to be established that would make a values history a permanent part of the person's medical record. If Mrs. M had completed a values history, Nurse B might have been able to identify the importance Mrs. M placed on truthtelling and thus lessen the ambiguity of whether to communicate that the morphine rate had been decreased.

Living Will

A second advance directive that increases patient autonomy during ethical decision-making is a living will (see box). Living wills have been used for more than 20 years but still seem to be poorly understood by the lay public. A living will is more specific than a values history since it includes specific

◆ SAMPLE LIVING WILL

DECLARATION UNDER ILLINOIS LIVING WILL ACT

This declaration is made this _____ day of _____ 19___.

I, ____________________________, being of sound mind willfully and voluntarily make known my desires that my moment of death shall not be artificially postponed.

If at any time I should have an incurable and irreversible injury, disease, or illness judged to be a terminal condition by my attending physician who has personally examined me and has determined that my death is imminent except for death delaying procedures, I direct that such procedures which would only prolong the dying process be withheld or withdrawn, and that I be permitted to die naturally with only the administration of medication, sustenance, or the performance of any medical procedure deemed necessary by my attending physician to provide me with comfort care.

In the absence of my ability to give directions regarding the use of such death delaying procedures, it is my intention that this Declaration shall be honored by my family and physician as the final expression of my legal right to refuse medical or surgical treatment and accept the consequences from such refusal.

Signed____________________

City, County and State of Residence____________________

The declarant is personally known to me and I believe the declarant to be of sound mind. I saw the declarant sign the declaration in my presence (or the declarant acknowledged in my presence that the declarant had signed the declaration) and I signed the declaration as a witness in the presence of the declarant. I did not sign the declarant's signature about for or at the direction of the declarant. At the date of this instrument, I am not entitled to any portion of the estate of the declarant according to the laws of interstate succession or, to the best of my knowledge and belief, under any will of declarant or other instrument taking effect at declarant's death, or directly financially responsible for declarant's medical care.

Witness____________________

Witness____________________

directions from the patient. The use of a living will is limited to rejecting life-sustaining medical treatments for terminally ill persons. Living wills are not legal documents in Canada but are recognized there at the physician's discretion. In the United States, living wills are legally recognized in 41 states. Some differences in wording and intent may occur from state to state. Despite these small differences, each state's living will includes the physical condition that determines when medical treatment should be withdrawn as well as the types of medical treatments that can be withdrawn.[9] These concepts are illustrated in the Illinois living will.

> If at any time I should have an incurable and irreversible injury, disease, or illness judged to be a terminal condition by my attending physician who . . . has deterimned that my death is imminent . . ., I direct that such procedures which would only prolong the dying process be withheld or withdrawn, and that I be permitted to die naturally with only the administration of medication. . .

A living will is helpful in guiding decision-making, but the living will does contain several deficiencies. First, the living will applies only to termination of medical treatment and does not identify what treatments are to be continued. Second, living wills generally apply only to terminal patients and not to persons in persistent vegetative states or with chronic conditions. Third, living wills are vague in describing what condition in which the patient must be before the living will is relevant. For instance, how close to death must the patient be before the living will may be implemented? Fourth, living wills are limited in delineating which interventions are to be withheld or which are to be continued, since wording is ambiguous. For example, criteria needs to be identified for determining whether a procedure or medication is delaying the dying process.[9] However, in the situation under consideration the presence of a living will could have guided Nurse B to continue the morphine at a rate sufficient to maintain comfort despite other physical changes.

Durable Power of Attorney

A third advance directive is a durable power of attorney for health care (see box). A durable power of attorney for health care (DPOA) indicates who should speak for the patient and make decisions on the patient's behalf in the event that the

◆ DURABLE POWER OF ATTORNEY FOR HEALTH CARE

Power of Attorney made this day of ________, 19___

1. I, the undersigned hereby appoint (insert name and address of agent)________________________________ as agent to act for me and in my name to make any and all decisions for me concerning my personal care, medical treatment, hospitalization and health care and to require, withhold or withdraw any type of medical treatment or procedure, even though my death may ensue. My agent shall have the same access to my medical records that I have, including the right to disclose the contents to others. My agent shall also have full power to make a disposition of any part or all of my body for medical purposes, authorize an autopsy and direct the disposition of my remains. (Neither the attending physician nor any other health care provider may act as your agent.)

2. The powers granted above shall be subject to the following rules or limitations (if none, leave blank):__________

____

(The subject of life-sustaining treatment is of particular importance. For your convenience in dealing with that subject some general statements concerning the withholding or removal of life-sustaining treatment are set forth below. If you agree with one of these statements, you may initial that statement; but do not initial more than one.)

(I do not want my life to be prolonged nor do I want
(life-sustaining treatment to be provided or continued if
(my agent believes the burdens of the treatment out-
(weigh the expected benefits. I want my agent to con-
(sider the relief of suffering, the expense involved and
___(the quality as well as the possible extension of my life in
(making decisions concerning life-sustaining treatment.

(I want my life to be prolonged and I want life-sustaining
(treatment to be provided or continued unless I am in a
(coma which my attending physician believes to be irre-
(versible, in accordance with reasonable medical stan-
(dards at the time of reference. If and when I have suffered
___(irreversible coma, I want life-sustaining treatment to be
(withheld or discontinued.

(I want my life to be prolonged to the greatest extent
___(possible without regard to my condition, the chances I
(have for recovery or the cost of the procedures.

Continued.

◆ DURABLE POWER OF ATTORNEY FOR HEALTH CARE—CONT'D

3. This power of attorney shall become effective on______

____

4. This power of attorney shall terminate on____________

____

5. If any agent named by me shall die, become legally disabled, resign, refuse to act or be unavailable, I name the following (each to act alone and successively, in the order named) as successors to such agent:

____

____

6. If a guardian of my person is to be appointed, I nominate the following to serve as such guardian (if same as agent, leave blank):____________________

7. I am fully informed as to all the contents of this form and understand the full import of this grant of power to my agent.

Signed____________________

Principal

The principal has had an opportunity to read the above form and has signed the form or acknowledged his or her signature or mark on the form in presence.

______________ Residing at __________________

Witness

(You may, but are not required to, request your agent and successor agents to provide specimen signature below. If you include specimen signature in this Power of Attorney, you must complete the certification opposite the signatures of the agents.)

Specimen signatures of agent (and successors)	I certify that the signature of my agent (and successors) is correct.
______________ (agent)	______________ (principal)
______________ (successor agent)	______________ (principal)
______________ (successor agent)	______________ (principal)

patient becomes incompetent. Besides appointing a proxy decision maker, the DPOA also allows the patient to document his preferences about aggressive care, medical procedures, and use of medications. The patient always makes the decision related to his care if competent.[12,13]

Competency is the ability to make a decision. Competency requires that the person be able to understand, be aware of choices, and make a choice that is reasonable and supported with rationale. A competent patient should be allowed to make his own health care decisions.[3,5,11] When a nurse bypasses a competent patient and consults instead with a family member or proxy decision maker, the nurse is violating the patient's right to autonomy.

Any health care professional can assess the patient's competency by documenting the patient's ability to identify options and provide consistent rationale for his decisions. The proxy decision maker acts only when the patient is incompetent to make decisions. When a patient is unable to make decisions, the nurse needs to consult the proxy decision maker for decisions and changes related to the patient's care.

For a durable power of attorney for health care to be used effectively, the patient needs to discuss his health care concerns and desires with the designated proxy decision maker. These conversations need to be held routinely and frequently. Ideally, the patient should keep the proxy decision maker updated about current health care treatment decisions or even include the proxy decision maker in the decision-making process. Thus the proxy decision maker would be knowledgeable about the patient's current health and decision rationale and would therefore be prepared to maintain the patient's wishes and treatment plan without notice. However, there is no way to guarantee that the proxy decision maker is actually making decisions as the patient would if competent. Thus a durable power of attorney for health care document could have assisted Nurse B by describing Mrs. M's wishes about pain medication and comfort and identifying who should be included in making the decision about the morphine infusion rate.

Medical Directives

A fourth advanced directive is a medical directive (see Figure 6-2). Medical directives should be used simultaneously

My Medical Directive

This Medical Directive expresses, and shall stand for my wishes regarding medical treatments in the event of illness should make me unable to communicate them directly. I make this Directive, being 18 years or more of age, of sound mind and appreciating the consequences of my decisions.

1. Cardiopulmonary Resuscitation—if on the point of dying the use of drugs and electric shock to start the heart beating, and artificial breathing.

2. Mechanical Breathing—breathing by a machine.

3. Artificial Nutrition and Hydration—nutrition and fluid given through a tube in the veins, nose, or stomach.

4. Major Surgery—such as removing the gallbladder or part of the intestines.

5. Kidney Dialysis—cleaning the blood by machine or by fluid passed through the belly.

6. Chemotherapy—drugs to fight cancer.

7. Minor surgery—such as removing some tissue from an infected toe.

8. Invasive Diagnostic Tests—such as using a flexible tube to look into the stomach.

9. Blood or Blood Products—

10. Antibiotics—drugs to fight infections.

11. Simple Diagnostic Tests—such as blood tests or x-rays.

12. Pain Medications, even if they dull consciousness and indirectly shorten my life.

FIGURE 6-2. Medical directives. (1). Copyright 1990 by Linda L. Emanuel and Ezekiel J. Emanuel. The authors of this form advise that it should be completed pursuant to a discussion between the principal and his or her physician, so that the principal can be adequately informed of any pertinent medical information, and so that the physician can be apprised of the intentions of the principal and the existence of such a document which may be made part of the principal's medical records.

Situation (A)

If I am in a coma or in a persistent vegetative state, and in the opinion of my physician and several consultants have no known hope of regaining awareness and higher mental function no matter what is done, then my wishes regarding use of the following, if considered medically reasonable, would be:

I want	I do not want	I am undecided	I want a trial; if no clear improvement stop treatment

FIGURE 6-2, cont'd. Medical directives. (2). This form was originally published as part of an article by Linda J. Emanuel and Ezekiel J. Emanuel, "The Medical Directive: A New Comprehensive Advance Care Document" in *Journal of the American Medical Association* June 9, 1989;261:3290. It does not reflect the official policy of the American Medical Association.

Continued.

Situation (B)

If I am in a coma, and I have a small likelihood of recovering fully, a slightly larger likelihood of surviving with permanent brain damage, and a much larger likelihood of dying, then my wishes regarding the use of the following, if considered medically reasonable, would be:

I want	I do not want	I am undecided	I want a trial; if no clear improvement stop treatment

FIGURE 6-2, cont'd. Medical directives.

Situation (C)

If I have brain damage or some brain disease which cannot be reversed and which makes me unable to recognize people or to speak understandably, **and I have a terminal illness,** such as incurable cancer which will likely be the cause of my death, then my wishes regarding use of the following, if considered medically reasonable, would be:

I want	I do not want	I am undecided	I want a trial; if no clear improvement stop treatment

FIGURE 6-2, cont'd. Medical directives. (3) Copies of this form may be obtained from the Harvard Medical School Health Letter, 164 Longwood Avenue, Boston, MA 02115 at two copies for $5 or five copies for $10; bulk orders also available.

Continued.

Situation (D)

If I have brain damage or some brain disease which cannot be reversed and which makes me unable to recognize people, or to speak understandably, **but I have no terminal illness,** and I can live in this condition for a long time, then my wishes regarding use of the following, if considered medically reasonable, would be:

I want	I do not want	I am undecided	I want a trial; if no clear improvement stop treatment

FIGURE 6-2 cont'd. Medical directives.

with a living will and durable power of attorney for health care. The medical directive assists the individual to think prospectively about a variety of possible health care scenarios concerned with persistent vegetative states and specifically document preferences about possible medical interventions. Therefore a medical directive can compensate for some of the deficiencies in a living will or durable power of attorney for health care.[9,10] Among the practical concerns in using an advance directive, a copy of each advance directive should be included in the patient's permanent health care record. The patient should keep the original document, and copies should be given to the holder of the durable power of attorney, significant other, and primary health care provider. In addition, the patient should present a copy of the advance directive upon admission to any health care facility. Therefore the nurse transferring a patient from one health care facility to another should include a copy of the advance directive in the transfer packet. If the patient does not have a copy of the advance directive with him when seeking health care, the patient need only complete a new form at that time. A nurse cannot assume an advance directive exists based on a verbal comment. A copy must be presented before the nurse is legally bound to carry out the specific directions in the advance directive.

If a health care professional does not agree to follow an advance directive, then the health care professional is legally obligated to transfer the patient's care to another health care professional who will agree to follow the advance directive. Not following a patient's advance directive, for example providing cardiopulmonary resuscitation (CPR) when no heroics were requested, is the equivalent of battery.

If a situation occurs where a health care professional is not honoring the advance directive and the patient's care has not yet been transferred, a competent patient or the proxy decision maker, if the patient is incompetent, should sign a refusal of treatment form (see box) for every undesired treatment. Therefore, if the patient were to have a cardiopulmonary arrest, the nurse would be legally supported for not initiating CPR even in the absence of a "do not resuscitate" order. Thus advance directives and refusal of treatment forms should be readily available at every health care facility.

Ideally, a patient should have a living will, a durable power of attorney for health care, and a medical directive to assist

◆ REFUSAL TO CONSENT

1. I have been advised by my physician, Dr. ______________ that the following procedure(s)/treatment(s) should be performed upon me: ______________________________

   ____
   procedure(s)/treatment(s)
2. My physician has explained to me, and I understand the following:
   A. The nature of the recommended procedure(s)/treatment(s).
   B. The purpose of and need for the recommended procedure(s)/treatment(s).
   C. The possible alternatives to the recommended procedure(s)/treatment(s) for which I similarly refuse consent.
   D. The probable consequences of not proceeding with the recommended procedure(s)/treatment(s) and/or alternatives.
3. I know that my failure to follow my physician's recommendations will endanger my life or health. I nonetheless refuse to consent to the proposed procedure(s)/treatment(s).
4. My reason for refusal is: ______________________________

   ____
5. I personally assume the risks and consequences of my refusal, and release for myself, my heirs, executors, administrators, or personal representatives, the physicians who have been consulted in my case and ______________ Hospital, its officers, agents, and employees from any and all liability for ill effects which may result from my refusal to consent to the performance of the proposed procedure(s)/treatment(s).
6. I acknowledge that I have read this document in its entirety and that I fully understand it.

CAUTION—THIS IS A RELEASE OF LIABILITY
READ BEFORE SIGNING

DATE: ______________ ______________________________

TIME: ______________AM/PM Signature of Refusing Party

WITNESS: **IF REFUSING PARTY IS OTHER THAN PATIENT**

______________________________ ______________________________

Signature of Witness Signature of Refusing Party

____

Relationship

with health care decisions when incompetent or during a terminal illness. If a patient desires to identify a new proxy decision maker to assume durable power of attorney for health care, such as after a divorce or death of the previous proxy decision maker, he can do so either by completing a form rescinding the previous DPOA (available in the state of Mississippi) or by tearing up the old form and completing a new document. The patient should remember to replace all outdated copies, and health care professionals should verify that an advance directive is current before honoring the directive.

In this scenario, Nurse B's ethical decision-making process was complicated by inadequate communication, which resulted in an ambiguity of roles and accountability for decision-making. This ambiguity created a new ethical question regarding veracity, which was further complicated by Nurse B's emotional involvement in Mrs. M's care. The presence of an advance directive might have provided Nurse B with guidance in proceeding with pain management. In addition, an advance directive might have prevented the sense of urgency that Nurse B experienced while deciding whether to inform Mrs. M's family about her actions.

◆ PROFESSIONAL STANDARDS

After a 20-year hiatus, Nurse C had returned to nursing practice on an acute care medical unit. Nurse C related the following ethical situation, which occurred during the evening shift.[7]

> I had a terminal cancer patient on a continuous morphine intravenous (IV) infusion. She had previously been on injections, but had been bolused and placed on the IV drip. After 2 hours, all her vital signs were cut in half. The B/P went from 130/80 to 70 systolic. I felt very uncomfortable. I knew absolutely that this patient was going to die. I did not want to continue the morphine at that rate and have the death occur just as a result of the morphine. So I talked with the charge nurse and she really disagreed with me. She said to call someone else since I was so new to this whole thing. I called the oncology unit because their nurses were more familiar with drips than we were. The oncology nurse said that the doctor had written the order so that nursing could titrate the rate according to our feelings. She said titrate meant either up or down. So I reduced the morphine rate. Later that evening, the patient seemed uncomfortable so I brought the rate back up again.

This scenario has many similarities with the situations described by Nurses A and B, such as fear of causing a patient's death with narcotics and limited knowledge about the patient's preferences regarding end-of-life treatment decisions. However, in this situation Nurse C's decisions and actions were directly influenced by a lack of knowledge regarding the administration of intravenous morphine. Rather than addressing the pharmacokinetics of morphine, which is beyond the scope of this chapter (see Chapter 7), the concepts of competency for professional practice will be addressed.

A basic premise for ethical professional behavior is that of professional competency. To be professionally competent, one must possess the knowledge and skills necessary to perform the duties of the assigned role. In an attempt to identify the nursing profession's obligations to society and, therefore, protect the public from exploitation, professional nursing organizations in both the United States and Canada have developed codes of ethics. For example, the American Nurses' Association[1] created the Code for Nurses (see box). This code identified the standards for ethical practice and provided a means for self-regulation.[2,8,14,16]

Criteria 6 of The ANA Code for Nurses[1] states, "The nurse exercises informed judgment and uses individual competence and qualifications as criteria in seeking consultation, accepting responsibilities, and delegating nursing activities to others." This criteria has clear implications for this ethical situation and illustrates the importance of having clinical and ethical resources available to nurses.

Although Nurse C sought assistance appropriately from the charge nurse, the charge nurse also did not appear to have the knowledge necessary to safely administer IV morphine. Since both nurses did not understand IV morphine infusions, the hospital may not have been thorough in the inservicing of staff and, therefore, has an obligation to reinservice the nurses before further IV narcotic infusions may be initiated on this unit. Until inservicing can take place, patients requiring IV pain control should be transferred to another nursing unit with the required expertise, such as the oncology unit. However, in defense of the charge nurse's administrative abilities, she did recognize Nurse C's and her own inexperience and provided permission as well as information so that Nurse C could seek appropriate assistance.

◆ ANA CODE FOR NURSES

1. The nurse provides services with respect for human dignity and the uniqueness of the client, unrestricted by considerations of social or economic status, personal attributes, or the nature of health problems.
2. The nurse safeguards the client's right to privacy by judiciously protecting information of a confidential nature.
3. The nurse acts to safeguard the client and the public when health care and safety are affected by the incompetent, unethical, or illegal practice of any person.
4. The nurse assumes responsibility and accountability for individual nursing judgments and actions.
5. The nurse maintains competence in nursing.
6. The nurse exercises informed judgment and uses individual competence and qualifications as criteria in seeking consultation, accepting responsibilities, and delegating nursing activities to others.
7. The nurse participates in activities that contribute to the ongoing development of the profession's body of knowledge.
8. The nurse participates in the profession's efforts to implement and improve standards of nursing.
9. The nurse participates in the profession's efforts to establish and maintain conditions of employment conducive to high-quality nursing care.
10. The nurse participates in the profession's efforts to protect the public from misinformation and misrepresentation and to maintain the integrity of nursing.
11. The nurse collaborates with members of the health professions and other citizens in promoting community and national efforts to meet the health needs of the public.

Nurse C seemingly accepted the assignment to administer morphine by continuous IV infusion without the necessary knowledge about the procedure and the terminology used in the physician's order. This ethical situation could have been prevented by a variety of methods. Upon reentering active nursing practice, Nurse C and the hospital shared a duty to assess Nurse C's clinical knowledge and skills and subsequently develop an education plan to ensure Nurse C's clinical proficiency. Also, the hospital's policy and procedure manual should have included information regarding the administration of continuous IV infusions.

Based on criteria 6 from the Code for Nurses (1985), the charge nurse was responsible for ensuring that Nurse C and the other nurses were competent to fulfill their patient assignments for the shift. The charge nurse also had an obligation to be aware of the type and acuity of nursing interventions for the shift. Similarly, Nurse C had a duty to independently and proactively inform the charge nurse at the beginning of the shift about her lack of knowledge of IV morphine infusions. Although Nurse C may not have acted prudently in accepting this assignment, she should, however, be commended for her critical thinking and courage to question the charge nurse's advice.

Thus, by following the criteria outlined in the Code for Nurses, this ethical situation could have been prevented.

◆ EMOTIONS

Another concern illustrated in this scenario is the influence of emotions on ethical decision-making. Nurse C commented about being uncomfortable with the situation and that feelings determined whether the morphine rate would be adjusted. This discomfort seems to be the cue by which Nurse C was able to identify the ethical situation. It is unclear whether Nurse C would have sought assistance with administering the morphine infusion if this discomfort related to the patient's impending death had not occurred. As nursing care becomes more complex, technology oriented, and shared with ancillary personnel, nurses may not be able to rely on personal beliefs or emotions when evaluating the moral appropriateness of a situation. Thus nurses need to develop the ability to recognize and discuss ethical situations using ethical principles and facts and not feelings and emotions. Opportunities need to be developed that will assist nurses to identify and discuss ethical concerns objectively rather than with subjective emotions and feelings.

◆ RECOMMENDATIONS FOR NURSING

No easy answers exist for preventing or resolving clinical ethical situations related to pain management. Therefore nurses should hesitate to accept the use of standardized ethical "recipes" because these standardized approaches negate patient autonomy and ignore the uniqueness of each patient's situation. Since no one right answer exists, nurses need to develop skills for dealing with the ambiguity inherent in ethical decision-making.

The majority of the obstacles to effective ethical decision-making identified previously could be controlled and possibly prevented with effective communication skills. Specifically, nurses need to develop and practice communication skills related to knowledge, personal experiences, and decision-making.

Nurses need to increase communication with each other by using already-established routes. The change-of-shift report needs to move beyond verbalizing physician orders to a point at which nurses can engage in critical thinking about the patient's care; teach one another about new drugs, treatments, or equipment; and communicate with each other about the nurse's role and responsibilities for decision-making.

Written care plans should be used to document data obtained from assessments, advance directives, and conversations. Patient preferences regarding how decisions should be made, the desired level of involvement significant others should assume, and the treatment goal, including evaluation criteria, should also be included in the written care plan.

Opportunities need to be established for nurses to deal with the emotional reactions associated with ethical decision-making and for sharing personal experiences. This may occur during nursing ethics discussions or staff meetings. The ideal time to constructively work through the emotional reactions associated with ethical decision-making is during or immediately after the ethical situation. Nursing managers and clinical nurse specialists need to make themselves known to and readily accessible to staff nurses, especially during night shifts and weekends. This may require daily walking rounds, an on-call schedule, and/or making telephones numbers available. Efforts are needed that move nurses beyond emotions to identifying and subsequently resolving the problem responsible for the emotional reaction, e.g., poor communication, lack of knowledge, or ambiguity about the patient's preferences.

Finally, nurses need to decide what role they desire to assume during ethical decision-making situations. If nurses desire to be active decision-makers, then nurses need to move beyond subjective reasoning based on feelings and be willing to assume accountability for their decisions. The move toward objective reasoning and decision-making will be facilitated as nurses become more skillful in identifying multiple options, developing a broad knowledge base, and communicating these options clearly.

◆ CONCLUSION

Despite efforts to increase ethical knowledge, communication, and decision-making skills, nurses will continue to experience ethical situations in the clinical setting. In fact, nurses may identify more ethical situations because of their increased awareness and knowledge. Thus nurses and nurse managers need to continue to support one another while developing the skills required to deal with future clinical ethical questions. However, as nurses do gain skill and confidence in clinical ethical decision-making, patients and their significant others will benefit from objective nursing care that facilitates patient autonomy and beneficence while managing the patient's pain.

REFERENCES

1. American Nurses' Association (1985). *Code for nurses with interpretive statements.* Kansas City, Mo: American Nurses' Association.
2. Bandman EL and Bandman B. (1985). *Nursing ethics in the life span.* Norwalk, Conn: Appleton-Century-Crofts.
3. Beauchamp TL and Childress JF. (1989). *Principles of biomedical ethics* (ed 3). New York: Oxford University Press.
4. Beauchamp TL and Walters L. (1982). *Contemporary issues in bioethics* (ed 2). Belmont, Calif: Wadsworth Publishing Company.
5. Chell B. (1988). Competency: what it is, what it isn't, and why it matters. In Monagle JF and Thomasma DC (eds), *Medical ethics: a guide for health professionals* (pp. 99-100). Rockville, Md: Aspen Publishers.
6. Curtin L and Flaherty MJ. (1982). *Nursing ethics: theory and pragmatics.* Bowie, Md: Robert J. Brady Company.
7. DeWolf MS. (1989a). Clinical ethical decision-making: a grounded theory method. *Dissertation Abstracts International, 50,*(11b), (University Microfilms No. 90-06, 043).
8. DeWolf MS. (1989b). Ethical decision-making. *Semin Oncol Nurs, 5*(2), 77-81.
9. Emanuel EJ and Emanuel L. (1990). Living wills: past, present, and future. *J Clin Eth, 1*(1), 9-19.
10. Emanuel LL and Emanuel EJ. (1989). The medical directive: a new comprehensive advance care document. *JAMA, 261,* 3288-3293.

11. Haddad AM. (1988). Determining competency. *J Gerontol Nurs, 14*(6), 19-22.
12. Lazaroof A and Orr W. (1986). Living wills and other advance directives. *Clin Geriatr Med, 2*(3), 521-534.
13. Lo B. (1988). The clinical use of advance directives. In Monagle JF and Thomasma DC (eds), *Medical ethics: a guide for health professionals* (pp. 209-216). Rockville, Md: Aspen Publishers.
14. Maloney MM. (1986). *Professionalization of nursing: current issues and trends.* Philadelphia: Lippincott.
15. Muyskens JL. (1982). *Moral problems in nursing: a philosophical investigation.* Totowa, NJ: Rowman and Littlefield.
16. Purtillo RB and Cassel CK. (1981). *Ethical dimensions in the health professions.* Philadephia: Saunders.
17. Rachels J. (1982). Active and passive euthanasia. In Beauchamp TL and Walters L (eds), *Contemporary issues in bioethics* (ed 2) (pp. 312-316). Belmont, Calif: Wadsworth Publishing.
18. Walters L. (1982). Euthanasia and the prolongation of life. In Beauchamp TL and Walters L (eds), *Contemporary issues in bioethics* (ed 2) (pp. 307-312). Belmont, Calif: Wadsworth Publishing.

7

Pharmacological Management

Judith A. Paice

IN THE WAR against pain, the primary weapons are pharmacological agents, and the battle is led by nurses. Because nurses have major responsibilities for the effective management of pain, nurses must understand the pharmacokinetics of analgesic agents, the mechanism of action of these drugs, their side effects, and the nursing care involved in administering these agents. The pharmacological approach includes nonsteroidal antiinflammatory drugs, opiate analgesics, and adjuvant and other drugs.

◆ PHARMACOKINETICS

Although hundreds of analgesic agents are already in clinical use, new analgesics are developed and introduced into clinical practice each day. An understanding of the underlying principles of pharmacology provides the nurse with the knowledge necessary to assess, plan, administer, and evaluate the response to a specific analgesic agent. These underlying scientific principles include the pharmacokinetics of analgesic agents and can be divided into three major phases: absorption, distribution, and excretion.[28]

Absorption

Once a drug (e.g., an oral tablet) is delivered into the body, it must be dissolved so that the drug may be absorbed into the circulation. The route of administration and formulation of the drug affect absorption. For example, liquid preparations are absorbed faster because they are already dissolved. The absorption of a drug is also influenced by the molecular size of the drug, its lipid solubility, its ionization (i.e., whether it has a positive, negative, or neutral charge), and other properties of the drug.

Drugs that have a very small molecular weight pass through membranes faster to reach the site of action more readily. Nitrous oxide has a very light molecular weight, and as a result has an almost immediate onset of action. Lipid-soluble, or lipophilic, drugs, such as fentanyl, can cross the fatty layers of membranes more easily. Drugs that are positively or negatively charged associate readily with water molecules and are described as water-soluble, or hydrophilic. An example of a hydrophilic drug is morphine.

Distribution

The dissolved drug is carried by red blood cells or plasma proteins throughout the body. Some tissues and organs that are exposed to the drug are not affected, but others serve as reservoirs to store the drug until a later time. Other tissues contain receptors that become bound by the drug. When a drug binds to its receptor, biochemical and physiological changes occur that are predictable and characteristic of that drug. Such a drug is called an agonist. Other drugs, antagonists, may block that receptor, preventing the agonist from binding. Opiate receptor binding by the agonist morphine, and blocking by the antagonist naloxone, are excellent examples of these processes and are explained in greater detail later in this chapter.

Elimination

Some drugs are taken up by the liver, converted into metabolites of the drug, and eliminated in the bile, where these products then reach the intestines. Upon reaching the intestines, these metabolites may be excreted in the feces or may be reabsorbed into the circulation. The kidney also serves to filter the drug and its metabolites, secreting them in the urine. In addition, some drugs may pass through the alveoli and are eliminated by the lungs. Finally, a variety of drugs are eliminated by sweat or saliva.

Diseases of the organ involved in the elimination of a drug

can lead to accumulation of the active drug or its metabolite. Most analgesic agents are eliminated by the liver or kidneys. Therefore, conditions such as cirrhosis, renal failure, or decreased functioning associated with aging may lead to accumulation of analgesic agents or their metabolites, leading to toxicity.[14] Normeperidine, a metabolite of meperidine, accumulates in persons with renal disease, causing significant side effects that include tremors, hallucinations, and seizures.[26]

◆ NONSTEROIDAL ANTIINFLAMMATORY DRUGS

The most widely used analgesic agents are the nonsteroidal antiinflammatory drugs (NSAIDs). The reasons for their popularity include their wide availability (usually obtained without a physician's order), their general lack of serious side effects, and their efficacy in relieving pain.

Mechanism of Action

Assume that damage to tissues occurs by some type of thermal, mechanical, or chemical trauma. This trauma causes cells to release chemicals, including potassium and histamine. Other substances also appear in the injured area, including bradykinin and prostaglandins. All of these chemicals trigger inflammation and can produce pain.[15]

Prostaglandins are produced when arachidonic acid is broken down by the enzyme cyclooxygenase, resulting in sensitization of free nerve endings and pain. But cyclooxygenase is inhibited by nonsteroidal antiinflammatory drugs (NSAIDs), which thereby prevent the breakdown of arachidonic acid and the formation of prostaglandins.[25,39] Therefore, NSAIDs are particularly effective in relieving pain associated with inflammation, as in musculoskeletal disorders (e.g., osteoarthritis), dysmenorrhea, and headache.[12] Other types of pain generally well controlled by NSAIDs include bone pain associated with bone metastases and pain related to trauma to peripheral tissues[30] (see Figure 7-1).

NSAIDs have an additional therapeutic effect. They act on the hypothalamus to reset the body's thermostat during febrile episodes, reducing the fever. This antipyretic effect is usually desirable; however, in some circumstances physicians may be monitoring temperature for fluctuations and alternative analgesics must be used.

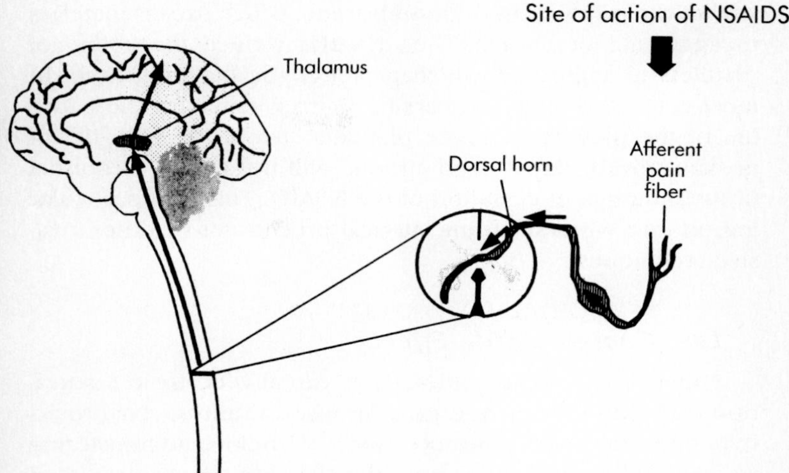

FIGURE 7-1. Pain pathway and the sites of action of analgesic agents.

Side Effects

Gastrointestinal Toxicity

Although prostaglandins cause pain and inflammation, they are also responsible for maintaining the mucous lining of the gastric mucosa.[60] Inhibiting the formation of prostaglandins diminishes the protective lining of the gastrum, leading to destruction of the gastric mucosa. Nonsteroidal antiinflammatory drugs, by their effect on prostaglandin synthesis, predispose individuals to gastrointestinal toxicity. This effect is exacerbated because many NSAIDs can directly damage the gastric lining. Thus the gastrointestinal effects of NSAIDs may range from nausea or "heart burn" to gastrointestinal bleeding. Strategies to prevent these toxicities include taking NSAIDs with meals, adding a mild antacid, or administering misoprostol (Cytotec). Misoprostol is a prostaglandin analogue that has been shown to protect against NSAID-induced ulcers. The major contraindication of this drug is that misoprostol's use in pregnant women is associated with spontaneous abortion.[51]

Bleeding Problems

NSAIDs inhibit cyclooxygenase and the resultant formation of prostaglandins.[49] In addition to their role in forming the protective mucosal lining of the stomach, prostaglandins are vital to the production of thromboxane, which causes platelets to aggregate or clump. Thus NSAIDs reduce the ability of platelets to aggregate, which prolongs the bleeding time. In most cases, this effect appears to be irreversible for the entire life of the platelet. Because platelets have a life span of approximately 10 days, bleeding time will not return to normal until 10 days after cessation of the NSAID. This is of particular importance when planning surgical procedures or other invasive techniques.

Less Common Side Effects

Other, less common side effects can also occur in association with these drugs: allergic responses, tinnitus, renal toxicity, and bone marrow suppression.[25,54] Before administering an NSAID, the nurse must consider the side effects associated with the specific drug, as well as any problems unique to the patient that may place the patient at risk for toxicities.

There are 10 major categories of NSAIDs, encompassing more than 25 drugs (see Table 7-1). These categories include the salicylates (acetylated and nonacetylated), para-aminophenol derivatives, proprionic acid derivatives, indole acetic acid derivatives, oxicams, pyrazolones, anthranilic acids, pyrrole-acetic acid derivatives, and phenyl-acetic acids.[25]

Commonly Used NSAIDs

Aspirin

Acetylsalicylic acid, aspirin, is the most widely used of the NSAIDs and serves as the standard of comparison for all the other NSAIDs.[38] Introduced in 1899, aspirin is effective in relieving mild to severe pain. It is available in a wide variety of formulations, including tablets, chewable tablets, enteric coated tablets, sustained release tablets, capsules, rectal suppositories, and topical cream.[46] A usual oral starting dose is 650 mg every 4 to 6 hours, increasing the dose by 325 mg to a total dose of 1300 mg every 4 hours. Unfortunately, increasing the dose also increases the potential for side effects.[25]

Aspirin use is associated with gastrointestinal toxicity and decreased platelet aggregation. Enteric coated tablets may limit the toxic effect on the stomach because the enteric coating prevents absorption until the drug reaches the small intestine. Another method that may protect the gastric lining is to

◆ **Table 7-1**
Nonsteroidal antiinflammatory drugs

Generic name	Trade name	Usual oral daily dosages
ACETYLATED SALICYLATES		
Acetylsalicylic acid (ASA)	Aspirin	650-1000 mg QID
NONACETYLATED SALICYLATES		
Choline magnesium trisalicylate	Trilisate	1500 mg BID
Diflunisal	Dolobid	500-1000 mg BID
Salsalate	Disalcid*	750 mg QID
PARA-AMINOPHENOL DERIVATIVES		
Acetaminophen	Tylenol	650-1000 mg QID
PROPRIONIC ACID DERIVATIVES		
Fenoprofen	Nalfon	200-600 mg TID or QID
Flurbiprofen	Ansaid	150-300 mg TID or QID
Ibuprofen	Advil, Motrin, Nuprin, Rufen	400-800 mg TID or QID
Ketoprofen	Orudis	50-75 mg TID or QID
Naproxen	Naprosyn	250-500 mg BID
Naproxen sodium	Anaprox	275 mg TID or QID
Tiaprofenic acid	Surgam	600 mg BID or TID
INDOLE ACETIC ACID DERIVATIVES		
Indomethacin	Indocin, Indocid	25-50 mg BID or TID
Sulindac	Clinoril	150-200 mg BID
OXICAMS		
Piroxicam	Feldene	20 mg QD
PYRAZOLONES		
Phenylbutazone	Butazolidin	100-200 mg TID
Oxyphenbutazone	Tandearil	100 mg TID or QID
Sulfinpyrazone	Anturan, Anturane	200-800 mg BID

*United States only.

Continued.

◆ **Table 7-1**
Nonsteroidal antiinflammatory drugs—cont'd

Generic name	Trade name	Usual oral daily dosages
ANTHRANILIC ACIDS		
Meclofenamate	Meclomen	200-400 mg TID or QID
Mefenamic acid	Ponstan	250 mg TID
Floctafenine	Idarac	200-400 mg TID or QID
PYRROLE-ACETIC ACID		
Tolmetin sodium	Tolectin	400-600 mg BID or TID
Ketorolac tromethamine	Toradol	15-30 mg IM QID (not available in oral formulations)
PHENYLACETIC ACID		
Diclofenac sodium	Voltaren	100-150 mg BID or TID

take the drug with food. As a result of the effect of aspirin on platelet function, the nurse must advise patients to stop taking aspirin for at least 10 days before any invasive procedure (e.g., surgery, dental extraction, blood donation).

Acetaminophen

Acetaminophen differs from other NSAIDs in that it does not inhibit cyclooxygenase and so has less antiinflammatory effect than other NSAIDs. Therefore it also lacks many of the side effects associated with prostaglandin inhibition, especially gastric irritation and increased bleeding times. Acetaminophen can be obtained without a prescription and is available in multiple formulations, including tablets, chewable tablets, capsules, liquids, and rectal suppositories.[46] The usual starting dose is 500 mg orally every 4 hours, increasing as needed to an absolute maximum of 4000 mg/day.[25]

Ibuprofen

Ibuprofen (Advil, Motrin, Nuprin) also inhibits cyclooxygenase, but this inhibition is reversible. Thus platelet function returns to normal more rapidly after ibuprofen is discontinued. In addition, gastrointestinal irritation occurs less frequently than with aspirin. Ibuprofen is currently available over the counter and is relatively inexpensive.

Indomethacin

Indomethacin (Indocin, Indocid) was introduced in 1963 for the relief of pain associated with rheumatoid arthritis. It has also been shown to be effective in the treatment of pain related to invasion of tumor into bone. Unfortunately, prolonged use is associated with significant side effects, including gastrointestinal toxicity, bleeding, and hypersensitivity reactions. Interestingly, the drug appears to be better tolerated when given at night. Thus a larger dose at night and a smaller dose during the day might obviate side effects.

Indomethacin is available in capsules, sustained release tablets, and rectal suppositories. A parenteral formulation is also available, but not for the management of pain.

Choline Magnesium Trisalicylate

Choline magnesium trisalicylate (Trilisate) has less effect on platelet aggregation than aspirin, making this group of NSAIDs particularly attractive for patients who might experience coagulopathies, especially persons with hematological disorders or cancer. Currently, the use of this drug requires a physician's prescription. The usual dose is 1000 mg three times daily. Because the tablets are quite large, the liquid form should be employed for patients with dysphagia.

Ketorolac Tromethamine

Ketorolac tromethamine (Toradol) is a parenteral NSAID intended for short-term IM use, such as postoperative pain relief. Ten mg of ketorolac tromethamine is approximately equianalgesic to 6 mg of morphine. The recommended postoperative dose is a 30 to 60 mg intramuscular loading dose followed by 15 to 30 mg IM every 6 hours, with a maximum total dose of 150 mg on the first day and 120 mg daily after that. Although attractive because it forgoes the effects of opiates, ketorolac trimethamine use can lead to side effects such as nausea, dyspepsia, gastrointestinal erosion and bleeding, altered platelet aggregation, and drowsiness. If given with an opiate, these drugs should not be mixed in the same syringe because ketorolac may precipitate.[41]

Each of the NSAIDs can be very effective in relieving pain; however, there is great variability in the way individuals respond to a particular drug. Therefore, if an individual does not respond to a reasonable trial of one drug, another drug might be used with good results. If several drugs are tried and moderate pain persists, opiate analgesics may be the next drugs of choice.

◆ NARCOTIC ANALGESICS

Narcotic analgesics, frequently referred to as opioid analgesics to denote their origins in the opium poppy, have been used since the third century BC. All opiates, including morphine, have the same mechanism of action and similar side effects.[26] Opiate analgesics are frequently categorized as weak or strong, to assist clinicians in choosing the appropriate drug for specific clinical situations.

Mechanism of Action

Unlike the NSAIDs, which primarily affect the periphery, opiate analgesics act in the central nervous system (CNS) to relieve pain (see Figure 7-1). Opiate analgesics, as well as endogenous opioids (e.g., enkephalin, endorphin), bind to opiate receptors that are distributed throughout the CNS and the gastrointestinal tract. When bound in the CNS, these receptors block the transmission of the painful, or nociceptive, message. There are several types of opiate receptors, including mu, delta, and kappa receptors; however, it is not certain which receptors other than mu may be effective in relieving pain. The opiate analgesics currently in clinical use work primarily at the mu receptor.[15]

Side Effects and Their Management

Sedation

Opiate analgesics may initially produce sedation, mental clouding, drowsiness, and difficulty concentrating.[26] This effect is dose-related, so that higher doses of opiate may cause extreme sedation. Tolerance usually develops to the sedative effect of opiates, so that over several days of drug administration, less sedation occurs. Also, patients may respond differently to different opiates, so that changing to another opiate may diminish the sedation.

Stimulants may be useful in combating sedation in persons who must receive chronic opiate therapy and in whom tolerance to the sedation does not develop after 1 week. For example, sedation may be offset by dextroamphetamine (Dexedrine) 2.5 to 10 mg or methylphenidate (Ritalin) 5 to 10 mg each morning.[1,4,18] The use of these stimulants must be weighed carefully, because they reduce appetite, of particular concern in persons with cancer or other chronic illness, and may lead to agitation, palpitation, headache, and dysphoria.

Constipation

The most common side effect of the opiate analgesics is constipation.[10] When given systemically, opiates bind to opiate receptors distributed throughout the CNS and the gastrointestinal tract. When binding occurs in the gastrointestinal tract, peristalsis decreases and intestinal secretions are reduced. These effects combine to create constipation. Unlike other side effects of opiate therapy, constipation tends to persist. The body develops tolerance to constipation slowly, if at all.

A bowel regimen must be initiated in persons who will be maintained on long-term opiate therapy.[35,47] These individuals must increase their fluid intake, add fiber and bulk-forming agents to their diet, increase their exercise regimen, and, if necessary, include daily stool softeners and laxatives in their list of medications. Prevention is imperative, as constipation can increase pain and in extreme cases, cause obstruction.

Another effect opiate analgesics are believed to have on the gastrointestinal tract is constriction of the common bile duct, causing an increase in biliary tract pressure. Patients with known gallbladder disease or with undiagnosed acute abdominal pain might experience biliary colic if given morphine or other morphine-like opiates. If biliary colic is of potential concern, meperidine or sublimaze (fentanyl) are alternative opiates that appear to have less effect on biliary pressure.[26]

Nausea and Vomiting

Opiates produce nausea and vomiting by stimulating the chemoreceptor trigger zone (CTZ). Once stimulated, the CTZ transmits messages to the vomiting center, which initiates the complex physiological responses that lead to nausea, retching, and vomiting.[26] In addition, the vestibular system, which is responsible for alerting the brain to changes in position and movement, adds input to the CTZ. Thus ambulatory patients receiving opiates appear to experience more nausea and vomiting than recumbent patients.[15]

To reduce the nausea and vomiting, patients can be pretreated with an antiemetic, such as prochlorperazine. In addition, during the first several days of opiate therapy, patients who experience chronic pain might be encouraged to remain in the recumbent position if ambulation increases their discomfort. The emetic potential of various opiate agents is controversial. Several experts suggest that to limit nausea it might be useful to change the opiate; however, there is no scientific evidence that at equianalgesic doses different opiates have different emetic potentials.[18] Tolerance to this emetic effect generally develops after several days of opiate therapy.

Respiratory Depression

Opiates can produce respiratory depression by acting on respiratory centers in the brain stem. Respiratory rate and volume are affected. Yet there are mechanisms within the body that counteract these depressant effects. As respiratory rate decreases and the depth of respiration becomes more shallow, carbon dioxide accumulates in the lungs and the bloodstream. The increasing CO_2 content within the blood stimulates the respiratory centers to increase the respiratory rate, counteracting the depressant effects of the opiate.[18]

Tolerance to this depressant effect generally develops by the time the patient has received several doses of the opiate. Thus respiratory depression occurs very rarely in persons receiving opiates over a long period of time. Persons at greatest risk for respiratory depression are those who are opiate-naive, or who have not recently received opiates. If respiratory depression does occur, it can be reversed by the narcotic antagonist naloxone (Narcan). Although the usual dose of naloxone is 0.4 mg, patients who are chronically receiving opiates should be given only enough naloxone to counteract the respiratory effects. The full 0.4 mg dose may precipitate severe opiate withdrawal, which includes agitation, rhinorrhea, diarrhea, and pruritis. Seizures may also occur if the patient has been receiving meperidine (Demerol). In addition, patients whose pain was being controlled by the opiate will again experience that pain. To easily titrate the naloxone and avoid administering more than necessary, one mixes naloxone with 10 cc of saline and delivers the drug slowly until respirations return to an acceptable rate.[36] The patient must be monitored frequently, as the half life of naloxone (about 30 minutes) is far less than the half life of most opiate analgesics. Thus repeated doses of naloxone at approximately hourly intervals are not unusual.

Urinary Retention

Opiate analgesics act directly to increase smooth muscle tone, especially that of the detrussor muscle of the bladder and the bladder sphincter.[26] This change in muscle tone results in urinary urgency and retention. The elderly and individuals with preexisting genitourinary abnormalities should be evaluated for difficulty with micturition. This is particularly important in those individuals who may experience changes in mentation and might not be aware of bodily functions. Catheterization may be necessary.

Pruritus

Opiates cause histamine release, which can create such effects as pruritus, flushing, and sweating. These effects may be reduced by the administration of an antihistamine such as diphenhydramine (Benadryl) or hydroxyzine hydrochloride (Atarax). Tolerance also develops to this side effect.

Categories of Opiate Analgesics

Opiate analgesics can be categorized according to their strength (weak opioids vs. strong opioids) or by their pharmacological composition (agonists vs. mixed agonist-antagonists) (see Table 7-2). Knowledge of these categories guides the clinical use of opiate analgesics.

Weak Opioids

Although all opiate analgesics have the potential to relieve equal levels of pain intensity at equianalgesic doses, some drugs require extremely large doses to equal a standard dose of morphine. These drugs are called weak opiates. Codeine is considered a weak opiate, because approximately 200 mg of oral codeine is equivalent to 60 mg of oral morphine (Table 7-2). Usual doses of codeine are much lower, starting at 15 to 30 mg orally every 4 hours. Codeine is a very effective drug in relieving minor pain, but is insufficiently strong to relieve moderate to severe pain.

Propoxyphene (Darvon) is also considered a weak opiate. Its effectiveness is controversial, and long-term use may lead to central nervous system toxicity caused by the accumulation of the metabolite norpropoxyphene.[38] Consequently this drug has little use in chronic pain management.

Oxycodone (Percodan, Percocet) is considered a moderately strong opiate. This drug, as well as codeine and hydrocodone, is usually formulated with aspirin or acetaminophen. As a result, patients must be cautioned to take only the amount prescribed or they run the risk of aspirin or acetaminophen overdosage.

Opiate Agonists

Strong opiates include morphine, hydromorphone, levorphanol, meperidine, methadone (United States), oxymorphone, and other agents with potent analgesic activity. Morphine, named after Morpheus, the Greek god of dreams, is the standard by which other opiates are measured. Morphine is a natural alkaloid of opium that is rapidly absorbed after oral or parenteral administration. Little morphine accumulates in the tissues: Almost all is excreted by the kidneys. Morphine is less lipophilic, or lipid soluble, than other opiates. Because membranes are composed of lipids, drugs that are lipid soluble cross over these membranes more rapidly. Thus when given subcutaneously, morphine has a slightly slower onset of action than other more lipid-soluble drugs.

Meperidine has a very short duration of action (2-3 hours), has poor oral bioavailability (50 mg po is approximately equal to 650 mg of aspirin), is irritating to subcutaneous tissue, and causes tremors and seizures with prolonged use resulting from the accumulation of the metabolite normeperidine.[27] In addition, meperidine causes disorientation, hallucinations, and mood changes. These effects occur most frequently in persons requiring high doses or extended periods of treatment, and in patients with renal dysfunction. Therefore, me-

◆ **Table 7-2**
Opiates

Generic name	Trade name	Equianalgesic dosages (mg) IM	po	Duration of action (hr)
WEAK AGONISTS				
Codeine		130	200	3-4
	Tylenol #1 = 7.5 mg with 300 mg acetaminophen			
	Tylenol #2 = 15 mg with 300 mg acetaminophen			
	Tylenol #3 = 30 mg with 300 mg acetaminophen			
	Tylenol #4 = 60 mg with 300 mg acetaminophen			
	Empirin #2 = 15 mg with 325 mg aspirin			
	Empirin #3 = 30 mg with 325 mg aspirin			
	Empirin #4 = 60 mg with 325 mg aspirin			
Propoxyphene	Darvon	—	500	3-4
	Darvocet-N 50 = 50 mg with 325 mg acetaminophen			
	Darvocet-N 100 = 100 mg with 650 mg acetaminophen			
	Darvon-N with ASA = 100 mg with 325 mg aspirin			
Hydrocodone		—	100	3-4
	Lortab = 5 mg with 500 mg acetaminophen			
	Lortab 7.5 = 7.5 mg with 500 mg acetaminophen			
	Vicodin = 5 mg with 500 mg acetaminophen			
	Vicodin ES = 7.5 mg with 500 acetaminophen			

Continued.

◆ **Table 7-2**
Opiates—cont'd

Generic name	Trade name	Equianalgesic dosages (mg) IM	po	Duration of action (hr)
Oxycodone	Roxicodone*	–	30	3-4
	Percodan = 5 mg oxycodone and 325 mg aspirin			
	Percocet = 5 mg oxycodone and 325 mg acetaminophen			
	Tylox* = 5 mg oxycodone and 500 mg acetaminophen			
STRONG AGONISTS				
Morphine		10	60 (20-30)	4
sustained release				8-12
Fentanyl	Sublimaze	0.05 (IV)	–	1½
Hydromorphone	Dilaudid	1.5	7.5	2-4
Levorphanol	Levo-Dromoran	2	4	4
Meperidine	Demerol	75	300	3-4 IM 12-16 oral

Methadone	Dolophine	10	20	3-5 (may be as long as 12-24 hours)
Oxymorphone	Numorphan	1	—	3-4
rectal		10		4-6
PARTIAL AGONIST				
Buprenorphine*	Buprenex	0.4	—	6
MIXED AGONIST-ANTAGONISTS				
Dezocine	Dalgan	10	—	3-4
Butorphanol	Stadol	2	—	3-4
Nalbuphine	Nubain	10	—	3-6
Pentazocine	Talwin	60	180	3

*United States only.

peridine is not an appropriate choice of narcotic for most patients and is strongly contraindicated for individuals requiring long-term pain therapy.

Mixed Agonist-Antagonist Drugs

Mixed agonist-antagonist drugs, when given by themselves, have agonist properties that bind the drug to opiate receptors to provide analgesia. However, when given in time proximity to agonists, antagonist components of the drug bind to the opiate receptors to block the effects of the agonist. This antagonist component of the drug acts in the same way that naloxone does to block the effects of the narcotic. The disadvantage of mixed agonist-antagonist drugs, such as pentazocine, butorphanol, and nalbuphine, is their ability to cause withdrawal in persons who are currently receiving pure agonist narcotics. Another disadvantage is the frequent occurrence of psychomimetic effects, including anxiety, nightmares, and hallucinations. Finally, most mixed agonist-antagonists are only available in parenteral formulations. As a result, these drugs are of limited use in chronic pain management.

New Methods of Opiate Delivery

Research has focused on providing new methods of delivering opiates. Many of these new methods are creative alternatives that circumvent potential obstacles that occur with previously used techniques. These include methods to deliver drugs when patients cannot take opiates orally and strategies that circumvent side effects associated with traditional routes.

Oral

Oral administration of opiates is one of the oldest methods of delivery and it remains the preferred route of delivery. This preference is based on ease of administration, reduced morbidity (absence of injection pain or hematomas and risk of cellulitis), and reduced cost (does not require purchase of syringes or needles). Most patients, including patients in the last 24 hours of their life, can receive adequate analgesia with oral medications.[17,33] Unfortunately, because the duration of action of most opiates is approximately 4 hours, patients with chronic pain have been forced to awaken several times during the night to medicate themselves for pain. For this reason, sustained release morphine tablets (MS Contin, Roxane) were developed. A special coating allows gradual breakdown of the drug, so that patients receive continuous relief over 8 to 12 hours.[31]

Another new method of oral opiate delivery is high-concentration liquid morphine. Available in concentrations of 20 mg morphine per ml, this formulation allows patients who can swallow only small amounts to continue taking the drug by mouth.

Transdermal

An alternative therapy for persons who cannot take oral medications is transdermal drug therapy.[37,21] Transdermal fentanyl (Duragesic) has recently been approved for use in chronic cancer pain patients who have previously been treated with opiates. The potential advantages of transdermal drug delivery are a relatively stable plasma drug level and the non-invasive nature of drug delivery. Each patch, available in 25, 50, 75, or 100 μg/hour, provides delivery of drug for 72 hours. Seventeen hours after removal of the patch, plasma levels of fentanyl drop by 50% and significant levels of drug may be found at 24 hours after removal.

Systemic side effects of transdermal fentanyl include nausea and vomiting, and somnolence. Local reactions to the patch include erythema and rash. Although transdermal drug therapy has been used for many years for the delivery of drugs such as nitroglycerine and scopalamine, more experience with transdermal fentanyl, and possibly other opiates, is needed. Specific questions that remain unanswered are the effects of hydration on absorption, as well as the influence of cachexia and reduced fat stores on drug availability.

Intravenous

The intravenous route is not new; however, this method of delivery is gaining greater acceptance.[7] The intravenous route provides more rapid onset of action and stable blood levels when delivered continuously, and precludes the need for painful injections. Patients obtain good relief with few side effects. Contrary to concerns about respiratory depression, Citron and colleagues[7] found that arterial blood gases remained at or near baseline levels. In addition to established safety, intravenous morphine can be delivered over extended time periods with relative ease via ambulatory infusion pumps.[13] Some experts suggest that the intravenous and intramuscular doses are equianalgesic; others recommend using 50% of the intramuscular dose when converting to the intravenous route.

Sublingual/Buccal

Little is known about the advantages of the sublingual (under the tongue) or buccal (between the cheek and gum) routes of opiate administration. These routes, already in use in Europe, benefit individuals who cannot swallow or who have a bowel obstruction.[3] Although opiates specially formulated for this use are not available in North America, very small volumes of liquid morphine may be placed in the sublingual or buccal space. Unfortunately, the taste of these formulations is not palatable for many patients. Pharmacists can manufacture troches with pleasing flavors to overcome this problem. Patients should be discouraged from swallowing the drug and should be advised not to eat or drink within 15 minutes of applying the drug. Because these routes bypass the liver on the first pass through the circulation (called the "first pass" effect), equianalgesic doses of drug should be based on parenteral doses.

Rectal

Although the rectal route is not new, this route is gaining acceptance and as a result, several opiates are now marketed in suppository form. Many pharmacists can formulate most opiates into suppository form. The rectal route is especially useful for patients who have dysphagia or nausea and vomiting. Rectal suppositories are also convenient to administer. When converting from the oral to the rectal route, the dose to be given rectally should be the same as a parenteral dose of drug. This is because of the "first pass" effect.

Subcutaneous

Although the subcutaneous route has been used extensively for many years, a new technique now being used incorporates subcutaneous catheters and infusion pumps for the administration of continuous subcutaneous narcotic.[9] The benefit of this approach is that patients without permanent venous access devices can receive continuous infusions of drug in the home setting. This is especially important for patients who can no longer take oral medications.

New, very small-gauged catheters are available to allow ease of administration (Figure 7-2). Family members can simply replace the needle if it becomes dislodged or requires changing. In fact, catheters may remain in place for 3 to 7 days or for even greater periods of time without negative effects. Indications for changing the catheter include site infection or poor drug absorption. Poor absorption is usually due to fibrosis at the insertion site and is evidenced by a decrease in analgesic effect. To reduce the potential for site fibrosis, high concentrations of opiate are necessary to allow delivery of adequate dose in a small volume of fluid.

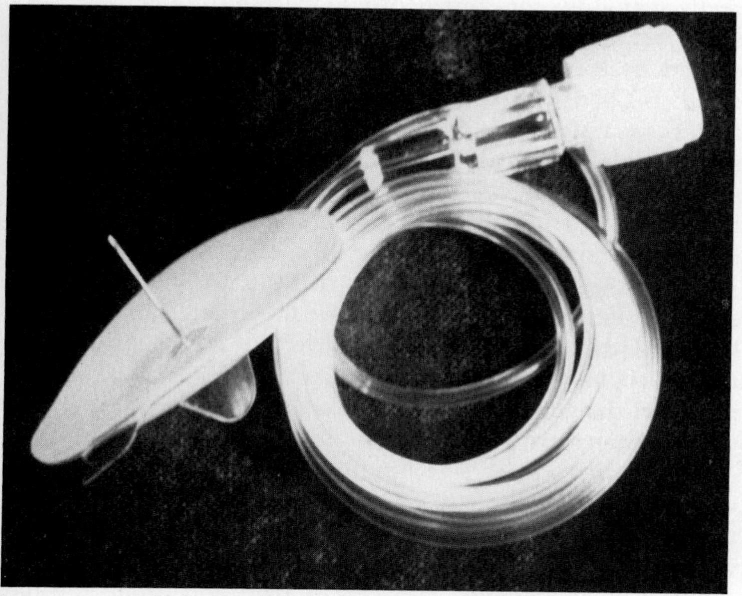

FIGURE 7-2. A needle designed for continuous subcutaneous infusion of analgesic agents (Auto Syring Sub-Q-Set Subcutaneous Infusion Set; Baxter Healthcare Corporation; Hooksett, NH).

Intraspinal Opiates

Another new method of delivery is the infusion of opiates and local anesthetics into the epidural or intrathecal (subarachnoid) space. As discussed earlier, undesirable side effects may occur when opiates are administered systemically, including sedation, constipation, nausea, and vomiting. These effects are due to binding of the drug to opiate receptors located throughout the brain and the gastrointestinal tract. The primary benefit of intraspinal opiate administration is the reduction of side effects seen with systemic opiates due to the direct action of the drug on opiate receptors in the dorsal horn of the spinal cord. As little drug enters supraspinal centers, few side effects, if any, occur. One example of the reduction in side effects, and a major benefit of these routes, is the lack of interference with bonding usually experienced by postcesarean mothers receiving conventional opiate therapy.[8]

The two sites of intraspinal delivery, epidural and intrathecal space, require significantly different doses of drug to achieve the same degree of analgesia. Their anatomical locations account for these differences. The intrathecal space directly surrounds the spinal cord. Opiates introduced into this space act quickly at the dorsal horn; very little drug is absorbed by blood vessels in that area. The epidural space, which is filled with fatty tissue and an extensive venous system, is separated from the spinal cord by the dura mater. This sheath serves as a barrier to drug diffusion, and the delay allows uptake of the drug into the systemic circulation through the venous plexus. Thus a higher dose of opiate is needed when the epidural route is used.

Many methods of delivering drugs into the intraspinal space are currently being used. External catheters allow either bolus injections or continuous delivery of the drug when attached to infusion pumps[6,16] (Figure 7-3). Because of the potential danger of infection, including meningitis, most external systems are placed epidurally so that the dural sheath can serve as a barrier (the intrathecal route has no such barrier). Because of the risk of infection, totally implanted systems have been developed. The Ommaya reservoir, indwelling venous access ports, and totally implanted pumps are currently used in patients with cancer pain and other chronic pain conditions[34,40,42,43,45] (Figures 7-4 and 7-5).

Although these routes have been used for many years in obstetrical pain with excellent results, information is needed

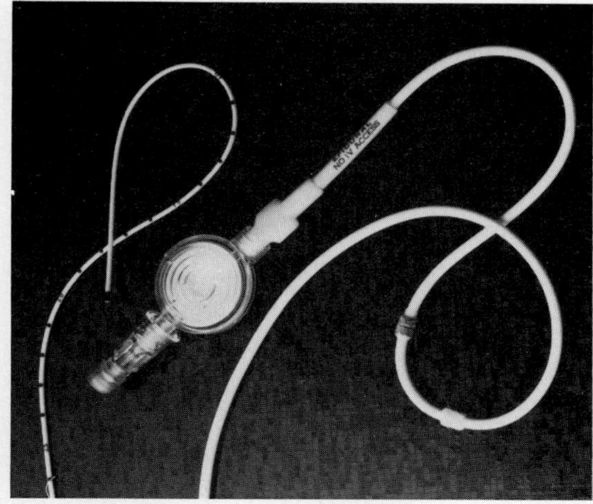

FIGURE 7-3. The Du Pen Long Term Epidural Catheter is associated with reduced site infection (Photograph courtesy of Davol Inc., a subsidiary of C.R. Bard, Inc. who hold Du Pen as a registered trademark).

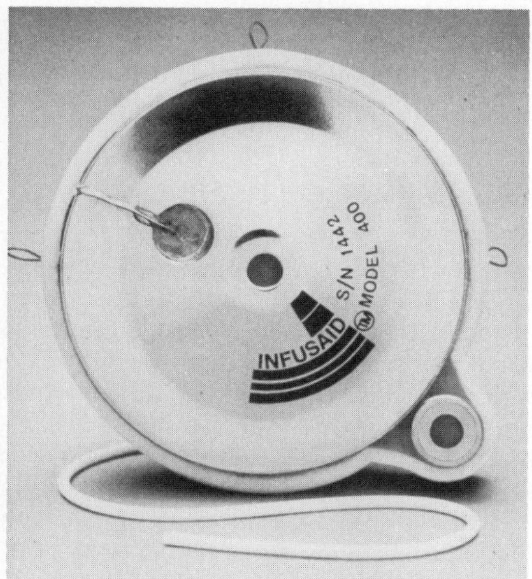

FIGURE 7-4. The Infusaid Model 400 implantable drug administration device delivers a continuous dose of drug (Infusaid Inc., Norwood, Mass).

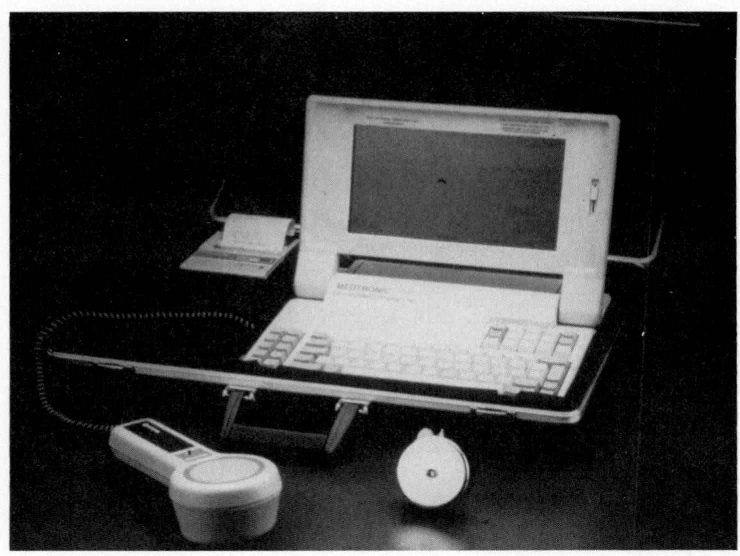

FIGURE 7-5. The SynchroMed Infusion System, including a pump, programmer, telemetry wand, and printer, can deliver continuous, bolus, or combination therapy (Medtronic, Minneapolis, Minn).

regarding the efficacy, morbidity, and costs of longer-term intraspinal therapy. Current studies indicate promising results.

Combining Opiates and NSAIDs

Because NSAIDs and opiates have different mechanisms of action, it is often useful to combine these agents. In fact, commercially available formulations that include both categories (e.g., codeine and acetaminophen) capitalize on these different mechanisms, providing analgesia while causing fewer side effects than if a higher dose of one drug were used.

The World Health Organization recommends a sequential, or three-step ladder, approach to the management of cancer pain (see Figure 7-6).[61] This approach, or modifications of this approach, might be applicable to types of pain other than cancer. Initial therapy begins with a NSAID (step 1). When the patient receives the maximum recommended dose of NSAIDs and continues to experience pain, one adds a weak opiate (step 2). The dose of the weak opiate is increased until relief is

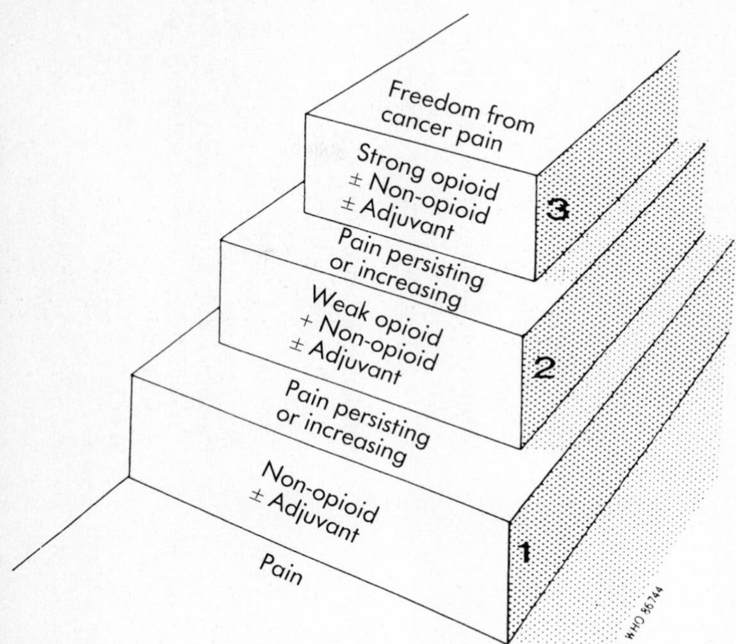

FIGURE 7-6. The analgesic ladder for cancer pain management proposed by the World Health Organization (From Cancer pain relief, 1986, and Cancer pain relief and palliative care, 1990, WHO, Geneva, Switzerland).

obtained, side effects occur, or the ceiling dose is reached. If an adequate dose of weak opiate does not provide relief, one changes to a stronger opiate (step 3). At any time during therapy, an adjuvant drug may be added.

◆ ADJUVANT DRUGS

Adjuvant drugs are defined as drugs that are primarily used for conditions other than pain relief.[61] These drugs include anticonvulsants, antidepressants, neuroleptics, anxiolytics, and corticosteroids (Table 7-3). It is important to note that these drugs do not replace NSAIDs or opiates, but merely serve to augment the pain relief associated with analgesics or to act as options for relief when adequate doses of analgesics fail.

◆ **Table 7-3**
Adjuvant analgesics

Generic name	Trade names	Suggested dosages	Side effects
ANTICONVULSANTS			
Phenytoin	Dantoin	100 mg BID	Rash, hirsutism, hypocalcemia, anemia
Carbamazepine	Mazepine, Tegretol	400-800 mg/day divided in 3 doses	Aplastic anemia
Clonazepam	Klonopin, Rivotril	1.5-6 mg day TID	Sedation, personality changes, irritability
ANTIDEPRESSANTS			
Amitriptyline	Amaril, Amiline, Amitril, Deprex, Elavil	10-300 mg/day	Anticholinergic effects: hypotension, dry mouth, sedation, urinary retention
NEUROLEPTICS*			
Chlorpromazine	ChlorProm, ChlorPromanyl, Largactil	10-25 mg TID	Extrapyramidal reactions: tardive dyskinesia, skin reactions, sedation, dry mouth
Haloperidol	Haldol, Novoperidol, Peridol	.5-20 mg BID	Same
Prochlorperazine	Compazine, Stemetil	5-10 mg TID	Same

ANXIOLYTICS*			
Diazepam	D-Tran, Diazemuls, E-Pam, Meval, Valium	5-10 mg TID	CNS depression
Hydroxyzine	Atarax, BayRox, Durrax, Multipax, Neucalm, Sedaril, Vistaril	25-50 mg every 4-6 hours	Sedation
CORTICOSTEROIDS			
Prednisone	Colisone, Deltasone, Winpred	5-30 mg TID or QID	Mentation changes Cushingoid features Diabetes
Prednisolone		10 mg TID	Same
Dexamethasone	Decadron	4 mg QD or higher in cases of increased intracranial pressure or spinal cord compression	Same

*Of little use in relieving pain. The primary indication of these drugs is in the relief of anxiety and nausea associated with opiate therapy.

Anticonvulsants

Anticonvulsants, including phenytoin (Dilantin) and carbamazepine (Tegretol), and clonazepam (Klonopin, Revotril) are believed to suppress spontaneous neuronal firing, which occurs after injury to the nerve. Therefore these drugs are useful in painful conditions associated with nerve damage. This includes trigeminal neuralgia and deafferentation pain (often described as stabbing in sensation).[20] Side effects include anemia and rash.

Antidepressants

Tricyclic antidepressants are useful in deafferentation or neuropathic pain conditions.[11,57] These types of pain are expressed as "tingling" or "burning" and are associated with conditions such as postherpetic neuropathy or diabetic neuropathy. The tricyclic antidepressants produce analgesia at doses below those necessary for alleviating depression. In addition, these drugs improve sleep.[2] Side effects include anticholinergic effects, such as orthostatic hypotension, dry mouth, and sedation.

Neuroleptics

Agents such as chlorpromazine (Largactil), prochlorperazine (Compazine, Stemetil), and haloperidol (Haldol) are not analgesics but are occasionally used to treat agitation that may occur during episodes of excruciating pain or to treat the nausea that may accompany narcotic therapy.[18] Extrapyramidal effects may occur.

Anxiolytics

Diazepam (Valium) is not an analgesic, yet may assist in reducing pain associated with muscle spasm.[2] One benefit of diazepam is that it can be given by several routes; orally, rectally, or parenterally. Diazepam does not provide an additive analgesic effect when combined with an opiate and in fact may increase side effects, such as sedation and hypotension. In addition, diazepam can lead to tissue damage at the injection site when given intramuscularly. Another anxiolytic, hydroxyzine (Vistaril), may provide an additive analgesic effect when combined with a narcotic. In addition, hydroxyzine has antiemetic and antispasmodic actions.

Occasionally, patients may experience severe agitation and restlessness, especially in terminal care. Midazolam (Versed), a benzodiazapine, may be used intravenously or subcutaneously to provide sedation. Patients should be monitored for respiratory depression. This drug should not be used in place of an opiate analgesic, rather as an adjunct when patients experience pain and agitation.[14]

Corticosteroids

Steroids have been shown to relieve pain associated with bone metastases, increased intracranial pressure, nerve compression, and spinal cord compression.[5,56] In addition, steroids elevate mood and stimulate appetite. Significant gastrointestinal side effects often preclude the use of steroids in conjunction with NSAIDs.

◆ OTHER ANALGESIC AGENTS

Capsaicin

Several analgesic agents do not fall under the categories previously described. A relatively new drug that is not considered an NSAID, opiate, or adjuvant drug, is capsaicin. Capsaicin is a naturally occurring substance derived from hot paprika or chili peppers and is currently available in two concentrations: 0.025% and 0.075%. Capsaicin appears to work by causing the release and depletion of substance P, an endogenous peptide active in pain transmission. As a result of this action, capsaicin appears to be effective in relieving pain associated with peripheral neuropathies, such as postherpetic neuralgia and diabetic neuropathy.[58]

Capsaicin is applied to the skin three to four times daily, with an optimal response achieved after 14 to 28 days. Side effects include burning and reddening of the skin. These side effects actually appear to dissipate after more frequent application of the drug. Patients must be cautioned to wash their hands immediately after application and to avoid contact of the drug with their eyes and with areas of broken skin.

Anesthetics

Other drugs that act as analgesics are anesthetic agents. Although these agents are usually used parenterally or as inhalants during invasive procedures, other delivery methods can also be used to provide analgesia. Anesthetic agents act by inhibiting the conduction of impulses along the neuron.

Viscous lidocaine is used for relief of pain in the mouth and esophagus and may facilitate the passing of nasogastric tubes. Patients must be instructed not to eat until the gag reflex has returned. Topical anesthetic jelly preparations aid in relieving pain associated with urinary catheterization, and rectal creams or suppositories with anesthetic components relieve pain related to hemorrhoids, fissures, or other rectal conditions. Anesthetic ointments can be applied to burns, abrasions, and insect bites to relieve discomfort. Many ointments combine small doses of anesthetic with steroids or other agents. Side effects of these topically applied anesthetics, although rare when used in limited doses, are associated with systemic absorption of the drug and include bradycardia and hypotension.[52,53]

Intraspinal anesthetics are commonly used in postoperative and cancer pain, either alone or in combination with an opiate such as fentanyl or morphine. Bupivacaine (Marcaine, Sensorcaine), a long-acting anesthetic, is frequently used in intrathecal or epidural infusions. Side effects include motor blockade and cardiac changes.

A specific anesthetic agent, nitrous oxide, has also been used in terminally ill adults and children. Fosburg and Crone[19] describe this application of inhalant anesthetic therapy as safe, easy to administer, and effective in relieving pain. More information is necessary regarding the efficacy and morbidity of this approach.

◆ PRINCIPLES OF PHARMACOLOGICAL NURSING THERAPY

A tremendous number of drugs are available in the war against pain, yet without nurses who are knowledgeable in the delivery of these drugs the battle is lost. Nursing care in the delivery of pharmacological agents is complex (see box). Ethical-decision making involved with issues of patients taking opioids is discussed in Chapter 6. Several principles guide the pharmacological nursing care of persons with pain.

Evaluate and Document Drug Efficacy

It is imperative to evaluate the success of pharmacological therapy for pain. Pain intensity ratings, such as the 0 to 10

◆ NURSING CARE IN THE DELIVERY OF PHARMACOLOGICAL AGENTS

1. Perform a complete pain assessment
2. Determine appropriate drug or drugs, as well as the schedule, route, and dose of these drugs
3. Prevent and manage side effects associated with analgesic therapy
4. Evaluate the effectiveness of the therapy and modify as needed
5. Teach patients, their family members, and colleagues about pain and its management
6. Document assessment data, therapies administered, and patient response
7. Act as patient advocate
8. Consult with experts as necessary

scale, should be obtained before administering the analgesic and at various intervals thereafter. This will provide objective data regarding the degree and duration of pain relief. This data must then be communicated, verbally and in writing through documentation in the patient's chart, to other members of the patient care team. Flow sheets are very useful in documenting the pain intensity, time of drug administration, respiration and blood pressure, and patient response to the analgesic.

The nurse should evaluate the patient's pain intensity before and each hour after administering the drug, particularly when starting a new drug, changing the dose or route, or treating patients in acute pain, such as in the postoperative period. If the pain intensity score remains above 0 (indicating the presence of pain) and the patient is not experiencing intolerable side effects, the nurse should increase the dose of the drug. If the patient is experiencing side effects, the nurse should employ measures to treat these effects or change to another drug. The nurse should continue to evaluate the pain intensity scores while titrating the dose of the drug until the patient achieves pain relief.

Assessment should continue well after the initial observation: It is the only mechanism available to evaluate the effectiveness of analgesic therapy. But assessment only provides information: The nurse must then act on that knowledge. If the patient is receiving inadequate relief, the nurse must seek changes in the prescription. And when responsible authorities do not respond to requests for change, the highest level of personnel must be approached.

Occasionally, patients may be reluctant to take opiate analgesics. The fact that patients refuse to take analgesics does not necessarily mean they do not have pain. It is important to correct patient-family misconceptions, particularly about addiction and tolerance (see Chapter 3). Nurses must define tolerance, physical dependence, and psychological dependence for patients and their support persons, and for colleagues.

Tolerance is the need for increasing doses of drug to maintain the original analgesic effect. Physical dependence is manifested as withdrawal symptoms when discontinuing a drug after repeated doses. Patients must be advised that although these two phenomena occur after opiate use, they do not signify addiction. Addiction, which is more appropriately called psychological dependence, is the "behavioral pattern of compulsive drug use, characterized by overwhelming involvement with the use of a drug, the securing of its supply, and a high tendency to relapse after withdrawal."[26] Patients fear addiction and, as a result, may take less drug than necessary.

Principles Associated With Determining the Appropriate Schedule, Route, and Dose

Although it is the legal domain of the physician to prescribe the drug, schedule, route, and dose, nurses provide essential input into these prescriptions and must interpret them in the clinical setting. Therefore it is essential that nurses understand the rationale and principles associated with choosing various schedules, routes, and dosages.

Schedule: Know the Correct Duration of Drug Action and Give the Drug Regularly

An around-the-clock (ATC) schedule, rather than prn administration, is most appropriate when patients have pain that lingers during the day.[1] The interval between doses is based on the duration of action of the drug being delivered. A drug with a duration of action of 4 hours should be given at least every 4 hours to preclude a reduction in therapeutic blood levels. Administering the next dose of drug only when the person is in pain (the prn approach) ensures the need for higher doses of analgesics and far more time for drug absorption. As a result, the individual remains in pain for an additional time. A "peak and valley" phenomenon occurs (see Figure 7-7) as the larger doses required result in side effects and overmedication. An ATC schedule obviates the extremes (undermedication and overmedication) while providing a more stable therapeutic plasma level of drug. In pain of longer duration, a combination of ATC dosing for baseline pain and prn dosing for intermittent increasing pain (breakthrough pain) may be necessary.[48]

Patient-controlled analgesia (PCA) is an innovative method of drug scheduling that allows patients to determine and act on their need for analgesia. Patients press a hand-held button, activating the infusion device to deliver a predetermined dose of opiate (Figure 7-8). The infusion device is programmed to deliver several doses of drug until a maximum dose is achieved. PCA has been used intravenously, subcutaneously, and epidurally in populations including postoperative patients, persons with cancer, post–cesarean section patients, and adolescents with sickle cell anemia.[29,50,55,59] Patients using PCA report greater satisfaction and better pain relief. Other benefits of PCA include improved pulmonary function

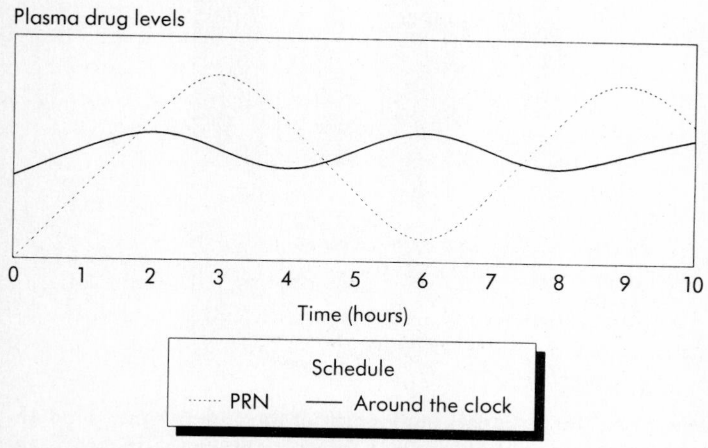

FIGURE 7-7. Plasma drug levels associated with prn vs ATC dosing.

tests and fewer pulmonary complications in postoperative patients.[22]

Route: The Oral Route is Preferred Whenever Possible

Although many routes are currently available to persons with pain, an important rule is, "If the gut works, use it." The oral route is preferred because it is convenient, is less costly than most other routes, and provides stable plasma levels of the drug.[1] The rectal route is a useful alternative when patients are unable to take oral medications.

Although the oral route is preferred, circumstances might preclude its use. These include bowel obstruction, ileus that accompanies the immediate postoperative period, periods before surgery or diagnostic procedures when patients must remain NPO, severe stomatitis secondary to chemotherapy, and many other situations. The most common alternative is currently the intramuscular route. The disadvantages of this route are variances in absorption, pain and bleeding at injection site (of particular concern in persons with thrombocytopenia or who are being treated with anticoagulants), and

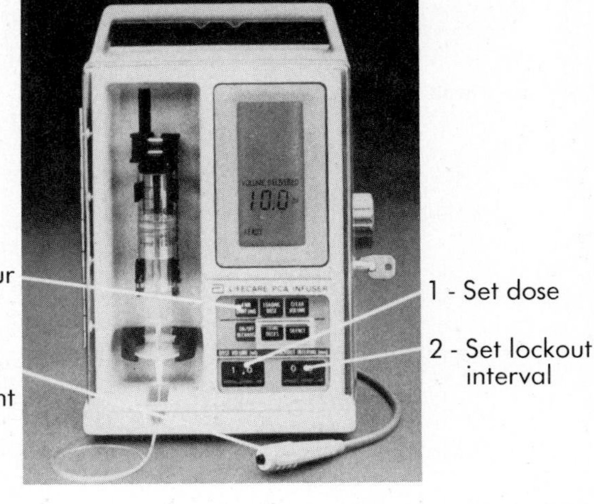

FIGURE 7-8. The essential components of the Patient Controlled Analgesia (PCA) pump (LifeCare PCA Infusor; Abbott Laboratories; Abbott Park, Ill).

shorter duration of action than the oral route. Other alternative routes include intravenous, subcutaneous, rectal, epidural, or intrathecal routes.

Dosage: Individualize to Meet the Patient's Needs

NSAIDs have maximum suggested dosages; the nurse should adhere to these recommendations to limit side effects. Opiates have no ceiling and can be gradually increased to very high dosages with few untoward effects. Dosages of greater than 10,000 mg/day of IV morphine have been reported with few adverse effects.[32,44]

Calculating the dosage of opiate may be difficult when changing route or drug (see box). Equianalgesic tables (see Table 7-2) and equivalency indexes assist in this calculation.[23]

◆ CONVERTING TO A DIFFERENT DRUG OR AN ALTERNATE ROUTE

1. Calculate the total narcotic dose over a 24-hour period (e.g., morphine 60 mg po every 4 hours is equal to 360 mg/24 hours)
2. Convert that dose to an equianalgesic dose of the new drug (e.g., morphine 30 mg po is approximately equivalent to hydromorphone 7.5 mg po). These equianalgesic doses can be found in Table 7-2. Divide equivalent dose of the old drug by the equivalent dose of the new drug (e.g., morphine 30 divided by hydromorphone 7.5 = 4). This provides a conversion factor.
3. Divide the actual dose of the old drug by the conversion factor (e.g., 360 divided by 4 = 90). Therefore, the 24-hour equivalent dose of hydromorphone is 90 mg po.
4. The next step requires incorporating the 24-hour dose into an appropriate schedule for that drug. Hydromorphone has a duration of action of 2-4 hours. Start by giving the drug every 4 hours (6 doses per day) and change the frequency based on the patient's response. Divide the 24-hour dose of the drug, 90 mg by 6 doses = 15 mg per dose. The new drug, dose, and schedule are hydromorphone 15 mg po every 4 hours.

In addition, a computer program is available to make calculations automatically.[24]

◆ CONCLUSION

Winning the battle against pain requires pharmacological therapy and the knowledge to use this therapy most appropriately. This knowledge includes understanding basic principles of pharmacology, the mechanism of action of the drug or drugs, potential side effects that may occur, and the nursing actions necessary to safely and effectively deliver the therapy. It is the nurse, through assessment, knowledge, and skill, who can best administer these pharmacological agents and provide analgesia to those in pain.

REFERENCES

1. American Pain Society. (1989). *Principles of analgesic use in the treatment of acute pain and chronic cancer pain* (ed 2). Skokie, Ill: The Society.
2. Baldessarini RJ. (1985). Drugs and the treatment of psychiatric disorders. In Gilman AG, Goodman LS, Rall TW, and Murad F (eds), *The pharmacological basis of therapeutics* (ed 7) (pp. 387-445). New York: Macmillan.
3. Bell MD, Mishra P, Weldon BD, et al. (1985). Buccal morphine—a new route for analgesia? *Lancet, 1,* 71-73.
4. Bruera E, Brenneis C, Paterson AH, and MacDonald RN. (1989). Use of methylphenidate as an adjuvant to narcotic analgesics in patients with advanced cancer. *J Pain Sympt Manag, 4,* 3-5.
5. Bruera E, Roca E, Cedaro L, Carraro S, and Chacon R. (1985). Action of oral methylprednisolone in terminal cancer patients: a prospective randomized double-blind study. *Cancer Treat Rep, 69,* 751-754.
6. Christensen FR. (1982). Epidural morphine at home in terminal patients. *Lancet, 1,* 47.
7. Citron ML, Johnston-Early A, Fossieck BE, et al. (1984). Safety and efficacy of continuous intravenous morphine for severe cancer pain. *Am J Med, 77,* 199-204.
8. Cohen SE and Woods WA. (1983). The role of epidural morphine in the post-cesarean patient: efficacy and effects of bonding. *Anesthesiology, 58,* 500-504.
9. Coyle N, Mauskop A, Maggard J, and Foley KM. (1986). Continuous subcutaneous infusions of opiates in cancer patients with pain. *Oncol Nurs Forum, 13,* 53-57.
10. Daniel EE, Sutherland WH, and Gogoch A. (1959). Effects of morphine and other drugs on motility of the terminal ileum. *Gastroenterology, 36,* 510-523.
11. Davar G and Maciewicz RJ. (1989). Deafferentation pain syndromes. *Neurol Clin, 7,* 289-304.

12. Dawood MY. (1981). Dysmenorrhea and prostaglandins: pharmacological and therapeutic consideration. *Drugs, 22,* 42-56.
13. Dennis EMP. (1984). An ambulatory infusion pump for pain control: a nursing approach for home care. *Cancer Nurs, 7,* 309-313.
14. DeSousa E and Jepson BA. (1988). Midazolam in terminal care. *Lancet, I,* 67-68.
15. Fields HL. (1987). *Pain.* New York: McGraw-Hill.
16. Findler G, Olshwang D, and Hadani M. (1982). Continuous epidural morphine treatment for intractable pain in terminal cancer patients. *Pain, 14,* 311-315.
17. Foley KM. (1985). The treatment of cancer pain. *N Engl J Med, 313,* 84-95.
18. Foley KM and Inturrisi CE. (1987). Analgesic drug therapy in cancer pain: principles and practice. *Med Clin North Am, 71,* 207-232.
19. Fosburg MT and Crone RK. (1983). Nitrous oxide analgesia for refractory pain in the terminally ill. *JAMA, 250,* 511-513.
20. Fromm GH. (1989). Trigeminal neuralgia and related disorders. *Neurol Clin, 7,* 305-319.
21. Gourlay GK, Kowlaski SR, Plummer JL, et al. (1989). The transdermal administration of fentanyl in the treatment of postoperative pain: pharmacokinetics and pharmacodynamic effects. *Pain, 37,* 193-202.
22. Graves DA, Foster TS, Baumann TJ, Batenhorst RL, and Bennett RL. (1983). Patient-controlled analgesia. *Ann Intern Med, 99,* 360-366.
23. Grossman SA and Sheidler VR. (1987). An aid to prescribing narcotics for the relief of cancer pain. *World Health Forum, 8,* 525-529.
24. Grossman SA and Sheidler VR. (1989). *The Johns Hopkins Oncology Center's narcotic conversion program.* Philadelphia: Lea & Febiger.
25. Insel PA. (1990). Analgesic-antipyretics and anti-inflammatory agents: drugs employed in the treatment of rheumatoid arthritis and gout. In Gilman AG, Rall TW, Nies AS, and Taylor P (eds), *Goodman and Gilman's The pharmacological basis of therapeutics* (ed 8) (pp. 638-681). New York: Pergamon Press.
26. Jaffe J and Martin W. (1990). Opioid analgesics and antagonists. In Gilman AG, Rall TW, Nies AS, and Taylor P (eds), *Goodman and Gilman's The pharmacological basis of therapeutics* (ed 8) (pp. 485-521). New York: Pergamon Press.
27. Kakio RF, Foley KM, Grabinski PY, et al. (1983). Central nervous system excitatory effects of meperidine in cancer patients. *Ann Neurol, 13,* 180-185.
28. Kalant H and Roschlau WHE. (1989). *Principles of medical pharmacology.* Toronto: BC Decker Inc.
29. Kane NE, Lehman ME, Dugger R, Hansen LE, and Jackson D. (1988). Use of patient-controlled analgesia in surgical oncology patients. *Oncol Nurs Forum, 15,* 29-32.
30. Kantor TG. (1982). The control of pain by nonsteroidal antiinflammatory drugs. *Med Clin North Am, 66,* 1053-1059.
31. Khojasteh A, Evans W, Reynolds RD, Thomas G, and Savarese JJ. (1987). Controlled-release oral morphine sulfate in the treatment of cancer pain with pharmacokinetic correlation. *J Clin Oncol, 5,* 956-961.
32. Lo SL and Coleman RR. (1986). Exceptionally high narcotic analgesic requirements in a terminally ill cancer patient. *Drug Exper, 5,* 828-832.

33. Lombard DJ and Oliver DJ. (1989). The use of opioid analgesics in the last 24 hours of life of patients with advanced cancer. *Pall Med,, 3,* 27-29.
34. Madrid JL, Fatela LV, Guillen F, and Labato RD. (1988). Intermittent intrathecal morphine by means of an implantable reservoir: a survey of 100 cases. *J Pain Sympt Manage, 3,* 67-71.
35. Maguire LC, Yon JL, and Miller E. (1981). Prevention of narcotic induced constipation. *N Engl J Med, 305,* 1651.
36. McCaffery M and Beebe A. (1989). *Pain: clinical manual for nursing practice.* St. Louis: CV Mosby.
37. Miser AW, Narang PK, Dothage JA, et al. (1989). Transdermal fentanyl for pain control in patients with cancer. *Pain, 37,* 15-21.
38. Moertel CG, Ahmann DL, Taylor WF, and Schwartau N. (1972). A comparative evaluation of marketed analgesic drugs. *N Engl J Med, 286,* 813-815.
39. Moncada S, Flower RJ, and Vane JR. (1985). Prostaglandins, prostacyclin, thromboxane A2, and leukotrienes. In Gilman AG, Goodman LS, Rall TW, and Murad F (eds), *The pharmacological basis of therapeutics* (ed 7) (pp. 660-673). New York: Macmillan.
40. Moulin DE and Coyle N. (1986). Spinal opioid analgesics and local anesthetics in the management of chronic cancer pain. *J Pain Sympt Manage, 1,* 79-86.
41. O'Hara DA, Fragen RJ, Kinzer M, et al. (1987). Ketorolac Tromethamine as compared with morphine sulfate for treatment of postoperative pain. *Clin Pharmacol Ther, 41,* 556-561.
42. Paice JA. (1986). Intrathecal morphine infusion for intractable cancer pain: a new use for implanted pumps. *Oncol Nurs Forum, 13,* 41-47.
43. Paice JA. (1987). New delivery systems in pain management. *Nurs Clin North Am, 22,* 715-726.
44. Paice JA. (1988). The phenomenon of analgesic tolerance in cancer pain management. *Oncol Nurs Forum, 15,* 455-459.
45. Penn RD and Paice JA. (1987). Chronic intrathecal morphine for intractable pain. *J Neurosurg, 67,* 182-186.
46. *Physicians' desk reference* (ed 43). (1989). Oradell, NJ: Medical Economics.
47. Portenoy RK. (1987). Constipation in the cancer patient: causes and management. *Med Clin North Am, 71,* 303-311.
48. Portenoy RK and Hagen NA. (1989). Breakthrough pain: definition and management. *Oncology, 3*(Suppl 8), 25-29.
49. Rapaport SI. (1985). Hemostasis. In West JB (ed), *Physiological basis of medical practice* (ed 11) (pp. 409-436). Baltimore: Williams & Wilkins.
50. Rayburn WF, Geranis BJ, Ramadei CA, Woods RE, and Patil KD. (1988). Patient-controlled analgesia for post-cesarean section pain. *Obstet Gynecol, 72,* 136-139.
51. Reynolds JEF. (ed). (1989). *Martindale: the extra pharmacopoeia.* London: The Pharmaceutical Press.
52. Ritchie JM and Greene NM. (1990). Local anesthetics. In Gilman AG, Rall TW, Nies AS, and Taylor P (eds), *Goodman and Gilman's The pharmacological basis of therapeutics* (ed 8) (pp. 311-331). New York: Pergamon Press.
53. Rowbotham MC and Fields HL. (1989). Topical lidocaine reduces pain in post-herpetic neuralgia. *Pain, 38,* 297-301.

54. Sandler DP, Smith JC, Weinberg CR, et al. (1989). Analgesic use and chronic renal disease. *N Engl J Med, 320,* 1238-1243.
55. Schechter NL, Berrien FB, and Katz SM. (1988). The use of patient-controlled analgesia in adolescents with sickle-cell crisis: a preliminary report. *J Pain Sympt Manage, 3,* 109-113.
56. Tannock I, Gospodarowicz M, Meakin W, et al. (1989). Treatment of metastatic prostatic cancer with low-dose prednisone: Evaluation of pain and quality of life as pragmatic indices of response. *J Clin Oncol, 7,* 590-597.
57. Watson CPN. (1989). Postherpetic neuralgia. *Neurol Clin, 7,* 231-248.
58. Watson CPN, Evans RJ, and Watt VR. (1988). Post-herpetic neuralgia and topical capsaicin. *Pain, 33,* 333-340.
59. White PF. (1988). Use of patient-controlled analgesia for management of acute pain. *JAMA, 259,* 243-247.
60. Whittle BJR and Vane JR. (1983). Prostacyclin, thromboxanes, and prostaglandins—actions and roles in the gastrointestinal tract. In Jerzy Glass GB and Sherlock P (eds), *Progress in gastroenterology* (pp. 3-30). New York: Grune & Stratton.
61. World Health Organization. (1986). *Cancer pain relief.* Geneva, Switzerland: The Organization.

8

Nonpharmacological Pain Management

Linda Edgar
Caroline M. Smith-Hanrahan

PHARMACOLOGICAL ANALGESIA REMAINS the most common method of pain management. Yet, despite the availability of numerous analgesic drugs, the prevalence and treatment of pain remain a major problem.[24,32,33,50] One possible reason is that pharmacological management of pain alone is often not adequate. Combinations of various treatment modalities that exert their effect at different levels of the peripheral and central nervous system often decrease nociception to a greater degree (see Chapter 2). In addition, pharmacological analgesics, particularly narcotics, are not appropriate for some patients. Several alternate therapies are now available to health professionals that involve some form of peripheral or central stimulation to manage pain. Varying degrees of success have been reported.

Nurses have traditionally focused on the whole person and family. Because nonpharmacological pain management techniques often involve a holistic approach, the nurse is uniquely prepared for effective use of these techniques. However, a recent study of medical, surgical, and oncology nurses revealed that although the nurses were familiar with many nonpharmacological techniques of pain management, they reported using most of these techniques less than 25% of the time.[35] Part of the reason for this underutilization may be a lack of adequate knowledge and/or skills necessary for implementation.

The purpose of this chapter is to provide an overview of the various nonpharmacological, research-based options that are available to nurses for the management of pain along with guidelines for their use. The authors have limited discussion to techniques that fall within the scope of nursing. All techniques meet the following criteria[138]:

1. The average nurse is qualified to use them effectively, although some special training may be necessary
2. They do not require special equipment that is not readily available
3. They do not interfere with any medical treatments the patient may be undergoing
4. They do not require the patient's official informed consent

As details of the techniques are beyond the scope of this chapter, comprehensive references are included to enable the reader to obtain more information regarding each technique.

Health professionals will undoubtedly continue to use pharmacological methods as the principal form of pain treatment. However, in selected patients, nonpharmacological techniques used alone or in combination with pain medications often provide a significant and improved form of pain relief.

◆ PERIPHERAL TECHNIQUES

In this chapter the term *peripheral technique* refers to any intervention involving stimulation of the skin to reduce pain. Several nonpharmacological techniques are available and can be used to treat a wide variety of acute and chronic pains. In this section the following interventions are discussed: cryotherapy, superficial heat, massage, acupressure, and transcutaneous electrical nerve stimulation (TENS). As pain is a unique, subjective experience, the clinician must implement various measures in different combinations to design the optimum program for each individual.

Cryotherapy

The application of cold to the body's surface to relieve pain has been practiced for centuries. However, surprisingly little formal evaluation of this concept has been undertaken.

Mechanisms of Action

Cooling can produce analgesia by several mechanisms. When applied to recently injured areas it can reduce the release of such pain-causing chemicals as lactic acid, potassium ions, kinins, serotonin, and histamine.[73] It also decreases lymph production and cell permeability, resulting in diminished edema formation[76] and subsequent pain reduction. Because these effects are mediated, at least in part, by vasoconstriction, more than just surface tissues can be affected.

Peripheral cold can slow the conduction velocity of the small unmyelinated nerve fibers, which conduct pain impulses from the periphery.[43,75] These small afferents also transmit impulses from the sensory nerve endings in muscle spindles constituting the stretch reflex, therefore reducing muscle tone and spasticity and hence pain.[75]

When acupuncture points, also called acupoints, are massaged with cold (ice massage), afferent stimulation is thought to activate brain stem mechanisms that are known to exert descending inhibitory influences on pain signals.[94] The afferent stimulation achieved with ice massage of an acupoint is thought to be of higher intensity than when other areas of the body surface are similarly treated. Therefore the analgesic effect is greater.[91]

Clinical Uses and Contraindications

Cryotherapy is particularly useful for initial posttraumatic pain, swelling, and muscle spasm.[76] It is also recommended for relief of pain associated with chronic ischemic ulcers.[128] Ice massage too has reportedly been helpful for a variety of pain types including musculoskeletal, myofascial, and acute dental pain.[94,95] Cryotherapy is contraindicated for patients with peripheral vascular disease with arterial insufficiency, Raynaud's phenomenon, cold allergy, paroxysmal cold hemoglobinuria, marked cold pressure response, or any indication of cold sensitivity.[37,75,77] Also, patients with heart disease and angina pectoris experience precordial pain when exposed to cold, which has been interpreted as a reflex vasoconstriction of the coronary arteries. Therefore cold therapy should be avoided for these patients.[74]

Guidelines for Use

Many methods of cold therapy are available to the nurse. Usually some type of cold pack or ice pack (wooden spatula placed in a cupful of water, frozen, and covered with a moist towel) is applied to the affected area. Contact time should be limited to 15 minutes per session to avoid frostbite.[43] With ice massage, a ice pack is massaged over the involved acupoints or painful area itself for no longer than 7 minutes.[94,95] For more detailed information regarding the many methods of cold application, we refer the reader to the excellent work of McCaffery and Beebe,[89] or Lehmann and De Lateur.[76]

Nursing's Role

Cryotherapy is often an effective analgesic. This therapeutic modality is inexpensive, requires little nursing time, and can easily be taught to the patient and/or the family. Therefore nurses have a responsibility to try this technique and, if successful, incorporate it into their patient's pain treatment program.

Superficial Heat

Like cold, the application of moist or dry heat to the body's surface has also been used for centuries to relieve pain.

Mechanisms of Action

Superficial heat can create analgesia by several means. Indirectly, once an inflammatory response has subsided, heat can reduce pain through a vasodilator effect. Vasodilation enhances blood flow, causing improvements in tissue nutrition and elimination of cellular metabolites that stimulate pain impulses.[91] It is thought that heat affects gamma fiber activity in the muscle, causing a decrease in the sensitivity of the muscle spindle to stretch. Heat also triggers pain-inhibiting reflexes through temperature receptors. Both of these actions result in relaxation of muscle spasm and an associated reduction in pain.[76] Elevation of the surface body temperature can also cause reactions distant from the site of temperature elevation. For example, superficial heat has been observed to relax smooth musculature of the gastrointestinal tract, which in turn reduces the pain of gastrointestinal cramps.[20]

Superficial heat also has direct influence on pain. Evidence suggests that the application of heat to a peripheral nerve or the skin increases the pain threshold in that area, although not as effectively as cryotherapy.[14] However, studies have shown that patients do prefer heat to cold.[39]

Clinical Uses and Contraindications

Heat is especially effective for muscle and joint pain.[134] However, because it increases swelling and the tendency to bleed, it is contraindicated after trauma. Also, moderate temperature increases have been shown to speed up the growth rate of malignancies. Therefore heat should not be applied to a malignancy site[77] unless, of course, the patient is terminal. Heating of tissues with inadequate circulation should also be avoided because elevated temperatures increase metabolic demands while tissue oxygenation remains inadequate. The combination of these reactions can lead to ischemic necrosis.[76] Because heat can burn, it should be used with caution over areas with impaired sensation or in patients with limited or no ability to communicate.[76]

Guidelines for Use

Superficial heat is commonly applied with hot water bottles, electric heating pads, moist towels, warm baths, infrared apparatus, or the summer sun.[91] Treatment should be limited to ½ hour 3 to 4 times per day to avoid thermal injury. McCaffery and Beebe[89] and Lehmann and DeLateur,[76] provide excellent descriptions of the various methods available for superficial heat application.

Nursing's Role

Like cryotherapy, heat is an effective analgesic and is inexpensive, simple to use, and not time consuming. Therefore, in appropriate cases, nurses should assess the effectiveness of this modality and incorporate it into the pain-treatment plan if it proves successful.

Massage

Lawrence, (as reported by White[137]) has defined massage as the "kneading, manipulation, or application of methodical pressure and friction to the body." This technique is instinctive, as it is a natural response to rub our own aches and pains. Hippocrates, in the fifth century B.C., was one of the first to describe massage as a therapeutic intervention.[137]

Mechanisms of Action

As with other nonpharmacological methods, little is known about the mechanism by which massage produces analgesia. In 1960, Jacobs[60] suggested that massage interrupts the pain cycle by two peripheral effects. The mechanical pressure of massage on superficial venous and lymphatic channels improves circulation directly, reducing the pain associated with edema. Second, massage causes capillary and, if strong enough, arteriole dilation through some unknown reflex mechanism. This further improves circulation.

More recently, Day, Mason, and Chesrown[36] evaluated the effect of massage on plasma beta-endorphin levels in 21 healthy adults before and after a 30-minute back massage. They found no significant differences in plasma beta-endorphin levels but recommended a similar study be carried out on those suffering acute or chronic pain. In 1989, Kaada and Torsteinbo[67] carried out such a study on 12 volunteers suffering from myalgia and various other types of pain. They noted a 16% significant increase in plasma beta-endorphins after 30 minutes of connective tissue massage, suggesting that the analgesic action of massage may be mediated, at least in part, by the release of endorphins. Surprisingly, to our knowledge, no work has been reported on the effects of massage on afferent nerve fiber stimulation and pain transmission in the spinal cord.

Clinical Uses and Contraindications

A recent review of the literature uncovered no randomized controlled clinical trials to assess the ability of massage to reduce pain. Anecdotal reports suggest that massage is applicable for most client populations. However, contraindications have not been fully delineated. Obvious indications for avoiding massage in the area of concern include conditions involving fractures, phlebitis, skin lesions, lacerations, and recent surgery or injury.[137]

Guidelines for Use

As a therapeutic intervention, massage consists of five basic movements or strokes used in sequence on the body's surface. White[137] has described these strokes. Briefly they are effleurage, pétrissage, friction, tapotement, and vibration. Joachim[63] demonstrates some massage techniques with step-by-step photographs. For more detailed information concerning the various massage techniques see Tappan,[127] or the American Massage Therapist Association.

Nursing's Role

Massage is an inexpensive, reasonably easy-to-learn technique but requires much time to perform. However, because of its simplicity, family members can carry out the treatment with relatively little instruction. At present, objective evidence of the therapeutic value of massage is scarce. Experimental studies now are needed concerning optimum forms, the best candidates, and the contraindications.

Acupressure

Acupressure developed in East Asia from the 3,000-year-old Chinese healing system of acupuncture.[13,127] This technique involves applying finger pressure to points that correspond to many of the points used in acupuncture.[127]

Mechanisms of Action

Little is known of how acupressure exerts its analgesic effect. Of the few quantitative studies, even fewer meet Western scientific standards. Histological studies of the acupoint have found that both the acupoint and its immediate surrounds are richly endowed with nerves, and pressure and stretch receptors.[57] Further, they are points of decreased electrical resistance,[13] suggesting that these areas are particularly susceptible to pressure and/or electrical stimulation. It has been hypothesized that acupressure stimulates pressure fibers, which belong to the larger, myelinated and rapidly conducting category of afferents. When stimulated, the pressure fibers function to "close" the gating mechanism in the spinal cord to impulses from the small unmyelinated and slower conducting nerve fibers that transmit pain impulses from the periphery.[13] Also, there is some evidence suggesting endorphins are released when specific acupoints are pressed.[55]

Clinical Uses and Contraindications

Many pain complaints have been treated with acupressure.[127,136] Anecdotal reports suggest that it is often moderately and sometimes spectacularly effective.[106] Clinically, Weaver[136] has reported good results when combining acupressure with progressive relaxation techniques (these will be discussed later in this chapter). Some of the pain types and the specific acupoint treated are listed in Table 8-1. (For a more complete listing of acupuncture points, some of which may be effectively treated with acupressure, see Chaitow[27] and Tappan.[127]) The only group for whom acupressure is contraindi-

◆ **Table 8-1**
Some pain types treated with acupressure and the specific acupoints used

Pain type	Acupoint	Anatomical location	Reference
Dental pain	Ho ku (LI-4)	First dorsal interosseus	(Penzer and Matsumoto, 1985)
Headache pain	Feng chi (GB-20)	Lateral to trapezius at occiput	(Ulett, 1982)
	Tai yang (EM-1)	At midpoint of line one finger breadth to lateral end of eyebrow and outer canthus of eye	(Ulett, 1982)
	Ho ku (LI-4)	First dorsal interosseus	(Ulett, 1982) (Joachim, 1984)

cated is pregnant women, because several acupoints are believed to have powerful oxytocic effects.[13]

Guidelines for Use

The location and probable etiology of the client's pain will determine which acupoints should be treated (see Table 8-1, Chaitow,[27] or Tappan[127] for a more complete listing of these).

A variety of acupressure techniques are taught in the West. Generally, the basic technique is as follows.

1. *Locate the specific acupoint.* Because acupoints exhibit a lower electrical resistance than the immediate surrounding areas, they can be located with commercially available electrical point locators.[13] However, it is reported that acupoints can be identified by touch. The acupoints are said to feel softer and more yielding than the adjacent skin surfaces, and finger pressure can elicit tenderness and/or pain.[106]
2. *Stimulate the acupoint.* Pressure can be applied with either a finger, thumb, or knuckle. Preferably, pressure is increased to the patient's level of tolerance.[127] Reference sources include Weaver,[136] Penzer and Matsumoto,[106] and Beggs.[13] Most therapists practice rotating the finger either slowly or briskly in a circular or spiral motion for anywhere from 15 seconds to 5 minutes.[106,127,136]
3. *Check for effectiveness.* After the treatment, assess the degree of relief and patient satisfaction. If the effect was not fully satisfactory, another point should be stimulated. In cases of extreme tenderness at the primary point, treating the same point on the contralateral side may be helpful.[13]

   For a more detailed guide to the various acupressure techniques, the reader is referred to Tappan.[127] For more information and a directory of authorized teachers, contact the Jin Shin Do Foundation, P.O. Box 1800, Idyllwild, CA 92349; (714) 659-5550.

Nursing's Role

Acupressure is a simple, safe, inexpensive and noninvasive technique that requires little time to learn or perform. As such, nurses familiar with the technique can use it in an attempt to reduce or alleviate pain. In addition, if the treatment proves effective, they can teach the specific technique to the patient in pain and/or his relatives.

Transcutaneous Electrical Nerve Stimulation (TENS)

The gate control theory[97] has generated a variety of methods to control pain, including TENS. Basically this treatment involves passing a mild electric current across the skin between two electrodes. By altering the stimulation parameters, several different types of TENS can be produced.

Mechanisms of Action

Evidence suggests that the various types of TENS exert their analgesic effect by one or a combination of two mechanisms. The first involves activating large-diameter, myelinated A beta fibers, closing the gate to pain impulses from the periphery.[98] The second mechanism appears to involve deep fiber activation,[41] followed by endorphin release in some cases.[114,115,116,118]

Clinical Uses and Contraindications

Clinicians and researchers have used TENS to treat a wide variety of both acute and chronic pain types. Collectively the findings suggest that TENS is an effective modality for some but not all pain types. For a listing of some of the acute and chronic pain types that have been treated successfully with TENS see Table 8-2.

Reports from the literature suggest that contraindications are few. TENS is not recommended for those with contact dermatitis or in early pregnancy[91] and should be used only with careful evaluation and extended cardiac monitoring for those with cardiac pacemakers.[29]

Guidelines for Use

TENS should be applied, as with all other techniques, only after a complete historical and physical evaluation of the client. In the United States and Canada, a physician's prescription is usually required for this treatment. Unwanted side

◆ **Table 8-2**
Some pain types that have responded positively to TENS

Pain type	References
Postoperative pain after the following types of procedures:	
Abdominal	(Ali, Yaffe, and Serrette, 1981; Hymes, Raab, Yonehiro, Nelson, and Printy, 1973; Smith, Guralnick, Gelfand, and Jeans, 1986; Sodipo, Adedeji, and Olumide, 1980)
Chest	(Klin, Vretzky, and Magora, 1984) (no control group)
Orthopedic	(Solomon, Viernstein, and Long, 1980)
Neurological	(Solomon, Viernstein, and Long, 1980; Schuster and Infante, 1980)
Labor pain (back only)	(Augustinsson et al, 1977; Thomas, Tyle, Webster, and Neilson, 1988)
Angina pectoris	(Mannheimer, Carlsson, Vedin, and Wilhelmsson, 1985; Mannheimer, Emanuelsson, Waagstein, and Wilhelmsson, 1989)
Dysmenorrhea	(Lewers, Clelland, Jackson, Varner, and Bergman, 1989; Mannheimer and Whalen, 1985; Neighbors, Clelland, Jackson, Bergman, and Orr, 1987)
Peripheral ischemia	(Kaada, 1982)
Trauma, e.g., fractured ribs	(Woolf, Mitchell, Myers, and Barrett, 1978)
Lower back	(Melzack, 1975; Melzack, Vetere, and Finch, 1983)
Phantom limb	(Finsen et al, 1988; Jeans, 1979; Melzack, 1975)
Peripheral nerve injuries	(Melzack, 1975)
Headaches	(Reich, 1989)

effects directly attributable to TENS are also rare and relatively minor.[144] The most common is contact dermatitis. This problem usually disappears when treatment is stopped, electrode gel changed, or electrode placement adjusted.[23,133,144]

The TENS unit consists of two to four electrodes connected by lead wires to a stimulator. The TENS stimulus consists of three parameters: intensity, frequency, and pulse width,

◆ **Table 8-3**
Stimulus parameters of the three more commonly used modes of TENS

Stimulus parameters	TENS mode		
	Conventional	**Acupuncture-like**	**Intense**
Intensity	To tolerable tingling sensation	To tolerable muscle contraction	Just below muscle contraction
Frequency (pulses/sec)	80-125	2-4 or a series of high frequency pulses delivered in bursts of 2-4/sec	125
Pulse Width (microseconds)	60-100	220-250	250

which can be adjusted on the stimulator to create the different types of TENS. The stimulus parameters of three of the more commonly used modes are shown in Table 8-3.

Successful treatment depends on adequately varying the stimulus parameters and electrode placement until the best results are achieved. There are many options for electrode placement, including site of pain, acupuncture points, spinal nerve roots, and contralateral side. For details of the technique the reader is referred to Berlant,[18] Mannheimer and Lampe,[86] Omura,[104] and Sjolund and Eriksson.[117]

Regardless of the type of pain being treated, TENS is rarely used alone but rather serves as an adjunct to other forms of pain management, such as medication. TENS does not require highly skilled and frequent nursing care to ensure effective use.[90] TENS units are expensive to purchase but cost little to maintain, provided they are not lost, stolen, or damaged.

Nursing's Role

Many facilities employ either TENS technicians or physiotherapists who provide the patient with the instrument and properly teach the patient to use it. As part of the pain management team, the nurse can recommend the use of TENS for specific patients. Nurses are the only caregivers available 24 hours a day, 7 days a week. Therefore they must be able to reinforce the instruction provided to the patient, assist the patient in experimenting with different settings and electrode placement sites, and trouble shoot.

◆ CENTRAL TECHNIQUES

Techniques involving central control are thought to exert their effect through alteration of sensory, evaluative, and/or affective factors. The interventions discussed in this section are: relaxation, cognitive strategies, imagery, music, distraction, and positive suggestion.

Relaxation

If we subscribe to an integrated view of pain and pain control, we can readily accept that pain is a complex, multidimensional phenomenon as suggested by Melzack and Wall[97] and Loesser.[81] One of the commonly occurring aspects of pain, especially chronic pain, is the production of the stress-response, which is associated with anxiety, tension, and muscle contraction. A wide variety of techniques categorized as self-regulating and self-control mechanisms are used for stressful conditions. It has long been established that, of these, relaxation training is one of the most often used adjunctive treatments for muscle tension and spasm, chronic sympathetic system arousal, and the fear and anxiety associated with pain. Relaxation training has been defined as a nonpharmacological technique to facilitate a relaxed state.[59] It has also been described as the "aspirin of behavioral medicine."[52] Although Jacobson[61] first developed relaxation training, his approach is very long and rarely used by nurses.

The most commonly used form of relaxation training is progressive muscle relaxation, which is associated with Benson[15] and Wolpe.[140] For an excellent training manual, we recommend one by Bernstein and Borkovec[19] or McCaffery and Beebe.[89]

Mechanisms of Action

Relaxation is characterized by decreased oxygen consumption, muscle tonus, and heart and respiratory rate, lowered arterial blood lactate, increased skin resistance, intense, slow alpha waves, and occasional theta activity in the brain.[15] The relaxation response may reduce distressing thoughts and feelings by reducing anxiety. As anxiety and relaxation produce opposite physiological results, clearly they cannot exist together.

Clinical Uses and Precautions

Literally hundreds of studies have been carried out in the area of relaxation. Some authors have compiled excellent reviews on the topic. We include in this group works by Chapman and Turner,[28] Turk, Meichenbaum, and Genest,[130] and Tan.[126] The sheer number of research studies completed on the use of relaxation training for pain control and the overall effectiveness that they have demonstrated, leads one to have confidence in relaxation training as a highly useful tool.

Nurses are well advised to read not only the research literature on relaxation, but also anecdotal case reports and descriptive clinical works such as that by Donovan,[38] Snyder,[121] and Johnson.[65] Relaxation training falls within the domain of nursing. Nurses who are interested in adding relaxation to their nursing interventions would do well to educate themselves through training and personal practice in these techniques. After all, besides increasing one's nursing skills, one also gains valuable stress management training for use in all aspects of life.

Knowing the pattern and intensity of the patient's pain is essential in deciding whether relaxation may be helpful. Patients with very mild pain may not be good candidates for relaxation training because they may not be motivated to expend the time and effort needed for learning. Patients with severe pain may require simpler or more other-directed techniques. Probably the best candidates are those with moderately severe acute or chronic pain that is not well controlled by analgesics, or is well controlled but with unwanted side effects, and patients undergoing procedural pain.

Guidelines for Use

Table 8-4 provides a brief overview of the most frequently used relaxation techniques. Although they appear to be different from one another, they have several characteristics in common, particularly the following four elements that are

◆ **Table 8-4**
Common types of relaxation techniques

Technique	Brief description
Progressive muscle relaxation	Active contraction and passive relaxation of gross muscle groups to contrast the two diametrically opposed states, often used with guided imagery[19]
Biofeedback	Information about physiological functions, such as blood pressure, is fed back to the patient so that the patient can alter the body's response in a more healthful way[21]
Hypnosis	An advanced state of relaxation in which patients are more receptive to suggestions[34]
Autogenic training	Suggestions made to oneself about warmth, heaviness, and other stages of physical relaxation while in a state of passive concentration[111]
Meditation	A form of structured or unstructured mental concentration in which the person, in a quiet state, focuses on a specific sound, object, or kind of breathing[17]
Yoga	An ancient art of health care consisting of meditation and gentle physical exercises
Focused or passive progressive muscle relaxation	Similar to progressive muscle relaxation but without the active contraction of groups[19]

thought to be essential to elicit the relaxation response according to Benson, Beary, and Carol[16]:

1. A quiet environment
2. A comfortable position that enhances decreased muscle tonus
3. A passive, "let it happen" attitude and an ability to disregard distracting thoughts and redirect them toward the technique
4. A mental device such as a word, sound, or phrase that can help shift thoughts from an external to an internal orientation

Adequate patient preparation is critical for the success of relaxation training. Since there has been so much attention in the lay literature on relaxation techniques, many patients have preconceived notions. Even if a patient does not raise doubts or seems uninformed about relaxation, time spent in preparatory discussion can contribute to its success. Although the exact words will depend on the sophistication of the patient, the level of cooperation, and the nature of the pain, the following guidelines may prove helpful.

First, one reassures patients that pain itself is a major contributor to stress, which in turn increases pain. One explains that stress is a normal reaction to pain and emphasizes that the use of behavioral approaches, such as relaxation, in no way suggests that pain is not real, but rather, that these approaches are used to lessen pain. Relaxation reduces pain in at least two ways—by diminishing the sensation of pain and by allowing the patient to control the intensity of his reaction to the pain. One should explain that relaxation is a personal resource for pain management that returns a sense of control to the patient. Some emphasis should be placed on the value of relaxation to prevent pain and as a useful resource in other aspects of life.

Some patients fear a loss of control when engaging in relaxation strategies The nurse should suggest that patients keep their eyes open if they are initially uncomfortable with the passive, "let it go" approach necessary for success. Indeed, as the patient relaxes and closes his eyes, the trainer has valuable feedback about the effectiveness of the technique. The trainer should remind patients that they maintain complete control over how much relaxation they allow themselves to experience. We instruct patients not to fall asleep while they are learning relaxation. Relaxation is a useful tool to prevent insomnia, but we recommend that it be learned while the patient is in an alert state. Patients who tend to fall asleep during relaxation practice can view their ability to sleep as an added incentive to continue relaxation. Every relaxation session ends with a slow, paced return to normal activities, to prevent any dizziness or orthostatic hypotension.

Patients need to practice at least three times a week until they are comfortable and familiar with the exercise. Patients in pain may use it two to three times daily. Using it more than three times daily seems to increase the feelings of loss of control and therefore is contraindicated. Limited regular practice will condition the relaxation response so that it will be accomplished more quickly.

Nursing's Role

Progressive muscle relaxation cannot be carried out by either the nurse or patient without considerable instruction and time. What nursing can accomplish within a brief time is creating an awareness of the technique and encouraging an interest in learning more about it. Giving the patient a list of a few centers that teach relaxation may be useful. Some of the shorter relaxation procedures, particularly deep breathing with focusing, involve only minutes at a time and no additional costs.

Cognitive Strategies

Long ago, Epictetus stated that people are distressed not by things, but by the views that they take of them. Today we know that cognitive factors contribute to an appraisal of the pain experience that influences not only the perception of pain but also the response to it.

The goal of directly altering the thoughts and appraisals that surround painful events is valued and supported by both researchers and clinicians. The effect of descending cortical impulses that affect the spinal cord, as proposed in the gate control theory of pain, is evident here. Cognitive strategies for pain control refer to techniques that influence pain through the use of one's thoughts or cognitions.

Mechanisms of Action

Ciccone and Grzesiak[30] stress their growing conviction that the psychological dysfunction that occurs with chronic pain is primarily the result of cognitive error. They received support for their view from a study by Smith, Follick, Ahern, and Adams[119] that found that subjects with chronic back pain who tended to misinterpret or otherwise misconstrue the meaning of their pain sensations tended to be more severely disabled. They emphasize that thinking is causally linked to behavior and emotion, and recall the classic report by Beecher,[11] who found that after wartime injury many soldiers were optimistic and even cheerful in the face of severe pain. Beecher concluded that injury was seen as a way out of the war, and perhaps a chance for personal safety once again. Thus the soldiers' thoughts strongly altered their perceptions of pain/trauma.

Another important factor in the cognitive approaches to pain is the evidence that one's perceived ability to successfully manage and tolerate pain leads to improved coping.[8]

Clinical Uses and Precautions

Cognitive strategies usually are proposed in a three-phased approach to implementation. The first stage is always to make patients become aware of their own thoughts about pain. In fact, the simple act of becoming aware of one's own thoughts is frequently an impetus to change. Patients can record the facts, thoughts, and feelings they have about pain so that they may become clear about whether it is a fact that is causing the distress or a thought emanating from the fact. Feelings result from the thought, not the fact. Although one may have little or no control over the facts in one's life, the individual has total control over the thoughts that are associated with every fact of life. Negative thoughts reduce tolerance to pain and make it much more difficult to handle.[68]

The second stage occurs when the patient begins to apply coping strategies and one or more new cognitive approaches to the pain experience.[135] With self-statement training the patient learns to substitute positive statements for negative ones. Burns,[26] Ellis,[40] and Beck[9] are leading clinicians and researchers in the field of cognitive theory. Burns identified a list of negative self-statements that illustrate distorted thinking. As examples of this kind of thinking, consider all-or-nothing statements, over-generalizations, statements disqualifying positive and overemphasizing negative experiences, and the inappropriate use of "should" statements. Any of these statements, when applied to painful sensations, tend to make the sensations more severe and harder to bear. Substituting more realistic and rational statements permits the patient to reframe his own experience in a less distressing way. With practice over time such positive self-statements become second nature and are able to enhance feelings of personal control and self-efficacy.

In the third stage, the patient needs to rehearse the cognitive strategies to become at ease and proficient with them. For example, a patient can rehearse by imagining how to use positive, rational thoughts during a painful or stressful situation. He may say to himself, "I'm able to manage this. It's not so bad. I've handled similar experiences in the past."

Cognitive appraisal, according to Lazarus and Folkman,[72] is the process by which an individual interprets information in terms of its significance for his or her well-being and evaluates its personal meaning. Thus an event is perceived as irrelevant, benign, challenging, or threatening (primary appraisal). Then the individual assesses how well he can deal with the event at hand (secondary appraisal). Patients with high self-efficacy (Bandura[6]) believe that positive change is possible and that they have the ability to make this positive change happen.

Other examples of cognitive appraisal and self-efficacy beliefs are self-statements such as, "You are doing fine, you're coping, just keep on top of the pain." For a comprehensive discussion of the concepts of cognitive reappraisal and self-efficacy that is beyond the scope of this chapter, the reader is referred to the works of Lazarus and Folkman[72] and Bandura.[6,8] Different authors use different labels for similar concepts or strategies. The reader is advised to bear with these inconsistencies.

Guidelines for Use

Whether the nurse's role is to suggest these strategies, to work directly with the patient on them, or to simply "plant seeds"[110] about contributing pain factors, the following guidelines may be useful.

1. The patient is the most significant person in the process.
2. It is essential to develop a collaborative team approach with the patient as captain. Patient centeredness and team collaboration are important whenever one treats pain and when cognitive approaches are to be employed.
3. The patient must always be in control of the process, since his feedback determines the next step. The patient is central to the pain, the process, and the control.
4. Encourage the patient to observe his own behavior and thought processes.
5. Help the patient identify cues in his environment that will prompt him to talk to himself differently.

6. If the patient is reluctant to "buy" into these approaches, suggest that he is actually enduring two kinds of pain, physical and emotional. Whether or not the physical pain can be readily eliminated, the other pains can be minimized.[30]

Nursing's Role

Although cognitive strategies look inherently simple, a considerable amount of time can be taken up in discussion about the role of thoughts in pain reduction. Further, this dialogue best occurs in blocks of time rather than in short periods of a few minutes each. Some of this discussion can certainly take place while the nurse is occupied with physical tasks or procedures.

Imagery

Although the focus of guided imagery as a therapeutic tool for pain control has seen renewed interest in recent years, imagery as a form of health promotion can be traced back thousands of years to ancient cultures. Imagery was defined according to Richardson[108] as a quasiperceptual event of which we are self-consciously aware and that exists for us in the absence of those stimuli that produce their genuine sensory or perceptual counterparts. Imagery, then, is a mental representation of reality or fantasy and may use all five senses in its creation.

The term *guided imagery* has been coined to reflect the purposeful development of an image or images for a specific goal—usually related to improving one's physiological processes, (pain, autonomic reactivity), mental state, self-image, performance, or behavior.[143] Guided imagery is generally preceded by some form of relaxation, which is thought to facilitate image development.

Mechanisms of Action

Support for the positive effects of guided imagery has emerged from the research on biofeedback training. Individuals have been shown to be able to control heart rate, skin temperature, blood pressure, and muscle tension through the process of biofeedback. When subjects were asked how they were able to bring about such physiological changes, they replied that they did so by imagining relaxing scenes and allowing themselves to relax.[92] Burish and Lyles[25] were able to document reduced nausea, vomiting, and distress in cancer patients after chemotherapy when their subjects practiced guided imagery and relaxation. Kiecolt-Glaser and Glaser[69] compared elderly subjects who used guided imagery with control group subjects who did not. The study group subjects had a lower heart rate at rest, slower respiration, and a significant improvement in the level of natural killer-cell activity. The link between pain management and guided imagery may be a function of an intermediary relaxation response and sense of well-being generated by the performance of guided imagery.

There are several reasons why guided imagery helps people deal with pain successfully. One explanation is that the distraction that results from focusing on a pleasant relaxing image adds to its effectiveness. Another is that patients who use guided imagery regain a sense of personal control and self-control, especially when they are encouraged and directed to create their own pleasant images. The relaxation that precedes and/or accompanies imagery also contributes to reduced muscle tension, anxiety, and pain.

Clinical Uses and Precautions

Perhaps the key function of guided imagery lies in its ability to alter how patients perceive the sensations of pain. Grimm and Kanfer[51] found that training in guided imagery produced longer tolerance and less self-reported pain than training in relaxation, although it has been suggested that relaxation and imagery strategies combine additively.[53] Malone and Strube,[83] in a review article of 109 published studies of nonmedical treatments for chronic pain, found that mood and the number of subjective responses consistently showed a greater response to treatment than did pain intensity, duration, or frequency. Their finding suggests that the benefit of psychological approaches to pain management lies in reducing the fear and depression associated with pain, rather than the pain itself. Donovan[38] has used guided imagery with success in several settings with patients suffering from phantom limb pain and aversiveness to cancer chemotherapy. Vines[132] explored the area of guided imagery in a well population. At least one half of the subjects reported being able to alter unpleasant physical symptoms such as pain during a root canal or with arthritis, and back pain.

Guided imagery varies in whether it is self-guided or other-guided. Other-guided imagery occurs when the nurse guides the imagery development explicitly by leading the patient through a prepared description of the scene to be imagined; self-guided imagery patients are instructed to use their own imagination to remember or create pleasant images. Researchers such as Worthington and Shumate[142] and Olness, Wain, and Ng[103] found client-generated, pleasant imagery to be a powerful and effective psychoanalgesic technique. Moran[100] tested these two methods on a sample of chronic pain patients and found that other-guided imagery was somewhat more effective. However, the imagery experience was presented only one time to the subjects. Kroger and Fezle[71] concluded that imagery techniques became more effective with repeated use, suggesting that practice is important to success. Guided imagery can be a particularly helpful strategy in conjunction with other pain management approaches for use in a wide range of acute and chronic pain states.

Guidelines for Use

It is often helpful for the nurse to know that there is no one right way to teach guided imagery or any other cognitive-behavioral intervention. Each nurse must learn and practice a technique so that she feels comfortable with it before employing it with patients. The nurse and the patient become partners in a collaborative relationship in selecting the imagery that the patient will develop, and when and how he will use it (see box).

Both the nurse and the patient need to be aware that guided imagery is a skill that needs to be learned and practiced at times when the patient is pain-free or nearly so. More than one session will be necessary to become proficient with the technique. There are some excellent reports of training techniques for interested readers in works by Turk, Meichenbaum, and Genest,[130] McCaffery,[88] and McCaffery and Beebe.[89]

There are two distinctly different approaches that imagery may take. One is in the direction away from the painful experience. This approach actually develops an "incompatible" image. It changes the situation into one in which pain is not

◆ SPECIFIC GUIDELINES FOR IMAGERY TECHNIQUES

1. Inquire about the patient's experience with images, so that you can build on his skills.
2. Enlist the patient's cooperation by explaining what imagery is, what it does, and its relation to pain control.
3. Present the technique as a self-control strategy that the patient will always have, to call on whenever and wherever he chooses.
4. Suggest applications for imagery in conjunction with other approaches to pain control, such as medications, deep breathing, or physiotherapy.
5. Use suggestions and permissive statements rather than firm commands. For example, use phrases such as, "You may feel," 'If you choose to you can," "You can let yourself think about . . ."
6. Avoid use in patients under psychiatric care, unless the physician's or psychologist's approval has been obtained.
7. Patients may be frightened by transient feelings of unreality when they begin. Use this phenomenon to help patients realize that their imagery is beginning the process of releasing tension, allowing them to experience feelings and emotions.
8. Avoid any image that would produce a contraindicated physiological effect, such as generating feelings of warmth in the abdominal area in a patient with an active gastric ulcer. Focusing on an image of a healing, sound body free of pain is a helpful alternative in instances where a possible negative effect is of concern.

present, allowing the patient to feel once more in charge of his feelings. This method is most frequently used by nurses and other health care professionals. A common example involves imagining a pleasant out-of-doors scene, such as a meadow, lake, or forest. Another approach imagery can take is described as transformational, because it is directed toward the pain. Specific strategies that patients have reported to be helpful are:

1. Converting the pain to nonpain, e.g., turning the painful area into ice, rushing water, trickles of sand, or pressure caused by imaginary animals sitting on the area.
2. Imagining the pain to be a color and then converting it

to another color, switching from a warm to a cool color, or vice versa.

3. Determining the pain level on a 0 to 10 horizontal scale, and then slowly moving the indicator lever to a slightly lower number, while breathing slowly and deeply with each incremental decrease in the pain rating.

Other useful techniques are found in McCaffery[88] and Bogin.[22]

Nursing's Role

Imagery is inexpensive and requires only small amounts of time. The effective use of imagery requires that the nurse have an open mind and a responsiveness to the patient's selection of images and how they can be adapted.

Music

Music has long been known for its soothing qualities. In recent years it has been the subject of many research studies. As a therapy, music is used to restore, maintain, and improve mental and physical health, according to the National Association for Music Therapy.[101] Music is a natural tool for nurses to use as an adjunct to pain management because of its ease of use and low cost. It is well suited to the practical demands of a wide range of health care settings.

Mechanisms of Action

Definitive explanations for the efficacy of music therapy are not currently known. It has been postulated that there may be a conditioned relaxation response or distraction effect because of enjoyable past associations. Another possible mechanism of action reported by Standley[124] is that auditory stimuli may directly suppress pain neurologically. Music can also encourage distraction or dissociation from unpleasant or painful stimuli through the development of imagery, increase the production of endorphins,[48] and serve as a cue for relaxation. All of these processes are well in keeping with our understanding of the mechanisms of the gate control theory. The potential of music as a practical measure has only begun to be recognized. According to Bailey,[5] the goals of music therapy in pain management are to improve the patient's comfort level, to assist him or her to regain a sense of perceived personal control, and to actively involve the patient in the management of his or her pain.

Clinical Uses and Precautions

Music-trained patients in an obstetrical study by Clark, McCorkle, and Williams[31] reported experiencing more support from their partner, less anxiety during childbirth, and decreased pain or discomfort. Hanser, Larson, and O'Connell,[54] Sammons,[109] and Geden, Lower, Beattie, and Beck[47] all found that many of the women in their studies had lowered mean pain responses and enhanced relaxation when they listened to music during labor and delivery.

Other studies have surveyed the helpful effects of music on chronic pain patients, and postoperative and hospitalized cancer patients.[4,80,139] Music therapy, like other nonpharmacological methods of pain control, is not meant to be used alone, nor is it meant to be used when pain is already at a peak intensity. Not all patients in pain wish to listen to music during or before painful episodes, and some find that they either cannot or do not wish to focus on the music.

When one discusses the use of music with patients, it is important to ascertain their experience with music, their skills or interest in different types of music, and their current listening abilities. Bailey suggests that patients generally fit into one of the following categories:

1. A music performer. The patient has played an instrument, sung in a choir, or even composed music.
2. A music listener. The patient has been an interested listener to music.
3. A music "event-er." The patient associates music with special events and does not ordinarily listen to music.

The most successful pain relief associated with music tends to happen when the music is carefully chosen according to the preferences of the patient. Not only can the music selection be tailored to the kind of music the patient enjoys, but it can also be selected to match the mood and the needs of the patient. For example, if a patient in pain is also feeling depressed or sad, music that supports that mood may be more acceptable at first, and the patient may then be able to progress into lighter melodies. We recommend instrumental over vocal selections.

Guidelines for Use

Although music is an easy-to-use modality, it is not enough to simply present the music to the patient and instruct the patient to listen to it. A clear set of instructions is required so that the patient will become an active participant in his or her own care. The following guidelines from McCaffery[88] are particularly helpful.

1. Listen only to the music.
2. Feel the music lifting you upward.
3. Let each measure rhythmically flow through your body and relax the muscles.
4. Let yourself float through the air with the melody.

It is best to introduce the patient to music therapy before pain becomes intense, or before commencing a painful procedure, such as wound packing.[2]

By encouraging the patient to become involved in the process of active listening, the nurse activates several other cognitive and mental strategies. The patient may conduct his or her own inner dialogue, which can focus attention onto more pleasant and relaxing images. Both the nurse and the patient can measure the effectiveness of music as a treatment modality for pain control by rating the level of distress caused by the pain on a 0-to-10 visual analogue or numerical scale before and after the listening session. Patients can then be encouraged to consider what strategies they might employ to increase the benefits at the next session. Some patients prefer to turn the volume up high during periods of severe pain, while others maintain it at a low level to ensure that they keep in tune with external events.

Changes in volume, attention to breathing, and variations in rhythm and tempo, plus the addition or deletion of movements such as toe or finger tapping, have been suggested and used successfully by patients.

Nursing's Role

The use of music requires some equipment, such as a portable cassette player and audio tape that may already be owned by the patient or be easily obtained from in-hospital resources. It can be readily explained to patients and family members, and mechanisms for its use (place, time, and a quiet setting) easily arranged.

Distraction

Almost everyone has used distraction at one time or another for pain relief. McCaffery has defined distraction as simply focusing attention on stimuli other than the pain sensation. Using that definition, almost any activity can qualify as distraction, from counting tiles on a ceiling to completing complex crossword puzzles. Much of the research on distraction has been carried out in laboratory settings.

Mechanisms of Action

Distraction may increase pain tolerance[113] or raise the perception threshold.[45] Distraction places pain at the periphery of awareness so that the patient can "tune out" the pain for the time distraction is being used. Whatever the exact mechanism may be, distraction does not make the pain disappear but makes it more tolerable.

Clinical Uses and Precautions

Distraction is useful for almost every type of pain, providing that an appropriate form of distraction has been chosen. Patients with chronic pain devise elaborate distraction activities that they use frequently throughout the day whether or not they are aware of it. Patients experiencing shorter episodes of acute pain also tend to benefit from receiving specific suggestions from the nurse. One of the most frequently used distraction techniques involves breathing exercises.[35] The use of breathing exercises combines the benefits of relaxation with the effectiveness of distraction. Slow, deep abdominal breathing is an easily learned and useful approach. The patient is directed to focus on his breathing by concentrating on the inhalations and exhalations. Although breathing techniques have been widely used in labor and delivery, and are a highly successful component of preparation for childbirth,[125] they are applicable to many other kinds of pain. Breathing techniques must be carefully explained and monitored during the learning process so that the patient does not breath too rapidly (not to exceed one breath per second) or too deeply. When teaching breathing techniques, the nurse should ensure that the exhalation phase is passive and relaxed, rather than forced.

Like all techniques, some disadvantages are associated with distraction. Others may doubt the existence or severity of pain if distraction is a successful intervention. However, the very fact that distraction works indicates that pain is present and has been only temporarily relieved. Distraction is fatiguing, and therefore is most useful for brief periods (less than 2 hours). Distraction requires energy and concentration, which results in a return of pain, irritability, and fatigue after its termination. However, the many benefits of distraction far outweigh the disadvantages, and an explanation of its efficacy and rationale should be provided to all patients in pain and their caregivers and family members.

Guidelines for Use

The types of distraction possible are limited only by the patient's or the nurse's creativity and ingenuity. Methods include rhythmic breathing, rocking, singing or humming, describing pictures or photos aloud, listening to music, and playing games. Humor is a highly successful distraction strategy that has been shown to improve the release of the body's natural endorphins.

Guidelines for using distraction have been adapted from McCaffery's excellent work on the subject (see box).[88,89]

Nursing's Role

Distraction is one area of pain management that particularly highlights the creativity of the nurse in combination with the abilities and preferences of the patient. While striving to suggest pleasant activities on which to focus, the nurse is also intent on giving the patient a sense of personal control over his situation. One of the rewards of the successful choice of a distraction strategy is the true collaborative process that precedes it. The nurse also needs to focus on making sure that the other members of the health care team are aware of the mechanisms of distraction, and especially that they know that the use of distraction does not mean that pain no longer exists. Rather, distraction has improved pain tolerance and temporarily made the qualities of the pain more acceptable to the patient. The nurse may suggest that an analgesic be admin-

◆ GUIDELINES FOR DEVELOPING AND USING DISTRACTION

1. Determine whether the patient has used distraction successfully for pain relief. If he has, try to utilize what he has done. If he has not, assess his interests and use them to give him choices or distraction strategies.
2. Explain the expected effects and limitations of distraction for pain relief. Most patients cannot use distraction for very long periods or as the only form of pain relief.
3. As pain increases in intensity, increase the complexity of the distraction; with high intensities of pain, decrease complexity.
4. Use several major sensory modalities, i.e., hearing, seeing, touching, and/or moving.
5. Avoid external or mental stimuli related to pain.
6. Include and emphasize rhythm.
7. Include a focus on breathing, unless the patient has respiratory difficulty.
8. Do not expect that perfection is necessary for success.

Modified from McCaffery M and Beebe A (1989): *Pain, clinical manual for nursing practice.* St. Louis: Mosby–Year Book Inc.

istered at the completion of the distraction exercise to encourage rest and comfort.

Positive Suggestion

The potential benefits of incorporating a positive, reassuring manner into one's practice to maximize the success of all interventions cannot be overemphasized. Positive suggestion as used here refers to the administration of any type of analgesia in combination with an explanation of its potential positive effects. Although this form of analgesia has been useful since medicine's beginnings, it remains a misunderstood treatment.[105]

Mechanisms of Action

As with many other nonpharmacological forms of pain management, the involved mechanisms are not fully understood. There is some evidence suggesting that endorphins mediate placebo responses when clinical pain (Evans,[42] Levine[78]) but not experimental pain is involved.[12,99]

Clinical Uses

Placebos are traditionally used in clinical trials as a control against which to judge the efficacy of other analgesics. Evidence has shown that in a variety of painful conditions a remarkably constant proportion (about one third) of patients obtain significant relief from placebos.[10,44] Gowdey[49] recently reviewed the list of pain disorders that have responded to placebos. These include pain associated with primary dysmenorrhea, chronic headache and migraines, rheumatoid and degenerative forms of arthritis, peptic ulcer, angina (with no demonstrable coronary artery disease), and cancer. Several studies also suggest that severe, steady postoperative pain often responds to placebo treatment.[10] Therefore these pain types may respond well to positive suggestion as well. More recently, Harrison[56] reported a significantly lower level of pain in a group of post–spinal surgery patients after medication administered by a nurse with an "empathetic" approach compared with a similar group receiving the same medication but from a nurse with a "nonempathetic" approach.

Guidelines for Use

The physical characteristics of an intervention (e.g., pill vs. injection), the environment in which it is given, and the patient-clinician relationship all appear important in determining the degree of response.[105] Therefore, health care workers need to recognize the potential benefits of incorporating a positive, reassuring manner in their routine practice, to maximize the success of all interventions.

Nursing's Role

Nurses are the health care workers who most frequently administer the various pain treatments. As such, the role they play in maximizing the effectiveness of these interventions through positive suggestion is crucial.

◆ SUMMARY

This chapter describes various nonpharmacological pain management strategies that are readily available to nurses. Their mechanisms of action, uses, contraindications, and methods of practice are reviewed. Although the mechanisms of these techniques are only partially understood, enough empirical evidence has accrued to demonstrate clinically significant effects for a variety of painful conditions. Nonpharmacological methods may not cure the pain, but they are usually effective, simple to apply, and easy to learn. These modalities can be used in combination with one another or with pharmacological agents to individualize treatment. The nurse has a responsibility to obtain a working knowledge of these strategies and to use them to decrease suffering and improve the quality of life for the victims of acute or chronic pain. Since each pain experience is not only individual but variable, the only practical clinical approach is to thoroughly assess each situation and then to apply creative interventions, followed by further assessments of pain relief and patient satisfaction. Such an ongoing cycle of individual and creative assessments and interventions will do much to achieve good pain control. With multimode therapy, no patient should have to suffer pain.

REFERENCES

1. Ali J, Yaffe C, and Serrette C. (1981). The effects of transcutaneous electric nerve stimulation on postoperative pain and pulmonary function. *Surgery, 89*(4), 507-512.
2. Angus JE and Faux S. (1989). The effect of music on adult postoperative patients' pain during a nursing procedure. In Funk SG et al (eds), *Key aspects of comfort: management of pain, fatigue, and nausea* (pp. 166-172). New York: Springer Publishing.
3. Augustinsson L, Bohlin P, Bundsen P, et al. (1977). Pain relief during delivery by transcutaneous electrical nerve stimulation. *Pain, 4,* 59-65.
4. Bailey LM. (1983). The effects of live music versus tape-recorded music on hospitalized cancer patients. *Music Ther, 2,* 17-28.
5. Bailey LM. (1986). Music therapy in pain management. *J Pain Sympt Manage, 1,* 25-28.
6. Bandura A. (1977). Self-efficacy: toward a unifying theory of behavioral change. *Psychol Rev, 84,* 191-215.
7. Bandura A. (1986). *Social foundations of thought and action: a social cognitive theory.* Engelwood Cliffs, NJ: Prentice-Hall.
8. Bandura A, O'Leary A, Taylor CB, Gauthier J, and Gossard D. (1987). Self-efficacy and pain control: opioid and nonopioid mechanisms. *J Pers Soc Psychol, 53,* 406-414.
9. Beck AT. (1976). *Cognitive therapy and emotional disorders.* New York: Meridian.
10. Beecher HK. (1955). The powerful placebo. *JAMA, 159,* 1602-1606.
11. Beecher HK. (1956). Relationship of significance of wound to pain experienced. *JAMA, 161,* 1609-1613.
12. Beecher HK. (1960). Increased stress and effectiveness of placebos and "active" drugs. *Science, 132,* 91-92.

13. Beggs D. (1980). Acupressure as a preventive measure, as a diagnostic aid and a treatment modality. *Am J Acupunct, 8(4),* 341-347.
14. Benson TB. (1973). The effects of therapeutic forms of heat and ice on the pain threshold of the normal shoulder. *Rheumatol Rehab, 13*(101), 100-105.
15. Benson H. (1975). *The relaxation response.* New York: William Morrow.
16. Benson H, Beary JF, and Carol MP. (1974). The relaxation response. *Psychiatry, 37,* 37-46.
17. Benson H and Klipper MZ. (1976). *The relaxation response.* New York: Avon Books.
18. Berlant SR. (1984). Method of determining optimal stimulation sites for transcutaneous electrical nerve stimulation. *Phys Ther, 64*(6), 924-928.
19. Bernstein DA and Borkovec TD. (1973). *Progressive relaxation training.* Champaign, Ill: Research Press.
20. Bisgard JD and Dye D. (1940). The influence of hot and cold application upon gastric and intestinal motor activity. *Surg Gynecol Obstet, 71,* 172-180.
21. Blanchard EB and Ahles TA. (1990). Biofeedback therapy. In Bonica JJ (ed), *The management of pain (vol 1)* (pp. 1722-1732). Philadelphia: Lea & Febiger.
22. Bogin M. (1982). *The path to pain control.* Boston: Houghton Mifflin.
23. Bolton L. (1983). TENS electrode irritation. *J Am Acad Dermatol, 8,* 134-135.
24. Bonica JJ. (1987). Importance of effective pain control. *Acta Anaesthesiol Scand, 31, S, 85,* 1-16.
25. Burish TG and Lyles JN. (1981). Effectiveness of relaxation training in reducing adverse reaction to cancer chemotherapy. *J Behav Med, 4* 65-78.
26. Burns DD. (1980). *Feeling good: the new mood therapy.* New York: William Morrow.
27. Chaitow L. (1983). *The acupuncture treatment of pain.* New York: Thorsons Publishers.
28. Chapman CR and Turner JA. (1986). Psychological control of acute pain in medical settings. *J Pain Sympt Manage, 1,* 9-20.
29. Chen D, Philip M, Philip PA, and Monga TN. (1990). Cardiac pacemaker inhibition by transcutaneous electrical nerve stimulation. *Arch Phys Med Rehab, 71,* 27-30.
30. Ciccone DS and Grzesiak RC. (1988). Cognitive theory: an overview of theory and practice. In Lynch N and Vasudevan S (eds), *Persistent pain: psychosocial assessment and intervention* (pp. 133-177). Boston: Kluwer Academic Publishers.
31. Clark ME, McCorkle RR, and Williams S. (1981). Music therapy-assisted labor and delivery. *J Music Ther, 18,* 88-100.
32. Cohen FL. (1980). Postsurgical pain relief: patient's status and nurses' medical choices. *Pain, 9,* 265-274.
33. Copp LA. (1986). Consensus: pain management ineffective. *J Prof Nurs, 2*(5), 272-274.
34. Crasilneck HB. (1979). Hypnosis in the control of chronic low back pain. *Am J Clin Hyp, 15,* 153-161.
35. Dalton JA. (1989). Nurses' perceptions of their pain assessment skills, pain management practices, and attitudes toward pain. *Oncol Nurs Forum, 16*(2), 225-231.

36. Day JA, Mason RR, and Chesrown SE. (1987). Effects of massage on serum level of beta-endorphin and beta-lipotropin in healthy adults. *Phys Ther, 67*(6), 926-930.
37. DeLateur B. (1974). The role of physical medicine in problems of pain. *Adv Neurol, 4,* 495-497.
38. Donovan MI. (1980). Relaxation with guided imagery: a useful technique. *Cancer Nurs, 3*(1), 27-32.
39. Donovan M, Dillon P, and McGuire L. (1987). Incidence and characteristics of pain in a sample of medical-surgical inpatients. *Pain, 30,* 69-78.
40. Ellis A. (1962). *Reason and emotion in psychotherapy.* New York: Lyle Stuart.
41. Eriksson M and Sjolund B. (1976). Acupuncturelike electroanalgesia in TNS-resistant chronic pain. In Zotterman Y (ed), *Sensory functions of the skin* (pp. 575-581). Oxford: Pergamon Press.
42. Evans FJ. (1974). The placebo response in pain reduction. *Adv Neurol, 4,* 289-296.
43. Everall M. (1976). Cold therapy. *Nurs Times, 72,* 144-145.
44. Fedele L. (1989). Dynamics and significance of placebo response in primary dysmenorrhea. *Pain, 36,* 43-47.
45. Fellner CH. (1971). Alterations in pain perceptions of multiple sensory modality stimulation. *Psychosomatics, 12,* 313-315.
46. Finsen V, Persen L, Lovlien M, et al. (1988). Transcutaneous electrical nerve stimulation after major amputation. *J Bone Joint Surg., 70-B(1),* 109-112.
47. Geden EA, Lower M, Beattie S, and Beck N. (1989). Effects of muscle and imagery on physiologic and self-report of analogued labor pain. *Nurs Res, 38*(1), 37-41.
48. Goldstein A. (1980). Thrills in response to music and other stimuli. *Physiol Psychol, 8,* 126-129.
49. Gowdey W. (1983). A guide to the pharmacology of placebos, *Can Med Assoc, 128,* 921-925.
50. Gray-Donald K, Abbott FV, Edgar L, Johnston CC, and Jeans ME. (1988). Prevalence of pain in hospitalized patients (abstract). In *Canadian Pain Society and American Pain Society Joint Meeting Abstracts* (p. 142). Toronto, Canada.
51. Grimm L and Kanfer FH. (1976). Tolerance of aversive stimulation. *Behav Ther, 7,* 593-601.
52. Grzesiak RC and Ciccone DS. (1988). Relaxation, biofeedback, and hypnosis in the management of pain. In Lynch NT and Vasudevan S (eds), *Persistent pain: psychosocial assessment and intervention* (pp. 163-188). Boston: Kluwer Academic Publishers.
53. Hackett G and Horan JJ. (1980). Stress inoculation for pain: what's really going on? *J Counsel Psychol, 27,* 107-116.
54. Hanser SB, Larson SC, and O'Connell AS. (1983). The effects of music on relaxation of expectant mothers during labor. *J Music Ther, 20*(2), 50-58.
55. Hare ML. (1988). Shiatsu acupressure in nursing practice. *Hol Nurs Pract, 2*(3), 68-74.
56. Harrison MP. (March 1988). *The effects of positive nursing behaviors on the patient perceived pain relief.* Paper presented at a national conference on research for practice—key aspects of comfort: management of pain, fatigue and nausea, Chapel Hill, NC.

57. Hou ZL. (1979). A study on the histologic structure of acupuncture points and types of fibres conveying needling sensation. *Chin Med J, 92,* 223-232.
58. Hyman RB, Feldman HR, Harris RB, Levin RF, and Malloy GB. (1989). The effects of relaxation training on clinical symptoms: a meta-analysis. *Nurs Res, 38*(4), 216-220.
59. Hymes AC, Raab D, Yonehiro E, Nelson G, and Printy A. (1973). Electrical surface stimulation for control of acute postoperative pain and prevention of ileus. *Surg Forum, 24,* 447-449.
60. Jacobs M. (1960). Message for the relief of pain: anatomical and physiological considerations. *Am Phys Ther Rev Assoc, 40*(2), 93-98.
61. Jacobson E. (1938). *Progressive relaxation.* Chicago: University of Chicago.
62. Jeans ME. (1979). Relief of chronic pain by brief, intense transcutaneous electrical stimulation—a double-blind study. *Adv Pain Res Ther, 3,* 601-606.
63. Joachim G. (1983). Step-by-step massage techniques. *Can Nurs, 79,* 32-35.
64. Joachim G. (1984). Acupressure: A self technique for relieving headache pain. *Can Nurs, 80,* 38-40.
65. Johnson J. (1984). Nonpharmacologic pain management in arthritis. *Nurs Clin North Am, 19,* 583-590.
66. Kaada B. (1982). Vasodilation induced by transcutaneous nerve stimulation in peripheral ischemia (Raynaud's phenomenon and diabetic polyneuropathy). *Eur Heart J, 3,* 303-314.
67. Kaada B and Torsteinbo O. (1989). Increase of plasma B-endorphins in connective tissue massage. *Gen Pharmacol, 20*(4), 487-489.
68. Kendall PC, Williams L, Pechacek TF et al. (1979). Cognitive-behavioral and patient education interventions in cardiac catheterization procedures: The Palo Alto Medical Psychology Project. *J Consult Clin Psychol, 47,* 49-58.
69. Kiecolt-Glaser J and Glaser R. (1987). Cited in Squires S. Visions to boost immunity. *Am Health, 6,* 54-61.
70. Klin D, Vretzky G, and Magora F. (1984). Transcutaneous electrical nerve stimulation (TENS) after open heart surgery. *J Cardiovasc Surg, 25,* 445.
71. Kroger WS and Fezle WD. (1976). *Hypnosis and behavior modification: imagery conditioning.* Philadelphia: JB Lippincott.
72. Lazarus RS and Folkman S. (1984). *Stress, appraisal, and coping.* New York: Springer Publishing.
73. Lee JM and Warren MP. (1978a). Clinical applications of cold for the musculoskeletal system. In *Cold therapy in rehabilitation* (pp. 69-75). London: Bell and Hyman.
74. Lee JM and Warren MP. (1978b). Precautions and contraindications. In *Cold therapy in rehabilitation* (pp. 81-86). London: Bell and Hyman.
75. Lehmann JF and DeLateur BJ. (1982a). Cryotherapy. In Lehmann JF (ed), *Therapeutic heat and cold* (ed 3) (pp. 561-602). Baltimore/London: Williams and Wilkins.
76. Lehmann JF and DeLateur BJ. (1982b). Diathermy and superficial heat and cold therapy. In Kruson FH, Kottke FJ, and Elwood PM (eds),

Handbook of physical medicine and rehabilitation (ed 2) (pp. 275-350). London and Philadelphia: Saunders.
77. Lehmann JF, Warren CG, and Scham SM. (1974). Therapeutic heat and cold. *Clin Orthop, 99,* 207-245.
78. Levine J. (1978). The mechanism of placebo analgesia. *Lancet, Sept 23,* 654-657.
79. Lewers D, Clelland JA, Jackson JR, Varner RE, and Bergman J. (1989). Transcutaneous electrical nerve stimulation in the relief of primary dysmenorrhea. *Phys Ther, 69*(1), 3-9.
80. Locsin RF. (1981). The effect of music on the pain of selected postoperative patients. *J Adv Nurs, 6,* 19-25.
81. Loesser JD. (1986). *Pain and its management: an overview.* Consensus Development Conference on the Integrated Approach to Management of Pain. Bethesda, Md: National Institutes of Health.
82. Ludwick-Rosenthal R and Neufeld RWJ. (1988). Stress management during noxious medical procedures: an evaluative review of outcome studies. *Psychol Bull, 104,* 326-342. Cambridge, Mass: Bullinger Publishing.
83. Malone MD and Strube MJ. (1988). Meta-analysis of non-medical treatments for chronic pain. *Pain, 34,* 231-244.
84. Mannheimer C, Carlsson CA, Vedin A, and Wilhemsson C. (1985). Transcutaneous electrical nerve stimulation (TENS) in angina pectoris. *Int J Cardiol, 7,* 91-95.
85. Mannheimer C, Emanuelsson H, Waagstein F, and Wilhelmsson C. (1989). Influence of naloxone on the effects of high frequency transcutaneous electrical nerve stimulation in angina pectoris induced by atrial pacing. *Br Heart J, 62,* 36-42.
86. Mannheimer JS and Lampe GN. (1984). *Clinical transcutaneous electrical nerve stimulation.* Philadelphia: FA Davis.
87. Mannheimer JS and Whalen EC. (1985). The efficacy of transcutaneous electrical nerve stimulation in dysmenorrhea. *Clin J Pain, 1,* 75-83.
88. McCaffery M. (1979). *Nursing management of the patient with pain* (ed 2). Philadelphia: JB Lippincott.
89. McCaffery M and Beebe A. (1989). *Pain, clinical manual for nursing practice.* St. Louis: Mosby–Year Book, Inc.
90. McCallum MID, Glynn CJ, Moore RA, Lammer P, and Phillips AM. (1988). Transcutaneous electrical nerve stimulation in the management of acute postoperative pain. *Br J Anaesthesiol, 61,* 308-312.
91. Mehta M. (1986). Current views of non-invasive methods in pain relief. In Swerdlow M (ed), *The therapy of pain* (ed 2) (pp. 115-131). Boston: MTP Press.
92. Melzack R. (1973). *The puzzle of pain.* New York: Basic Books.
93. Melzack R. (1975). Prolonged relief of pain by brief, intense transcutaneous somatic stimulation. *Pain, 1,* 357-373.
94. Melzack R, Guite S, Gonshor A. (1980). Relief of dental pain by ice massage of the hand. *Can Med Assoc J, 122,* 189-191.
95. Melzack R, Jeans ME, Stratford JG, and Monks RC. (1980). Ice massage and transcutaneous electrical stimulation: comparison of treatment for low-back pain. *Pain, 9,* 209-217.
96. Melzack R, Vetere P, and Finch L. (1983). Transcutaneous electrical nerve stimulation for low back pain. *Phys Ther, 63*(4), 489-493.

97. Melzack R and Wall PD (1965). Pain mechanisms: a new theory. *Science, 150,* 971-979.
98. Melzack R and Wall PD. (1984). *The challenge of pain.* Suffolk, Great Britain: Chaucer Press.
99. Mihic D and Binkert E. (1978). Is placebo analgesia mediated by endorphin? *Pain Abstr, 1,* 19.
100. Moran KJ. (1989). The effect of music on adult postoperative patients' pain during a nursing procedure. In Funk SG et al (eds), *Key aspects of comfort: management of pain, fatigue, and nausea* (pp. 160-165). New York: Springer.
101. National Association for Music Therapy. (1977). *Music therapy as a career.* Lawrence, Kan: National Association for Music Therapy.
102. Neighbors LE, Clelland J, Jackson JR, Bergman J, and Orr J. (1987). Transcutaneous electrical nerve stimulation for pain relief in primary dysmenorrhea. *Clin J Pain, 3*(1), 17-22.
103. Olness K, Wain JH, and Ng L. (1980). A pilot study of blood endorphin levels in children using self-hypnosis to control pain. *Devel Behav Pediatr, 1*(4), 187-188.
104. Omura Y. (1988). Basic electrical parameters for safe and effective electro-therapeutic (electro-acupuncture, TES, TENMS [or TEMS]), TENS and electro-magnetic field stimulation with or without drugs. *Acupunct Electrother Res, 12,* 201-225.
105. Pasternak SJ and Paris PM. (1988). Placebo therapy. In Paris PM and Stewart RD (eds), *Pain management in emergency medicine* (pp. 501-510). Norwalk, Conn: Appleton & Lange.
106. Penzer V and Matsumoto K. (1985). Acupressure in dental practice: magic at the tips of your fingers. *J Mass Dent Soc, 34(2),* 71-72, 74-75.
107. Reich BA. (1989). Non-invasive treatment of vascular and muscle contraction headache: a comparative longitudinal clinical study. *Headache, 29*(1), 34-41.
108. Richardson A. (1969). *Mental imagery.* London: Routledge and Kegan Paul.
109. Sammons LN. (1984). The use of music by women during childbirth. *J Nurs-Midwif, 29*(4), 266-290.
110. Scandrett S. (1985). Cognitive reappraisal. In Bulechek GM and McCloskey JC (eds), *Nursing intervention: treatment for nursing diagnoses* (pp. 49-57). Philadelphia: WB Saunders.
111. Schultz JH and Luthe W. (1969). Autogenic methods. In Luthe W (ed), *Autogenic therapy: vol. 1.* New York: Grune and Stratton.
112. Schuster G and Infante M. (1980). Pain relief after low back surgery: the efficacy of transcutaneous electrical nerve stimulation. *Pain, 8,* 299-302.
113. Scott DS and Barber TX. (1977). Cognitive control of pain: effects of multiple cognitive strategies. *Psychol Rec, 2,* 373-383.
114. Sjolund BH. (1988). Peripheral nerve stimulation suppression of C-fiber-evoked flexion reflex in rats. *J Neurosurg, 68,* 279-283.
115. Sjolund B and Eriksson M. (1976). Electro-acupuncture and endogenous morphines. *Lancet, 13,* 1085.
116. Sjolund BH and Eriksson BE. (1979). The influence of naloxone on analgesia produced by peripheral conditioning stimulation. *Brain Res, 173,* 295-301.

117. Sjolund BH and Eriksson MBE. (1985). *Relief of pain by TENS* (pp. 1-116). Chichester, Great Britain: Wiley and Sons.
118. Sjolund B, Terenius L, and Eriksson MBE. (1977). Increased cerebrospinal fluid levels of endorphins after electroacupuncture. *Acta Physiol Scand, 100,* 382-384.
119. Smith TW, Follick MJ, Ahern DK, and Adams A. (1986). Cognitive distortion and disability in chronic low back pain. *Chron Ther Res, 10,* 201-210.
120. Smith CM, Guralnick MS, Gelfand MM, and Jeans ME. (1986). The effects of transcutaneous electrical nerve stimulation on post-cesarean pain. *Pain, 27,* 181-193.
121. Snyder M. (1984). Progressive relaxation as a nursing intervention: an analysis. *Adv Nurs Sci, 6*(3), 47-53.
122. Sodipo J, Adedeji S, and Olumide O. (1980). Postoperative pain relief by transcutaneous electrical nerve stimulation (TENS). *Am J Chin Med, 8*(1-2), 190-194.
123. Solomon RA, Viernstein MC, and Long DM. (1980). Reduction of postoperative pain and narcotic use by transcutaneous electrical nerve stimulation. *Surgery, 87*(2), 142-146.
124. Standley JM. (1986). Music research in medical/dental treatment: meta-analysis and clinical applications. *J Music Ther, 23*(2), 56-122.
125. Stevens RJ and Heide F. (1977). Analgesic characteristics of prepared childbirth techniques. *J Psychosom Res, 21,* 429-438.
126. Tan SY. (1982). Cognitive and cognitive-behavioral methods for pain control: a selective review. *Pain, 12,* 201-228.
127. Tappan FM. (1988). *Healing massage techniques* (pp. 1-347). Norwalk, Conn: Appleton & Lange.
128. Tepperman PS, De Zwirek CB, and Chaircossi AL. (1977). Pressure zones: prevention and step up management. *Postgrad Med, 62,* 83-89.
129. Thomas IL, Tyle V, Webster J, and Neilson A. (1988). An evaluation of transcutaneous electrical nerve stimulation for pain relief in labour. *Aust J Obstet Gynaecol, 28,* 182-189.
130. Turk DC, Meichenbaum D, and Genest M. (1983). *Pain and behavioral medicine: a cognitive behavioral perspective.* New York: Guilford Press.
131. Ulett GA. (1982). *Principles and practice of physiologic acupuncture* (pp. 209-210). St. Louis: Warren H. Green.
132. Vines SW. (1988). The therapeutics of guided imagery. *Hol Nurs Pract, 2*(3), 34-44.
133. Wall PD. (1985). The discovery of transcutaneous electrical nerve stimulation. *Physiotherapy, 71*(8), 348-350.
134. Wallace KG and Hays J. (1982). Nursing management of chronic pain. *J Neurosurg Nurs, 14(4),* 185-191.
135. Wells N. (1987). Cognitive-behavioral strategies in pain management. *J Royal Soc Health, 107*(3), 92-94.
136. Weaver MT. (1985). Acupressure: an overview of theory and application. *Nurse Pract, 10*(8), 38-40.
137. White JA. (1988). Touching with intent: therapeutic massage. *Hol Nurs Pract, 2(3),* 63-67.
138. Witt JR. (1984). Relieving chronic pain. *Nurse Pract, 9,* 36-38.
139. Wolfe DE. (1978). Pain rehabilitation and music therapy. *J Music Ther, 4,* 162-168.

140. Wolpe J. (1958). *Psychotherapy by reciprocal inhibition.* Stanford: Stanford University Press.
141. Woolf CJ, Mitchell D, Myers RA, and Barrett GD. (1978). Failure of naloxone to reverse peripheral transcutaneous electro-analgesia in patients suffering from acute trauma. *S Afr Med J, 53,* 179-180.
142. Worthington EL Jr and Shumate M. (1981). Imagery and verbal counseling methods in stress inoculation training for pain control. *J Counsel Psychol, 28*(1), 1-6.
143. Zahourek RP. (1988). *Relaxation and imagery: therapeutic tools for communication and intervention.* Philadelphia: WB Saunders.
144. Zugerman C. (1982). Dermatitis from transcutaneous electrical nerve stimulation. *J Am Acad Dermatol, 6,* 936-939.

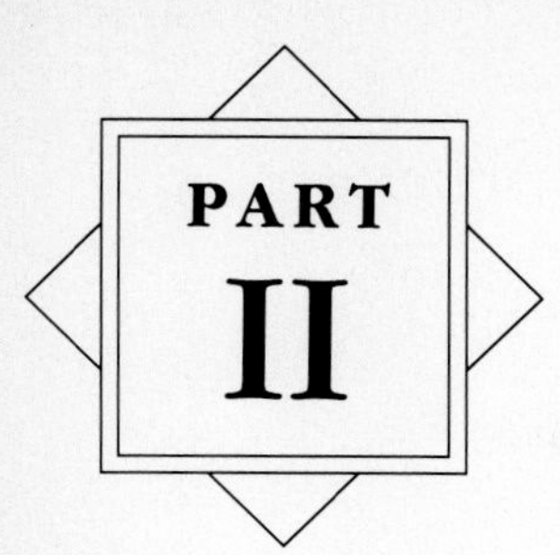

DEVELOPMENTAL DIFFERENCES IN PAIN MANAGEMENT

9

Pain in Infants

Celeste Johnston
Bonnie Stevens

◆ INTRODUCTION

Pain is a complex, subjective, and elusive phenomenon that presents special problems in assessment and management in the infant or neonate. Early studies of pain in the neonate supported the notion that neonates were incapable of feeling pain because their responses were thought to be decorticate.[90] It was also assumed that infants were incapable of remembering a painful event and therefore were unable to express their pain in a meaningful way.[79,95] Recent evidence has demonstrated that neurological development of pain pathways, as well as cortical and subcortical centers necessary for pain perception, are well developed late in gestation, and therefore the neonate is quite capable of experiencing pain.[43,107]

Although pain research has flourished in recent years, the knowledge about the measurement and management of pain in infants is sparse in comparison with the knowledge of pain in older children[88] and adults.[11,14] There is a lack of validated measures of pain in infants. Furthermore, in infants born prematurely, there is essentially no understanding of the pain expression at various stages of premature development. This paucity of knowledge and lack of understanding results in infrequent administration of analgesia or anesthetic agents during a number of painful invasive procedures, including surgery.[4,12,57,111,112]

Theoretical Understanding of Pain in Infants

As pain is a complex subjective experience, its existence must be inferred by others. Several definitions of pain exist,* but many specify that pain is what and where the patient says it is. Obviously infants cannot use language to say that they are in pain (the word infant comes from the Latin *infans,* meaning incapable of speech). Therefore current definitions are not particularly useful in understanding pain in infants, and other ways of looking at pain must be considered. This may be accomplished by considering relevant pain theories that may be applicable to this young age group.

Gate Control Theory

The gate control theory[92,93] is based partly on the accumulation of physiological evidence and partly on assumptions derived from psychological and clinical observations. The physiological basis of this theory is described in detail in Chapter 2.

Melzack[93] describes the three components of pain as intensity, sensory, and affective. Although he acknowledges that intensity is "the salient dimension of pain" (p. 2), he also writes that "describing pain solely in terms of intensity is like specifying the visual world only in terms of light flux without regard to pattern, color, texture, or the many other dimensions of visual experience." As for the evaluative component of pain, Melzack writes, "Pain has a unique, distinctly unpleasant, affective quality that differentiates it from sensory experiences such as sight, hearing, and touch. It becomes overwhelming, demands immediate attention, and disrupts ongoing behavior and thought. To consider only the sensory features of pain and ignore its motivational and affective properties is to look at only part of the problem, and not even the most important part at that" (p. 3).

Aspects of this pain theory require special consideration if applied to the infant because of the limited understanding of early sensory, cognitive, and emotional development. For example, we do not know if newborns and infants experience different sensory features of pain. Is there an unpleasantness about pain that includes the evaluative component? Are infants capable of remembering painful incidents? The answers

* References 16, 61, 72, 87, 95, 122.

to these questions concern the development of specific emotional responses in infants. Although the strength of the gate control theory is its attention to the sensory (neurophysical), perceptual (psychological), and evaluative components of the individual's pain experience, it does not incorporate the development of specific responses in the infant and how these responses would influence his pain experience. Some developmentalists believe that pain, as a specific emotional response, exists from birth[62,127] but others[105,134] find the model of a stress arousal continuum more appropriate for studying pain in infants.

Emotional Specificity Model

Those who support this model believe that pain is a specific emotional response that exists from birth and that there is a particular constellation of facial and/or cry patterns for pain that is unique and discrete from other emotional states. This model proposes that there is survival value in the uniqueness of the cry and facial behaviors; that is, a helpless infant in pain will cry in a particular manner or show a particular face that will signal to the caretaker that he is in pain and needs assistance. In Izard's work,[64] babies showed facial expressions of emotions, including pain, that were identifiable by adults. Their conclusion was that discrete emotional expression exists and can be measured in infants. However, many infants showed blends of expression (e.g., anger and pain) that did not fit the specific constellations of one particular emotion. These blends are problematic clinically because there will still be questions about which emotion the infant is expressing.

Stress-Arousal Model

In the model of stress-arousal,[76] stress is directly associated with arousal. In infants, arousal is reflected in varying states on a continuum from quiet sleep to active wakefulness and finally, crying. The underlying belief of this conceptualization is that the infant's level of arousal depends on the degree of stress. This, in turn, elicits from the caregiver an adaptive response commensurate with the level of infant arousal.[121] Clinically, this conceptualization of infant pain is reflected in increased sympathetic activity (e.g., in increased heart rate) and also behaviorally in increased body movements, facial action, and crying. Not only does the amount of crying increase in this model, but characteristics of the cry that particularly elicit caregiver attention are a reflection of increased innervation to the vocal tract.[47] For example, infants who are stressed from a traumatic birth have cries that are perceived by caregivers as more urgent and arousing. These cries alert the caregiver to attend to them more promptly than nonstressed infants. Cries that are high-pitched, harsh, tense, and perceived as urgent by adult listeners have been reported as characterizing the most stressed state of pain.[39a,67,68,104,134] (See Table 9-1 and section on Behavioral Approaches, Crying.)

Parallel Sensory–Emotional Processing Model

Leventhal and Everhart[78] have proposed a parallel processing model of pain. This model is based on the point of view that emotions contribute to the subjective experience of pain. Their assumption is that processing of the sensory or physical properties of a noxious stimulus occurs at the same time as processing of emotional properties, such as feelings of distress. For example, when an infant is subjected to an acute painful stimulus, it is assumed that parallel processing will lead to observable behavioral outcomes such as crying, facial grimacing, body thrashing, and autonomic responses.[26] This model would ultimately provide for making assessments of the

◆ **Table 9-1**
Infant pain cries

Stimulus situation	Pain cry characteristics	References	Date
Hunger	Arousing	Zeskind et al	1986
Medical problems	Arousing	Boukydis	1985
Immunization	Intense, high pitched, jittery	Johnston and O'Shaughnessy	1988
Immunization	High pitched, tense, harsh	Fuller	1991
Heel lance	High pitched	Grunau and Craig	1987
Circumcision	Intense, high pitched, jittery	Porter, Porges, and Marshall	1988

infant's pain state based on more than one behavioral dimension.[69,102]

Nociception Rather than Pain

After a thorough review of the research on pain in fetuses and newborns, Anand and Hickey[6] suggested that *nociception* may be a more correct word than *pain* when referring to neonates. Nociception is the detection of a painful stimulus in the peripheral nerve endings and the transmission of information of the site of painful stimulation to the brain.[87a] Nociception does not involve the affective or evaluative component of pain. Nociception involves both the nervous system, where pain signals are generated and processed, and the endocrine system, which governs the chemical response to pain signals. Anand and Hickey point out that there is now considerable evidence that the fetal nervous system is sufficiently mature by 20 weeks' postconceptual age to experience nociception. Furthermore, it appears that the neurotransmitters that enhance pain perception are being produced earlier than endogenous opiates, which attenuate nociception. Fetuses may therefore have enhanced nociception or an increased ability to perceive pain.[2]

This notion of enhanced nociception in the neonate is supported by the work of Fitzgerald, Shaw, and MacIntosh.[34] Their study was carried out to increase the understanding of the consequences of excessive handling and pain-producing procedures undergone by preterm infants. The cutaneous flexor reflex has been shown to be particularly well correlated with sensory input[130] and can be evoked only by noxious skin stimulation in adults where, as a defense mechanism, the adult withdraws a limb from an offending stimulus.[115] Fitzgerald et al[34] demonstrated a decreased cutaneous flexor reflex threshold in premature infants less than 30 weeks' gestational age. Clinically, this finding supports the idea that premature infants may, in fact, experience increased nociception given the same stimulus as older infants.

In summary, there are exciting discoveries in the physiological properties of pain and some interesting theoretical prospects in the emotional response to pain in the young infant. For older infants, however, emotional development may precede language development or the ability to label discrete emotions. Pain, with its sensory and affective components, in the way they are described by Melzack,[91] may indeed exist in preverbal children. Dunn[29] reports that infants have developed the capability of intentional crying well before 1 year of age, and Levy[79] reports anticipatory fear of painful stimuli at 6 months of age. Issues related to the development of pain in infants as an experience more complex than nociception, require much greater study to establish a more definitive understanding that would have systematic clinical implications.

◆ ASSESSMENT OF PAIN IN THE INFANT

Assessment and management of pain is of particular importance to all health professionals, especially nurses. Yet nurses experience much ambiguity surrounding the meaning of physiological and behavioral signals given by infants in painful situations. Unfortunately, physiological responses to pain in neonates may not be present or may differ from responses to other stressors in the infant's world. Beyer and Byers[13] suggest that nurses can neither infer pain from signs of autonomic arousal nor rule out pain in the absence of autonomic arousal.

Many myths/misconceptions lead to uncertainty about pain in infants and are often the principal cause of poor assessment and ineffective management. Therefore the exploration of erroneous beliefs about pain and assessment approaches is important to the development of meaningful interventions.

Evidence of Pain in the Neonate

One prevalent myth is that infants do not experience or respond to pain (see Chapter 3). Research in the 1940s has shown that infants respond to cutaneous sensory stimulation during the early weeks of gestation. Gleiss and Stuttgen[45] have further demonstrated that infants have peripheral nerve endings capable of nociception. The density of these nerve endings increases between 26 and 32 weeks' gestation. More recently, Fitzgerald et al[34] have shown that although infants respond to painful stimuli at a slower rate than adults, about one fifth the adult rate, they certainly *do* respond.

The lack of myelinization is another much-quoted reason for the inability of the infant to experience pain. Yet from gate control theory[91,92] it is known that pain impulses are carried by C fibers, which are not myelinated. Therefore the lack of myelinization does not imply lack of function in the peripheral nerves, although the conduction speed of nerves is slower. Considering the shorter distance to the central nervous system in a tiny infant, it appears reasonable that pain messages can be transmitted.

The presence of an immature central nervous system is another common reason given for the infant's inability to experience pain. Yet we now know that neurotransmitters appear as early as 8 to 10 weeks' gestation,[20] and by 20 weeks the cerebral cortex is completely developed, making cutaneous sensory perception possible. Nerve tracts continue to develop between 22 and 30 weeks. Some recent work does suggest that descending pain pathways may not be functionally developed until some time after birth.[33] Premature neonates may therefore be particularly sensitive to aversive procedures because of the immaturity of descending inhibitory pain control mechanisms.

Thus, although it is clear that infants are capable of many physiological and behavioral responses to painful stimuli, these responses differ from those of adults. There is a need for nurses to redefine pain as it is experienced in infants.

The Effect of Pain in Infants

Some clinicians believe that even if the infant does experience pain, the pain will not have any harmful effect. Pain is intimately associated with the stress response and causes elevations in heart rate and blood pressure, plus the release of adrenal stress hormones, which may ultimately lead to protein wasting, mobilization of substrate from energy stores, electrolyte imbalances, and impaired immune function.[73] Anand et al,[6] in a study of infants undergoing patent ductus arteriosis (PDA) ligation procedure, demonstrated that infants who received pain-relieving medication had a much lower incidence of complications than those who received anesthetic alone. In a further study by Anand and Hickey,[7] there was also a higher mortality rate in babies who received less potent analgesia. This study has major importance in suggesting that pain may be harmful to infants when they are vulnerable or in high-risk situations.

In summary, there is evidence to support the assumption that infants experience pain, respond to pain in certain ways, and may suffer needless consequences because of pain. The next step in dispelling the myths/misconceptions about pain in infants and rectifying the current mismanagement of pain in infants, is to better assess their pain.

Assessment of Pain in Infants

Pain assessment in the infant is difficult because of underdeveloped language and comprehension skills, a paucity of measurement tools, and a number of other intervening reactions to stressful situations.[10,72,119] No specific clinical or laboratory parameters have been identified as unique to the pain experience of either adults or children unable to verbalize. Infants have a limited repertoire of responses that serve highly differentiated sensory systems and therefore the absence of a response does not indicate a lack of pain.[38] Pain assessment is further hampered in sick infants or neonates by such factors as gestational age, intubation, restraints, alterations in states of consciousness, and the influence of certain drugs.

Two major approaches to the measurement of pain in infants have been utilized: physiological responses and behavioral responses.* Although many of the measures within these approaches give us some information about the infant in pain, it appears that a multidimensional approach is needed as no single assessment tool has adequate sensitivity and specificity.[102]

A few research studies have incorporated more than one type of measure,[17,69,105] but typically, a single approach such as behavioral (e.g., Grunau and Craig[50]) or physiological (e.g., Williamson and Williamson[129]) has been used to assess pain in the infant.

Physiological Approach

Various physiological indices have been associated with the stress of acute pain in adults, older children, and infants. These physiological reactions all indicate the activation of the sympathetic nervous system and commonly include increases in heart rate, systolic and diastolic blood pressure, respiratory rate, and palmar sweating; decrease in oxygen saturation and vagal tone; and rapid fluctuations in intracranial pressure. Table 9-2 summarizes the results of studies utilizing various physiological parameters.

---

* References 6, 25, 32, 36, 50, 59, 67, 97, 104, 106, 132.

◆ **Table 9-2**
Physiological assessment of infant pain

Measure	Pain Event	Results	Reference
Heart rate	Circumcision	Increase	Owens and Todt, 1984
	Immunization	Brief (6-second) decrease followed by increase of 30 bpm	Johnston and Strada, 1986
	Heel lance	Increase	Field and Goldson, 1984
	Heel lance	Increase	Booth et al, 1989
Vagal tone	Circumcision	Initial increase followed by decrease	Porter et al, 1988
Transcutaneous oxygen	Circumcision	Decrease	Williamson and Williamson, 1983
	Circumcision	Decrease throughout and after procedure	Rawlings et al, 1980
Transcutaneous oxygen	Heel lance	Decrease	High and Gorski, 1985
Palmar sweating	Heel lance	Increase	Harpin and Rutter, 1982
Palmar sweating	Heel lance	Increase	Gedaly-Duff, 1990
	Injection		
Intracranial pressure	Heel lance	Rapid fluctuations	Stevens and Johnston, 1991

Although these physiological measures tend to show consistent results in relation to pain, they are not specific to pain. Furthermore, there is considerable variation among infants, with some showing greater changes than others. The more recently reported measure of palmar sweating needs more investigation before it can be used as a clinical tool.

Hormonal and biochemical changes in response to pain have also been demonstrated in infants undergoing stressful procedures in earlier work[9,53] and more recently by Anand and his colleagues.[4,5,6] The stress response to pain from surgery in newborns (i.e., the relationship to hormonal responses and the subsequent clinical changes; Anand et al,[5,7]) is shown in Figure 9-1.

The most important finding in Anand's work[5,7] is that this stress response can be attenuated by the use of opioid analgesic agents such as fentanyl or sufentanil. Among babies who had received these opioids, there were fewer clinical complications and better recovery from surgery.

Behavioral Approaches

Predictable patterns of behavior in response to acute pain have also been observed in healthy babies and could be utilized as indicators of pain in clinical situations. The behavioral aspects of infant pain that have been studied in the most detail are facial expression, crying, and body movements.

Facial Expression

In the late 1800s, Charles Darwin[28] first described the facial expression of pain in infants. His description included a face that had "eyes firmly closed so that the skin around them is wrinkled, and the forehead is contracted into a frown. The mouth is widely open with the lips retracted in a peculiar manner, which causes it to assume a squarish form, the gums or teeth being more or less exposed" (p. 147).

More than a century later, two other facial expression coding systems that corroborate Darwin's description were proposed.[63,50]

Izard's[63] system is based on scoring of three areas of a still (i.e., photographed) face (brow, eyes, mouth), which represent discrete emotional expressions in particular combinations (see Figure 9-2). The "pain" configuration has the brows

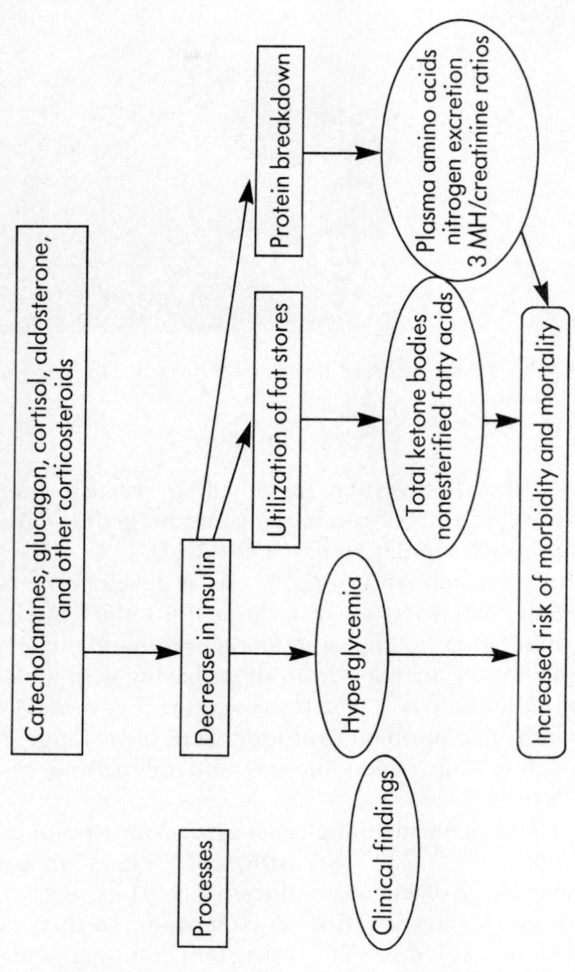

FIGURE 9-1. Hormonal response to pain in infants.

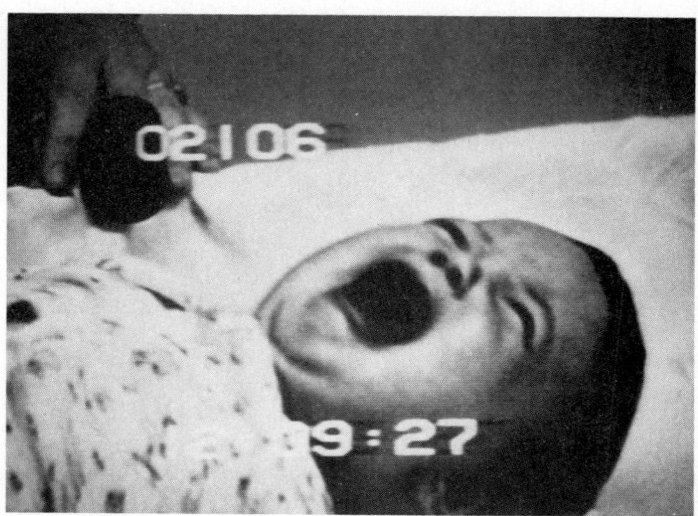

FIGURE 9-2. Facial expression of healthy 4-month-old infant seconds after receiving injection.

lowered and drawn together, bulge and/or vertical furrows between brows, nasal root broadening and bulged, eye fissure tightly closed, and angular squarish mouth.

In contrast, Grunau and Craig[50,51] have developed a facial coding system that is based on facial actions (i.e., a moving face or video). This coding system differentiated newborns who were having an injection from those having gentian violet applied to the umbilicus.[52] The facial actions that most distinguished pain from a nonpain condition were brow bulge, eyes squeezed tightly shut, open mouth, and deepening of the nasolabial furrow.

Recent studies have included facial expression as one index of pain in infants.[25,26,50,51,69] Johnston and Strada,[69] in a multidimensional study of infant pain, found facial expression to be the most consistent response to pain, more so than heart rate or crying, across babies. This consistent response suggests a clinical usefulness to a facial response assessment approach.

Grunau and Craig[50] also examined whether behavioral expression of pain varied with sex and sleep/wake patterns in 140 healthy newborns. Results from this study suggested that awake-alert but inactive infants responded with the most facial activity (see Figure 9-2). Infants in quiet sleep showed the least facial activity and had the longest latency to cry. Most recently, Grunau and Craig[51] studied facial and cry responses to invasive and noninvasive procedures. In this study, significant effects were found for total face activity, latency to facial movement, and latency to cry. It was concluded that facial expression, in combination with short latency to onset of cry, may be a sensitive and specific indicator of pain.

In summary, examining facial expression appears to be a promising way of assessing pain in infants. To date, however, studies have been primarily limited to assessing response to acute pain in healthy children and newborns. There is a need to explore facial expression in high-risk infants and for pain of longer duration before this indicator can be utilized in a wide variety of clinical situations.

Crying

Infants of many species cry or give a distress vocalization in response to painful stimuli. In the past 25 years, cry analysis has been used to augment the diagnosis of medical problems such as chromosomal abnormalities,[125] endocrine disturbances,[99] hyperbilirubinemia,[126] hypoglycemia,[128] asphyxia,[96] bacterial meningitis,[100] herpes simplex virus encephalitis,[128] and hydrocephalus.[97] Cry analysis has also been suggested as a possibility for predicting infants at risk for sudden infant death syndrome (SIDS).[46,48] Cries of infants suffering from fetal malnutrition[71] or fetal growth problems[132] are different from those of low-risk normal infants. Cries may also predict developmental outcome.[76]

The underlying assumption in the interpretation of cries of normal and abnormal infants is that cry production is a result of complex physiological mechanisms and that the lack of neurological integrity will result in abnormal vocalizations.[47] Following this assumption, it could be thought that pain might induce sufficient stress so that the normal infant becomes briefly disorganized physiologically and produces an atypical high-pitched cry. Crying can be considered a graded signal that reflects the continuum of an infant's state of arousal. The extent of the arousal is reflected in the cry, and this degree of arousal is also perceived by the caregiver.[134] Caregivers may use the gradations of the cry and the context in which the level of arousal occurs (e.g., feeding) to define the baby's emotional state.[105]

The analysis of infant crying is improved by the use of spectrographic or visual representations of the cries (see Figure 9-3). Spectrographs can be created rapidly by computers, and some features can be computer derived, but others still require subjective visual examination.

Parameters of infant crying that have been studied fall into the domains and categories described in Table 9-3.

The original cry research was pioneered by a Scandinavian group.[128] Since that time, other studies have compared pain cries with other types of cries (see Table 9-4).

Although a specific, absolutely identifiable pain cry does not seem to exist any more than an absolutely identifiable facial expression of pain, the features that would characterize the most stressed state (i.e., pain) along a stress-arousal continuum are a cry that is high-pitched, tensed, harsh or non-voiced, and intense.[67]

Body Movements

McGraw[90] first described body movements in response to pain from pinstick. More recently, Craig, McMahon, Morrison, and Zaskow,[22] in studying infants and toddlers from 2 to 24 months of age receiving routine immunization, corroborated earlier work by McGraw[90] that the incidence of anticipatory fear and touching of the site increased with age. They also reported kicking and thrashing of legs and a rigid torso as part of the body response to pain exhibited by most of the children. Johnston and Strada,[69] using the scoring system of Craig et al,[22] described an initial extension and tensing of limbs and torso followed by flexion and thrashing of limbs after immunization in 2-month to 4-month babies.

In an additional study using precise measures of newborn body movement after heelstick, Franck[36] was able to quantify body response to acute pain. She observed the presence of a swiping movement by the unaffected leg against the affected leg in 7 of the 10 babies. This movement may reflect the infants' attempts to touch the affected site. This ability had not previously been observed in such young infants.

In summary, the assessment of infant pain appears to be still underdeveloped. It does not seem appropriate to assess only one aspect of a complex phenomenon such as pain, because no single approach captures the response or is spe-

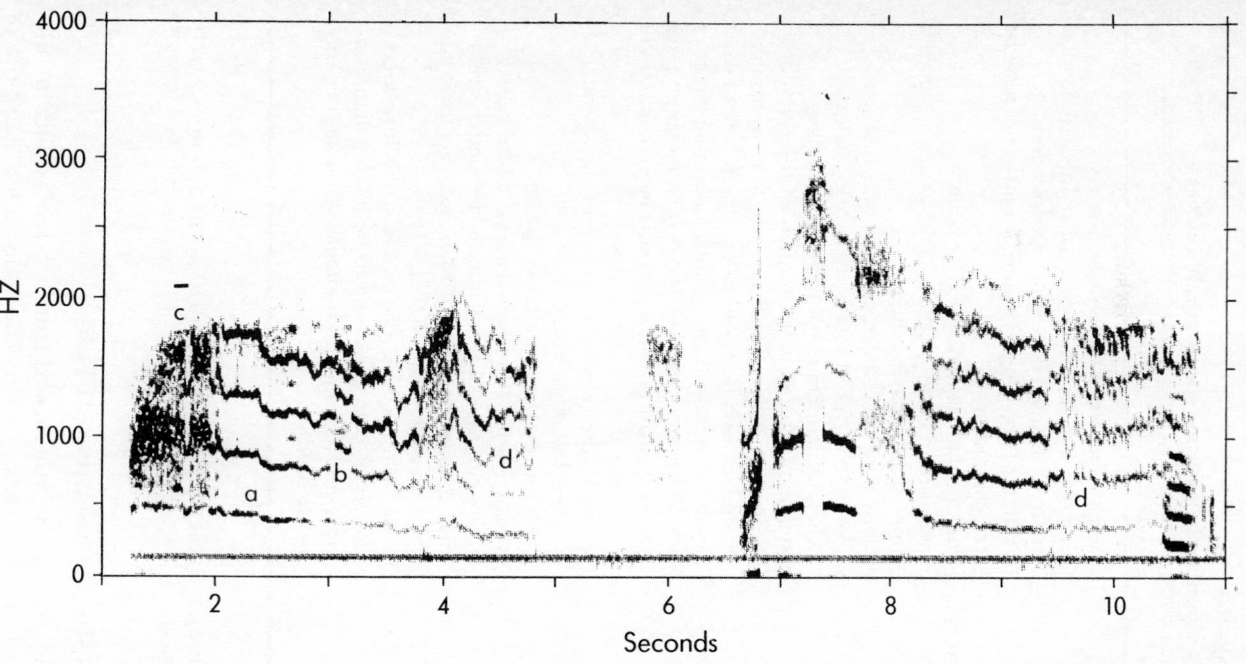

FIGURE 9-3. Spectrograph of infant pain cry. *a*, F_O is seen as bottom line; *b*, melody is falling; *c*, dysphonia; *d*, jitter.

◆ **Table 9-3**
Cry characteristics from spectograph analyses

Domain	Features
Time	Latency: time from stimulus to first cry
	Duration of cry episode: bout of crying with less than 30 seconds between cry expirations
	Duration of cry: length of time sound is heard from cry expiration
Frequency	Fundamental frequency (F_0) or pitch: measure of cycles per second (Hz) and is heard as how high or low pitched
	Melody pattern: changes in pitch over one cry expiration; typical infant cry is rising-falling, whereas pain cry tends to be flat or falling
	Phonation: reflects the periodicity of the cry and is heard as a continuum from pure tone to harsh soundless hiss or dysphonia: pain cries tend to sound more harsh and grating than nonpain cries
	Jitter or vibrato: rapid up and down change in pitch; this is heard as shakiness and is more common in pain cries than nonpain cries
	Tenseness: the relative frequency of the sound energy; the more energy at higher frequencies, the more tense the cry
	Formants: areas of frequency range which reflect resonance of the vocal tract; an infant under stress may change the shape of the vocal tract and thus the formants
Intensity	Measured in decibels (db) and heard as how loud the cry is; pain cries tend to be louder than nonpain cries, assuming an infant has enough energy to cry loudly

cific enough. Rather a multidimensional approach needs to be developed.

Nursing Assessment of Pain

Craig, Grunau, Whitfield, and Linton[21] have studied neonatal nurses' assessments of pain. They concluded that 90% of infants were evaluated by their primary nurse as having some pain during the nurse's shift. They also stated that the most

◆ **Table 9-4**
Comparison of infant pain cries with other infant cries

Pain cry characteristics	Reference
Higher pitched, more intense than anger or fear	Johnston and O'Shaughnessy, 1988
More intense in higher frequencies than hunger	Fuller and Horii, 1988
Higher pitched, more intense during invasive part of circumcision procedure	Porter et al, 1986
Lower pitched than hunger	Zeskind et al, 1985
More intense than hunger or fussiness, same tenseness as hunger	Fuller, 1991

commonly reported signs of pain were attempts to cry, facial grimacing, body movements, hypoxia, color changes, increased heart rate, respiration, tachypnea, tachycardia, and bradycardia. Nurses can and do interpret the presence of physiological and behavioral changes, such as tachycardia, high-pitched crying, facial grimacing, and limb thrashing, in combination with contextual cues, such as procedures, as indications of the infant's pain state. If a nurse goes through a mental checklist, noting behavioral as well as physiological parameters, then she will be in a better position to answer the question of whether the infant is in pain. Caution should be used, however, in using a checklist. At this time, there is no available, valid checklist, although current research is promising.

Knowledge of the normal developmental or maturational process of premature and term infants is useful when assessing pain. Infant development tools, such as the Brazelton neonatal assessment scale, have been used to monitor behavioral changes of the baby during painful procedures.[86]

Individualized parameters for assessing pain should be established based on the infant's behavioral and physiological responses, age, and underlying condition. Once these parameters are chosen, they should be used as a basis for frequent evaluation and should be included in a nursing care plan. In this way, perceptions about an infant's response to and tolerance of painful stimuli will be supported by clinical evidence. Documentation of the individual parameters should be specific and as precise as possible. The usual narrative format of nursing documentation does not reflect identification of trends or changes in patterns of parameters used to assess pain.[38] An alternative may be the use of a pain flow sheet.[118] This instrument can provide a concise summary of information related to the child's pain experience across time. If kept in an accessible location, a pain flow sheet can provide the needed basis for multidisciplinary communication related to the ongoing management of the infant's pain.

◆ MANAGEMENT OF PAIN IN INFANTS

Management of pain in infants is controversial and has often been inadequate and sparse. The results of a survey presented to the Association of Pediatric Anaesthetists in March, 1986, showed that although 85% of those surveyed believed that newborn babies felt pain, only about 5% used opioid analgesics, and few used local anesthetic blocks on any regular basis.

Recent attention has focused on the issue of infant pain and reports of babies undergoing surgery without benefit of anesthesia.[116] Concern over this practice has prompted the American Academy of Pediatrics to issue a statement regarding the use of anesthesia for neonates.[1] In addition, Booker[18] pleads that, assuming that babies do experience pain, we do all we can to decrease their suffering by providing postoperative analgesia and supporting research into new and safe methods of effective analgesia.

There are two major categories of pain managment, pharmacological and nonpharmacological. Although there is little research in either area in infants, what is known will be reviewed under these categories.

Pharmacological Approach

Research has consistently demonstrated that children receive few opioids postoperatively[30,120] and fewer analgesic medications than adults after the same type of surgery.[15,30,109]

In a more recent and broader survey of pain management in neonatal intensive care units across North America, Franck[37] found that medication was ranked sixth in methods used to manage infant pain. Medication was rated behind such methods as pacifier, position changes, and tactile stimulation.

The use of analgesic medication was rated as "none" or "rare" in 44% of the units with infants undergoing major abdominal surgery and 83% of units with infants undergoing PDA repairs. Koh[74] refers to an even lower level of analgesic treatment in other parts of the world. Major reasons given for this undermedication of infants are the lack of valid, sensitive, standardized approaches to measure the effects of the management strategy, the fears of addiction and respiratory depression, and the lack of knowledge concerning the physiological effects of opiate pain relief in neonates.

Recent studies have been directed at the use of opiates in infants. The national survey by Franck[37] indicated that this approach is correct since the most widely used drug in neonatal units surveyed was morphine, followed by meperidine; acetaminophen was only third. Other drugs utilized for pain relief included fentanyl and chloral hydrate.

The effect of opioid pain relief on infant outcomes has not been studied until recently. In a landmark study by Anand et al,[7] a randomized clinical trial of fentanyl anesthesia in conjunction with nitrous oxide and curare versus nitrous oxide and curare without fentanyl in infants undergoing PDA repair demonstrated a significant decrease in the stress response in the fentanyl group. Most notably, there were postoperative complications in the control group but none in the fentanyl group. After these findings, three groups of infants scheduled for cardiac surgery were randomly assigned to receive: (1) halothane (nonanalgesic anesthetic) intraoperatively and morphine postoperatively, (2) sufentanil intraoperatively and morphine postoperatively, or (3) sufentanil both intraoperatively and postoperatively.[7] Results of this study corroborated the earlier findings. More importantly, the mortality rate in the halothane-morphine group was at the expected level (30%) but there were no deaths in the sufentanil groups. The work of Anand and his colleagues demonstrates that stress response in infants undergoing cardiac surgery can be attenuated by management with opioids.

Morphine

Morphine is the standard for analgesia against which all other opioids are measured.[131] Although morphine kinetics have been studied in infancy[74a,82] and throughout the childhood years,[124] the effects of morphine administration on newborn infants have not been studied until recently.

Infants 1 month of age or older appear to have clearance levels of opioids at least equivalent to those of adults.[82] Therefore concerns about the use of opioids in infants 1 month of age or older should be similar to concerns nurses have for adults who are unable to communicate verbally.

In infants less than 1 month of age, however, a prolonged elimination half-life and decreased clearance of morphine has been reported.[24,81,82,124] Thus these very young infants will attain higher serum concentrations with continuous infusions that will decline more slowly with discontinuation of the infusion. These physiological differences may account for the increased sensitivity to respiratory depression that is also seen in infants less than 1 month of age.[70,82] Possible explanations for this increased sensitivity in young infants may be related to differences in opiate receptors and/or the blood brain barrier as well as the pharmacokinetics of the drug.[131]

These young infants should not be denied the benefit of opioid analgesia, but they do require closer monitoring. If an infant requires opioid analgesia outside an intensive care unit or recovery room, the use of an apnea monitor will assist nurses in monitoring the infant's respiratory rate. If respirations decrease, then the infant's condition and dose of the drug should be carefully reassessed before administration of the next dose of the drug.

The use of morphine and other opioid analgesics also causes concern about the risks of psychological and physiological addiction. Studies of opioid addiction in infancy have concentrated primarily on the phenomenon of perinatal addiction and infrequently address iatrogenic habituation to opioid analgesics.[35,83,94] Although this issue requires further research, it should not preclude the use of opioids when their use is warranted.[110]

Meperidine

Meperidine (Demerol) is a synthetic opioid that is commonly used for infants preoperatively in preparation for anesthesia or as a treatment for postoperative pain. It is a potent analgesic with pharmacokinetic properties similar to those of morphine. The most significant difference between meperidine and other opioid analgesics is the production of the metabolite normeperidine, as discussed in Chapter 7.

Fentanyl

Fentanyl is another frequently used potent opioid agent that until recently was used most commonly as an anesthetic for neonatal surgery.[108,131] Fentanyl and its analogs are now often used as an analgesic agent for short procedures, such as bone marrow aspiration, because of its rapid onset and brief duration of action. A potential side effect of fentanyl is chest muscle rigidity, which is most commonly observed after high bolus doses of the drug are administered.[131] This effect may make respiration/ventilation difficult or impossible. However, it can be reversed through the administration of muscle relaxants, such as pancuronium bromide, or an opioid antagonist such as naloxone.[1a,44]

Slower clearance and longer elimination half-life have also been reported with the use of fentanyl[65] and sufentanil in the neonatal period,[49] which like other narcotics produce problems for the infant under 1 month of age. Conversely, the greater clearance of fentanyl in infants older than 3 months results in lower plasma concentration and may allow these babies to tolerate more drug without respiratory depression.[58,117]

Nonopioid and Adjuvant Drugs

Nonopioid drugs (such as acetylsalicylic acid (aspirin) and acetaminophen) play a limited role in pain relief in infants and, according to Franck's 1987 survey,[37] rate lower in usage than opioid drugs. Acetaminophen (which is available in liquid and rectal suppositories) is a common over-the-counter preparation that is often used for mild pain in infants. Acetylsalicylic acid is rarely used because of concerns of the development of Reye's syndrome in children with viral infections and its adverse effects on platelet aggregation. It might be used in preference to acetaminophen when its antiinflammatory properties are desired, as in rare instances of arthritis in infants.

Other groups of medications are often used with neonates to assist the opioid analgesics in pain control or to moderate activity and excitement, promote drowsiness or sleep, and decrease anxiety. Drugs used for this purpose fall into the categories of barbiturates, benzodiazepines, and miscellaneous agents, including sedatives such as chloral hydrate, phenothiazides such as chlorpromazine, antihistamines, and CNS depressants. With the exception of chlorpromazine, which has a weak potentiating analgesic effect, the use of these drugs has generally not been shown to provide pain relief.

Nurses are in an excellent position to assist other health professionals and families to overcome their concerns and hesitancies about using opioid analgesics to manage pain in infants. Although physicians prescribe the medications, it is often nurses who suggest what drugs to give and when and how often to administer them. If nurses can learn to recognize the infant's pain cues and teach parents to recognize and report them, the delay between the onset of pain and its relief can be minimized. Since analgesics are most effective when given before pain reaches its peak, the use of regular interval doses or continuous IV infusion of opioid analgesics is highly recommended.

Nonpharmacological Approach

There have been several reports of nonpharmacological measures used by pediatric and neonatal intensive care nurses to manage pain in the infant. These include positioning and swaddling; holding and rocking; providing tactile stimulation, music, vocalization, diaper changes, nourishment, and pacifiers; and decreasing environmental stimulation.[27,31,37,85,113] Few studies, however, have scientifically evaluated the effectiveness of these simple, noninvasive, and inexpensive approaches to diminishing pain in infants. Table 9-5 lists some of the interventions that have been studied.

When simple and brief procedures, such as heelstick, are carried out on infants, it is possible that nonpharmacological approaches may help decrease the infant's pain or perhaps assist in coping with that pain. It is unlikely, however, that these procedures alone would be sufficient to deal with the more intense and prolonged pain associated with lumbar punctures, bone marrow aspirations, chest-tube insertions, surgery, or circumcision.[85a] More research is required on the effectiveness of nonpharmacological approaches alone and in combination with other nonpharmacological and pharmaco-

◆ **Table 9-5**
Nonpharmacological interventions to control pain in infants

Intervention	Pain situation	Observed outcome	Reference
Pacifier	Postcircumcision	Decreased HR	Gunnar et al, 1981
	Heel lance	Decreased HR	Field and Goldson, 1984
Carrying	Normal crying	Decreased crying	Hunziker and Barr, 1986
Music	Circumcision	Less increase in HR	Marchette et al, 1989
Transcutaneous electrical nerve stimulation (TENS)	Arterial puncture	Less increase in HR	Froese-Fretz, 1990
Sucrose	Heel lance	Decreased crying	Blass and Hoffmeyer, 1991
	Circumcision		
Music, pacifier intrauterine sounds	Circumcision	No change in physiological parameters	Marchette et al, 1991

logical methods to increase knowledge of pain reduction in infants and neonates.

Implications for Nursing Infants in Pain

For nurses in neonatal and newborn environments, assessment and management of infant pain represents a monumental challenge. As Franck[38] states:

"Relief of suffering is a major goal of nursing care. Nurses caring for nonverbal patients must develop specialized skills needed to assess pain and communicate their assessments to other nurses, physicians, and parents. Through collaborative efforts, pain relief for these patients can be achieved" (p. 65).

The assessment of infant pain through physiological, biochemical, and behavioral approaches has been reviewed in detail in this chapter. With increased knowledge of pain indicators, nurses can accurately collect data on pertinent cues during stress-producing situations. In piecing this data together nurses can begin to develop an overview of how a particular infant responds to pain.

In the short term, untreated pain may result in an acute stress response that may have many harmful effects for the infant, and thus the nurse caring for the infant needs to protect him from needless stress.

The long-term effects of infant pain must also be considered by the nurse. According to Tyson,[123] there is growing belief that a baby's initial experiences may affect the development of attitudes, fears, anxieties, conflicts, wishes, expectations, and patterns of interaction with others. It may well be that nurses who understand the long-term effects of pain can contribute to the medical and development status of the newborn by minimizing or alleviating their painful experiences.[110]

Nurses and physicians often share feelings of frustration stemming from the apparent lack of interest shown by each other in assessing or managing the infant's pain. Each group may have biases and misconceptions about infant pain and about the other's ability to accurately assess and manage it. These impediments can only be changed through optimal communication, education, and research about the responses of infants to pain. Accurate and precise assessment of the physiological and behavioral parameters in objective terms can enhance nurses' credibility and successful communication with the physician concerning pain management. If the physician is reluctant to prescribe analgesia, the nurse may suggest a trial (e.g., for 24 to 48 hours) treatment to determine whether the treatment produced any improvement in the pain. The health professionals involved should agree on specific assessment parameters. If medication is prescribed, nurses must take responsibility to ensure that the appropriate dose of analgesia is administered on a regular basis (not prn), not only to treat observable pain but also to prevent pain from reaching maximum intensity. Clearly defined evaluation criteria for the infant's response to analgesia will serve to minimize the effects of multiple caregivers and the "yo-yo" effect resulting from frequently changing medication orders.[38]

Parents are also very concerned about the pain that their infants may be experiencing during invasive procedures. This concern has been evident in the recent publication of reports by parents who believe that their infant's suffering did not receive adequate attention from the medical profession.[75] Networks have been established between parents and professionals concerned about painful procedures that take place in the NICU environment. Parents are being encouraged to ask whether particular procedures will be painful and what pain management measures will be employed.[55,56] Butler[19] has also developed a list of questions for parents and health professionals to use to heighten awareness of infant pain at local health care institutions.

Parents are often very anxious about the perceived pain that their infant may endure and are only too aware of his dependence on his caregivers. Parents need to know of the sincere intent of those caring for their child to minimize infant suffering. They must also be encouraged to voice their feelings and concerns about their infant's pain experience and concerns about the competence of caregivers involved in managing their child's pain.

Parents are often particularly anxious about their infant receiving opioid drugs because of intense media attention to addiction and/or tolerance. Nurses may need to convince parents of the necessity of these analgesics to diminish pain.

Generally, parents should be included in discussions concerning assessment and management of their child's pain (or potential pain) with health care professionals. Parents have the right to withold consent for invasive procedures if they are not satisfied with the use of pain prevention or reduction measures. If parents participate in discussions of their child's pain and its management, they are better equipped to assist with comfort measures and the ongoing evaluation of the pain experience. More important, they become perhaps the best advocate for their child.

◆ SUMMARY

There is evidence that infants and neonates do experience pain and that the associated stress of a painful experience may have both short-term and long-term effects. Although knowledge of assessment and management of infant pain lags that in other age groups, there has been a recent burgeoning of research and literature aimed at increasing this knowledge.[8,89]

Clinicians have the daily dilemma of managing the infant in pain and often struggle with personal biases, myths and misconceptions, a lack of reliable and valid assessment tools, controversial management approaches, and ineffectual collaboration among health professionals and parents.

The need to reduce pain in infants so that they can grow and develop without using their energies for coping with the pain is basic. As Lucretius[80] wrote in the first century BC, "Nature cries aloud for nothing else but that pain may be kept far sundered from the body, and that, withdrawn from care and fear, she may enjoy in mind the sense of pleasure."

REFERENCES

1. American Academy of Pediatrics Committees on Fetus and Newborn and Drugs, Sections on Anesthesiology and Surgery (1987). *Neonat Anesth Ped,* 80, 446.

1a. American Academy of Pediatrics, Naloxone dosage and route of administration for infants and children: addendum to emergency drug doses for infants and children (1990). *Peds* 86, 484–485.

2. Anand KJS. (July 1990). Pain and its effects on the human neonate. Paper presented at the First International Symposium on Pediatric Pain, Seattle.

3. Anand KJS. (June 1989). Pain in the neonate: myths and realities. Keynote address at the First European Conference on Pain in Children, Maastricht, The Netherlands.

4. Anand KJS and Aynsley-Green A. (1988). Measuring the severity of surgical stress in newborn infants. *J Pediatr Surg, 23,* 297-305.

5. Anand KJS, Brown RC, Causon RC, et al. (1985). Can the human neonate mount an endocrine and metabolic response to surgery? *J Pediatr Surg, 20,* 41-48.

6. Anand KJS and Hickey PR. (1987a). Pain and its effects in the human neonate and fetus. *N Engl J Med, 317,* 1321-1347.

7. Anand KJS and Hickey PR. (1987b). Randomized trial of high-dose sufentanil anesthesia in neonates undergoing cardiac surgery: effects on the metabolic stress response. *Anesthesiology, 67,* 502A.
8. Anand KJS and McGrath PJ. (In press) *Pain in infants.* Amsterdam: Elsevier.
9. Anders TF, Sachar EJ, Kream J, Roffmarg H, and Hellman L. (1971). Behavioral state and plasma cortical response in the human newborn. *Pediatrics, 46,* 530-537.
10. Aradine CR, Beyer JE, and Tompkins JM. (1988). Children's pain perceptions before and after analgesia: a study of instrument construct validity and related issues. *J Pediatr Nurs, III*(I), 11-23.
11. Barr RG. (1982). Pain tolerance and development change in pain perception. In Levine MD, Carey WB, Crocker AC, and Gross RT (eds), *Developmental behavioral pediatrics* (pp. 505-511). Philadelphia: WB Saunders.
12. Bettes EK and Downes JJ. (1984). Anesthetic considerations in newborn surgery. *Semin Anesth, 3,* 59-74.
13. Beyer J and Byers ML. (1985). Knowledge of pediatric pain: state of the art. *Child Health Care, 13,* 150-159.
14. Beyer JE and Levin CR. (1987). Issues and advances in pain control in children. *Nurs Clin North Am, 22,* 661-676.
15. Beyer JE, DeGood D, Ashley L, and Russell GA. (1983). Patterns of post operative analgesic use with adults and children following cardiac surgery. *Pain, 17,* 71-81.

15a. Blass EM and Hoffmeyer LB. (1991). Sucrose as an analgesic for newborn infants. *Peds* 87, 215-218.

16. Bond MR. (1984). *Pain: its nature, analysis and treatment.* London: Churchill Livingstone.
17. Booth JC, McGrath PA, Brigham MC, Frewen TC, and Whittall S. (1989, June). Pain in infants: distress responses to repeated noxious stimuli. Paper presented at the First European Conference on Pain in Children. Maastricht, the Netherlands.
18. Booker PD. (1987). Postoperative analgesia for neonates (Editorial). *Anaesthesia, 42,* 343-345.
19. Butler NC (1988). How to raise professional awareness of the need for adequate pain relief for infants. *Birth, 15*(1), 38-41.
20. Charnay Y. (1989, June). Ontogenesis of some peptidergic neuronal systems in the human spinal cord: a morphological approach. Paper presented at the First European Conference on Pain in Children, Maastricht, The Netherlands.
21. Craig KD, Grunau RVE, Whitfield MF, and Linton J. (1989, June). Neonatal intensive care: nurses' evaluation of pain. Paper presented at the First European Conference on Pain in Children, Maastricht, The Netherlands.
22. Craig KD, McMahon RJ, Morison JD, and Zaskow C. (1984). Developmental changes in infant pain expression during immunization injections. *Soc Sci Med, 19,* 1331-1337.
23. Deleted in proofs.
24. Dahlstrom B, Bolme P, Feychting H, Noack G, and Paalzow L. (1979). Morphine kinetics in children. *Clin Pharmacol Ther, 26,* 354.
25. Dale JC. (1986). A multidimensional study of infants' responses to painful stimuli. *Pediatr Nurs, 12*(7), 27-31.

26. Dale JC. (1989). A multidimensional study of infants' behaviors associated with assumed painful stimuli: phase II. *J Pediatr Health Care, 3,* 34-38.
27. D'Apolito K. (1984). The neonate's response to pain. *Am J Mat Child Nurs, 9,* 256-257.
28. Darwin CR. (1872). *The expression of emotion in man and animals.* Chicago: The University of Chicago Press, 1965.
29. Dunn J. (1977). *Distress and comfort.* Cambridge: Harvard University Press.
30. Eland JM and Anderson JE. (1977). The experience of pain in children. In Jacox AK (ed), *Pain: a source book for nurses and other health professionals.* Boston: Little, Brown.
31. Field T and Goldson E. (1984). Pacifying effects of nonnutritive sucking on term and preterm neonates during heelstick procedures. *Pediatrics, 74,* 1012-1015.
32. Fisicelli VR, Karelitz RM, Fisicelli RM, and Cooper J. (1974). The course of induced crying activity in the first year of life. *Pediatr Res, 8,* 921-928.
33. Fitzgerald M and Kotzenburg M. (1986). The functional development of descending inhibitory pathways in the dorsolateral funiculus of the newborn rat spinal cord. *Dev Brain Res, 24,* 261-270.
34. Fitzgerald M, Shaw A, and MacIntosh N. (1988). The postnatal development of the cutaneous flexor reflex: a comparative study in premature infants and rat pups. *Dev Med Child Neurol, 30,* 520-526.
35. Flandermeyer AA. (1987). A comparison of the effects of heroin and cocaine abuse upon the neonate. *Neonat Net, 6,* 42-47.
36. Franck LS. (1986). A new method to quantitatively describe pain behavior in infants. *Nurs Res, 35,* 28-31.
37. Franck LS. (1987). A national survey of the assessment and treatment of pain and agitation in the neonatal intensive care unit. *J Ob Gyn Neonat Nurs, 16,* 387-393.
38. Franck LS. (1989). Pain in the nonverbal patient: advocating for the critically ill neonate. *Pediatr Nurs, 15*(1), 65-68.
39. Froese-Fretz A. (1990). The use of a transcutaneous electrical nerve stimulator (TENS) to decrease the pain associated with arterial punctures in newborn infants. Poster presented at the First International Symposium on Pediatric Pain, Seattle.

39a. Fuller BF. (1991). Acoustic discrimination of three types of infant cries. *Nurs Res* 40:156-160.

40. Fuller BF and Horii Y. (1988). Spectral energy distribution in four types of infant vocalizations. *J Com Dis, 21,* 111-127.
41. Fuller BF, Conner DA, and Horii Y. (1990). Potential acoustic measures of infant pain and arousal. In Tyler DC and Krane EJ (eds), *Advances in pain research and therapy* (vol. 15, pp. 137-145). New York: Raven Press, Ltd.
42. Gedaly-Duff V. (1989). Palmar sweat index (PSI) use with children in pain research, *J Pediatr Nurs, 4,* 3-8.
43. Gillies FJ, Shankle W, and Dooling EC. (1983). Myelinated tracts: growth patterns. In Gillies FJ, Leviton A, and Dooling EC (eds), *The developing human brain: growth and epidemiologic neuropathy.* Boston: John Wright.
44. Gilman AG et al. (1985). *Goodman and Gilman's the pharmacological basis of therapeutics* (ed 7). Toronto: Collier MacMillan Canada.

45. Gleiss J and Stuttgen G. (1970). Morphologic and functional development of the skin. In Stave U (ed), *Physiology of the perinatal period* (vol 2, pp. 889-906). New York: Appleton-Century-Crofts.
46. Golub HL. (May/June 1988). Interview with Steven Nadis. *Tech Rev MIT.*
47. Golub HL and Corwin MJ. (1985). A physioacoustic model of the infant cry. In Lester BM and Boukydis C (eds), *Infant crying: theoretical and research perspectives* (pp. 59-82). New York: Plenum Press.
48. Golub HL and Corwin MJ. (1982). Infant cry: a clue to diagnosis. *J Pediatr Surg, 69,* 197-201.
49. Greeley WJ and deBruijn NP. (1987). Changes in sufentanil pharmacokinetics within the neonatal period. *Anesth Analg, 66,* 1067-1072.
50. Grunau RVE and Craig KD. (1987). Pain expression in neonates: facial action and cry. *Pain, 28,* 395-410.
51. Grunau RVE and Craig KD. (1990). Facial activity as a measure of neonatal pain expression. In Tyler DC and Krane EJ (eds), *Advances in pain research and therapy* (pp. 147-155). New York: Raven Press.
52. Grunau RVE, Johnston CC, and Craig KD. (1990). Facial and cry responses to invasive and non-invasive procedures in neonates. *Pain 42,* 295-305.
53. Gunnar ME, Fisch RO, Korsvik S, and Donhowe JM. (1981). The effects of circumcision on serum cortisol and behavior. *Psychoneuroendocrinology, 6,* 269-275.
54. Harpin VA and Rutter N. (1982). Development of emotional sweating in the newborn infant. *Arch Dis Child, 57,* 691-695.
55. Harrison H. (1983). *The premature baby book.* New York: St. Martin's Press.
56. Harrison H. (1987). Pain relief for premature infants. *Twins, July/August,* 10, 11, 53.
57. Hatch DJ. (1987). Analgesia in the neonate. *Br Med J, 284,* 920.
58. Hertzka RE, Fisher DM, Gauntlett IS, and Spellman M. Are infants sensitive to respiratory depression from fentanyl? (Absract). *Anesthesiology, 67,* A512.
58a. High A and Gorski PA. (1985). Recording environmental influences on infant development in the ICN: womb for improvement. In Gottfield A and Gaiter JL (eds), *Infants stress under intensive care,* Baltimore: University Park Press.
59. Hindmarsh KW, Sankaran K, and Watson VG. (1984). Plasma beta-endorphine concentrations in neonates associated with acute stress. *Dev Pharm Ther, 7,* 198-204.
60. Hunziker UA and Barr RG. (1986). Increased carrying reduces infant crying: a randomized controlled trial. *Pediatrics, 77,* 641-648.
61. International Association for the Study of Pain, Subcommittee on Taxonomy. (1979). Pain terms: a list with definitions and notes on usage. *Pain, 6,* 249-252.
62. Izard CE. (1982). *Measuring emotions in infants and children.* Cambridge: Cambridge University Press.
63. Izard CE. *The maximally discriminative facial movement coding system (MAX).* (1979). Newark, NJ: University of Delaware Instructional Resources Center.
64. Izard CE, Huebner RR, Risser D, McGinnes GC, and Dougherty LM. (1980). The young infant's ability to produce discrete emotional expressions. *Dev Psychol, 16,* 132-140.

65. Johnson KL, Erickskon JP, Holley FO, and Scott JC. (1984). Fentanyl pharmacokinetics in the pediatric population. (Abstract). *Anesthesiology, 61,* A441.
66. Johnston CC. (July 1988). Infant crying: in search of the pain template. Paper presented at the First International Symposium on Pediatric Pain, Seattle.
67. Johnston CC. (1989). Pain assessment and management in infants. *Pediatrician, 16,* 16-23.
68. Johnston CC and O'Shaughnessy D. (1988). Acoustical attributes of pain cries: distinguishing features. In Dubner R, Gebbart GF, and Bond MR. (eds), *Advances in pain research and therapy* (pp. 336-340). Vol 5. New York: Raven Press.
69. Johnston CC and Strada ME. (1986). Acute pain response in infants: a multidimensional description. *Pain, 24,* 373-382.
70. Johnstone RE, Jobes DR, Kennell EM, Behar MG, and Smith TC. (1974). Reversal of morphine anesthesia with naloxone. *Anesthesiology, 41,* 361-367.
71. Juntanen K, Sirvo P, and Michelsson K. (1978). Cry analysis of infants with severe malnutrition. *Eur J Pediatr, 128,* 241-246.
72. Katz ER, Kellerman J, and Siegel SE. (1981). Anxiety as an effective focus in the clinical study of acute behavioral distress. *J Consult Clin Psychol, 49*(3), 470-471.
73. Kehlet H. (1986). Pain relief and modification of the stress response. In Cousins MJ and Phillips GD. (eds), *Acute pain management* (pp. 49-75). New York: Churchill Livingstone.
74. Koh THHG. (1987). Anesthesia and analgesia in newborn babies and infants. *Lancet, i,* 1090.
74a. Koren G, Butt W, Chinyanga H, Soldin S, Tan Y, and Pape K. (1985). Postoperative morphine infusion in newborn infants: assessment of disposition characteristics and safety. *J Pediatr, 1:7,* 963-967.
75. Lawson JR. (1987, October 31). Letter to the editor. *Lancet,* 1033.
76. Lester BM. (1984). A biosocial model of infant crying. In Lipsitt LP (ed), *Advances in infancy research,* Vol 3 (pp. 167-212). Norwood, NJ: Ablex.
77. Lester BM and Zeskind PS. (1979). The organization and assessment of crying in the infant at risk. In Field TM, Sostek AM, Goldberg S, and Shuman HH (eds), *Infants born at risk* (pp. 121-144). New York: Spectrum.
78. Leventhal H and Everhart D. (1979). Emotion, pain, and physical illness. In Izard CE (ed), *Emotions in personality and psychopathology* (pp. 263-335). New York: Plenum.
79. Levy DM. (1960). The infant's earliest memory of innoculation: a contribution to public health procedures. *J Genet Psychol, 96,* 3-46.
80. Lucretius. (1952). The nature of things (translated by Munro HAJ). *Great Books of the Western World,* Vol 12. Chicago: University of Chicago Press.
81. Lynn AM, Opheim KE, and Taylor DC. (1984). Morphine infusion after pediatric cardiac surgery. *Crit Care Med, 12,* 863.
82. Lynn AM and Slattery JT. (1987). Morphine pharmacokinetics in early infancy. *Anesthesiology, 66,* 136-139.
82a. McGrath PA. (1990). *Pain in children: nature, assessment, and management*, New York: Guilford Press.
83. Maguire DP and Maloney P. (1988). A comparison of fentanyl and morphine use in neonates. *Neonat Net, 7,* 27-31.

84. Maloni JA, Stegman CE, Taylor PM, and Brownell CA. (1986). Validation of infant behavior identified by neonatal nurses. *Nurs Res, 35,* 133-138.

85. Marchette L, Main R, and Redick E. (1989). Pain reduction during neonatal circumcision. *Pediatr Nurs, 15*(2), 207-210.

85a. Marchette L, Main R, Redick E, Bagg A and Leatherland J. (1991). Pain reduction interventions during neonatal circumcision. *Nurs Res* 40:241-244.

86. Marshall RE, Stratton WC, Moore JA, and Boxerman SB. (1980). Circumcision: effects on newborn behavior. *Infant Behav Dev, 3*(2), 1-14.

87. McCaffery M. (1972). *Nursing management of the patient with pain.* Philadelphia: Lippincott.

87a. McGrath PA. (1990). *Pain in children: nature, assessment, and management,* New York: Guildford Press.

88. McGrath PJ and Johnson GC. (1988). Pain management in children. *Can J Anesth, 35,* 107-110.

89. McGrath PJ and Unruh AM. (1987). *Pain in children and adolescents.* New York: Elsevier.

90. McGraw MB. (1941). Neural maturation as exemplified in the changing reactions of the infant in pin prick. *Child Dev, 12,* 31-42.

91. Melzack R. (1983). *Pain assessment and management.* New York: Raven Press.

92. Melzack R and Wall P. (1965). Pain mechanisms: new theory. *Science, 150,* 971-979.

93. Melzack R and Wall P. (1983). *The challenge of pain.* New York: Basic Books.

94. Merker L, Higgins P, and Kinnard E. (1985). Assessing narcotic addiction in neonates. *Pediatr Nurs, 11,* 177-181.

95. Merskey H. (1970). On the development of pain. *Headache, 10,* 116-123.

96. Michelsson K. (1971). Cry analysis of symptomless low birth weight neonates and of asphyxiated newborn infants. *Acta Paediatr Scand Supp, 216,* 10-45.

97. Michelsson K, Kaskinen H, Aulanko R, and Rinne A. (1984). Sound spectrographic analysis of infants with hydrocephalus. *Acta Paediatr Scand, 73,* 65-68.

98. Michelsson K, Raes J, Thoden CJ, and Wasz-Hockert O. (1982). Sound spectrographic analysis in neonatal diagnostics: an evaluative study. *J Phonet, 10,* 79-80.

99. Michelsson K and Sirvo P. (1976). Cry analysis in congenital hypothyroidism. *Folia Phoniat, 26,* 40-47.

100. Michelsson K, Sirvo P, and Wasz-Hockert O. (1977). Sound spectrographic cry analyses of infants with bacterial meningitis. *Dev Med Child Neurol, 19,* 309-315.

101. Obrist PA, Light KC, and Hastrup JL. (1982). Emotion and the cardiovascular system: a critical perspective. In Izard CE (ed), *Measuring emotions in infants and children* (pp. 299-316). Cambridge: Cambridge University Press.

102. Owens ME. (1984). Pain in infancy: conceptual and methodological issues. *Pain, 20,* 213-230.

103. Owens ME and Todt EH. (1984). Pain in infancy: neonatal reaction to heel lance. *Pain, 20,* 77-86.

104. Porter FL, Miller RH, and Marshall RE. (1986). Neonatal pain cries: effect of circumcision on acoustic features and perceived urgency. *Child Dev, 57,* 790-808.

105. Porter FL, Porges SE, and Marshall RE. (1988). Newborn pain cries and vagal tone: parallel changes in response to circumcision. *Child Dev, 59,* 495-505.

106. Rawlings DJ, Miller PA, and Engle RR. (1980). The effect of circumcision on trancutaneous PO_2 in term infants. *Am J Dis Child, 134,* 676-678.

107. Rizvi T, Wadhwa S, and Bijlani V. (1987). Development of spinal substrate for nociception. *Pain,* (supp), *4,* 195.

108. Robinson S and Gregory GA. (1981). Fentanyl-air-oxygen anesthesia for patent ductus arteriosus in preterm infants. *Arch Analg, 60,* 331-334.

109. Schecter N, Allen D, and Hanson K. (1986). Status of pediatric pain control: a comparison of hospital analgesic usage in children and adults. *Pediatrics, 77,* 11-15.

110. Shapiro C. (1989). Pain in the neonate: assessment and intervention. *Neonat Net, August,* 6-21.

111. Shaw EA. (1982). Neonatal anesthesia. *Hosp Update, 8,* 423-434.

112. Shearer MH. (1986). Surgery in the paralyzed unanesthetized newborn. *Birth, 13,* 79.

113. Sheredy C. (1984). Factors to consider when assessing responses to pain. *Mat Child Nurs, 9,* 250-252.

114. Sherman M. (1927). The differentiation of emotional responses in infants. *J Comp Psychol, 7,* 265-284.

115. Sherrington CS. (1898). Experiments in examination of the peripheral distribution of the fibers of the posterior roots of some spinal nerves. Part II. *Philos Trans R Soc Lond (Biol), 190,* 45-186.

116. Should infants have surgery without anesthesia? (April 12, 1987). *Parade Magazine,* pp. 18-19.

117. Singleton MA, Rosen JI, and Fisher DM. (1987). Plasma concentrations of fentanyl in infants, children and adults. *Can J Anesth, 34,* 152-155.

118. Stevens BJ. (1991). Development and testing of a pediatric pain management sheet. *Pediatr Nurs, 16*(6), 543-548.

119. Stevens BJ, Hunsberger M, and Browne G. (1987). Pain in children: theoretical, research and practice dilemmas, *J Pediatr Nurs, May,* 154-167.

119a. Stevens B and Johnston CC. (1991). Premature infants response to pain: a pilot study. *Nursing Quebec 11,* 6, 90-95.

120. Swafford LI and Allen D. (1968). Pain relief in the pediatric patient. *Med Clin North Am, 48*(4), 131-162.

121. Tronick E, Als H, and Brazelton TB. (1977). Mutuality in mother-infant interaction. *J Comm, 7,* 74-79.

122. Tursky B, Jammer LD, and Friedman R. (1982). The pain perception profile: a psychophysical approach to the assessment of pain report. *Behav Ther, 13,* 376-394.

123. Tyson P. (1984). Developmental lines and infant assessment. In Call JD, Galenson E, and Tyson RL (eds), *Frontiers of infant psychiatry* (pp. 121-124). New York: Basic Books.

124. Vandenberghe H, MacLeod S, Chinyanga H, Endrenyi L, and Soldin S. (1983). Pharmcokinetics of intravenous morphine in balanced anesthesia studies in children. *Drug Metab Rev, 14,* 887-903.

125. Vuorenkoski V, Lind J, Partanen TJ, et al. (1966). Spectrographic analysis of cries from children with maladie du cri du chat. *Ann Paediatr Fenn, 12,* 174-180.
126. Wasz-Hockert O, Koivisto M, Vuorenkoski V, and Lind J. (1971). Spectrographic analysis of pain cry in hyperbilirubinemia. *Bio Neonate, 17,* 260-271.
127. Wasz-Hockert O, Lind J, Vuorenkoski V, Partanen T, and Valanne E. (1968). *The infant pain cry: a spectrographic and auditory analysis.* London: Spastics International.
128. Wasz-Hockert O, Michelsson K, and Lind J. (1985). Twenty-five years of Scandinavian cry research. In Lester BM and Boukydis CFZ (eds), *Infant crying: theoretical and research perspectives,* (pp. 83-104). New York: Plenum Press.
129. Williamson PS and Williamson RN. (1983). Physiologic stress reduction by a local anesthetic during newborn circumcision. *Pediatrics, 71,* 36-40.
130. Woolf CJ. (1986). Functional plasticity of the flexion withdrawal reflex in the rat following peripheral tissue injury. *Adv Pain Res Ther, 9,* 193-210.
131. Yaster M and Deshpande JK. (1988). Management of pediatric pain with analgesics. *J Pediatr, 113,* 421-429.
132. Zeskind PS and Lester BM. (1978). Acoustic features and auditory perception of the cries of newborns with prenatal and perinatal complications. *Child Dev, 49,* 580-589.
133. Zeskind PS and Lester BM (1981). Cry features of newborns with differential fetal growth. *Child Dev, 52,* 207-212.
134. Zeskind PS, Sale J, Maio ML, Huntington L, and Weiseman JR. (1985). Adult perceptions of pain and hunger cries: a synchrony of arousal. *Child Dev, 56,* 549-554.

10

Clinical Judgment in Assessing Children's Pain

Nancy O. Hester
Roxie L. Foster
Judith E. Beyer

KNOWING WHEN A child has pain is an important responsibility for nurses; however, the lack of clear objective criteria for determining the presence and absence of pain in children makes it difficult for nurses to fulfill this responsibility. To make clinical judgments of pain, nurses must rely on a multiplicity of cues, some of which are vague and elusive. Pain cues may be misinterpreted because they are similar to other physiological (e.g., stress) or psychological (e.g., separation anxiety) responses. Additionally, cues may be misunderstood because they are child-specific. Recognition of the difficulties inherent in knowing about children's pain led to research on this phenomenon. The purpose of this chapter is to present guidelines for clinical judgment in assessing pain in children. They are based on a definition of pain as a human experience and on research findings related to measurement of pain, cues used by nurses in the assessment process, and personal factors that may influence the nurse's clinical judgment.

◆ PAIN AS A HUMAN EXPERIENCE

Pain is a unique human experience. Defining pain as a human experience suggests that *pain brings with it the child's physical condition, developmental level, gender, psychologi-*

cal condition, personal concerns, background meanings, family issues, culture, emotions, reflective thoughts, and environment.[14,66,147] This perspective on pain delineates a number of factors that could influence children's interpretations of and responses to pain, thus accounting for the individual nature of the experience.

Studies of children's understanding of the word *pain* in relation to their developmental level help establish the importance of viewing pain as a unique human experience. In a study of children 5 through 14 years of age, younger children understood what pain meant but described pain more concretely than did older children.[47] Similarly Ross and Ross[117] found that children 5 through 12 years of age understood the word *pain.* In contrast, other researchers concluded that children under 6 years of age rarely understood the word *pain* and tended to use the words hurt and owie.[33,37,60,61] Research findings appear to differ depending on the setting in which the study occurred: Young children who were *not hospitalized* understood the word *pain,* but young children who were *hospitalized* did not. The results from two studies[57,61] suggest that some hospitalized children as old as 12 years do not understand the word *pain* (see Figure 10-1).

Children who do not understand the word *pain* may deny their pain if asked, "Do you have any pain?" To avoid this problem, researchers and clinicians must clarify with the child and family the words the child uses to communicate about pain.

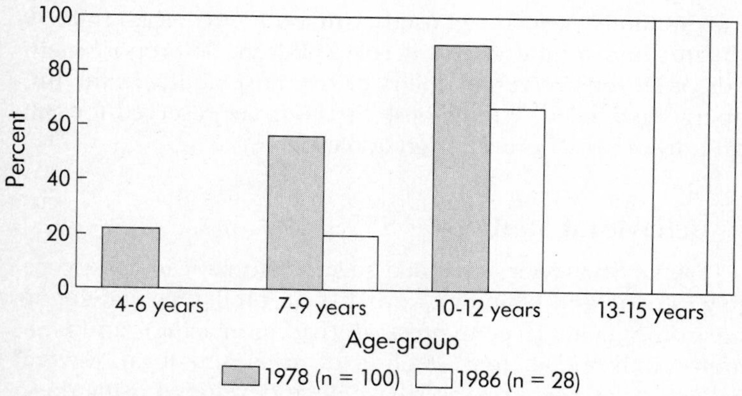

FIGURE 10-1. Understanding of the word *pain* by hospitalized children.

In addition to age or developmental level and hospitalization, family issues may also influence a child's experience of pain. A vivid example of the effect of a father's illness on the child's response to pain is illustrated in this quote from a 10-year-old girl who was hospitalized for a leg fracture[56]:

> When I have pain, it's hard on my mom because my dad has MS. She has to take care of him . . . So when I get hurt, I feel guilty sometimes because that puts more pressure on my mom and she has to work a lot harder to take care of both of us.[56]

A 7-year-old girl, hospitalized for diabetes, expressed her concern about the family financial situation[57]:

> I don't like . . . them to think that I'm really, really sick and spend all their money.

Factors such as these explain why pain is different for individual children. Hence, in assessing a child's pain, a nurse must consider which of the child's background variables may affect the pain experience. However, researchers have yet to determine how background variables might affect children's pain.

◆ MEASUREMENT OF PAIN

The development and testing of methods to measure pain in children have been the primary foci of child pain research. The methods generally fall into one of three categories: behavioral, physiological, and self-report. Behavioral and physiological methods have been used with both preverbal children (infants and toddlers) and verbal children. Self-report methods often require verbal ability or cognitive ability at the preoperational level[109]; thus these methods are reserved for children from preschool through adolescence.

Behavioral Methods

Primary behaviors assumed to indicate pain include vocal (e.g., crying and whining), verbal (i.e., intelligible statements regarding pain), facial expression (e.g., grimacing), and large motor movements (e.g., flailing of arms and legs). Several behavioral observation tools have been developed using these indicators singularly or in combination. Most of the studies using these tools, however, have been conducted with children undergoing painful procedures (e.g., immunizations, bone marrow aspirations, venipunctures, circumcisions), and the findings may not be applicable to children with acute or chronic pain.*

Behavioral Indicators

Research findings pertinent to each of the commonly used behavioral indicators provide a context for understanding the relevance of behaviors for measuring pain. Of importance is the specificity of the behavior in relationship to the presence and degree of pain.

Vocal and verbal behavior. Crying, one type of vocal behavior, has received a significant amount of attention, particularly in regard to preverbal children. Often the presence or absence of crying signifies to caregivers whether an infant is in pain. Several studies that focused on crying as an indicator of pain suggested that infants cry when they undergo medical procedures: heel lances,[39,42,108] needle sticks,[24] and circumcision.[67,97,150] Levy[86] concluded that by 6 months of age infants remember painful events and cry in anticipation of events such as immunizations.

Crying, however, is also associated with other conditions such as hunger, fear, and anger. Recognition of the ambiguity of crying as an indicator of pain led researchers to address the question, "Is there a pain cry?" Wolff[151] characterized a pain cry as a pattern of respiratory inspiration followed by expiratory crying. However, this description lacked specificity in distinguishing a pain cry from other cries.

To determine if a pain cry exists and, if so, whether it can be distinguished from other types of cry, researchers have measured various acoustic attributes (e.g., pitch, jitter, shimmer) of cries. The findings across researchers conflict. Wasz-Hockert, Michelson, and Lind,[146] Fuller, Horii, and Connor,[46] and Fuller, Connor, and Horii[45] concluded that a distinguishable pain cry exists and that certain attributes (particularly pitch and tenseness) of pain cries are discernible by mothers or by trained listeners. Johnston and O'Shaughnessy[77] agreed that tenseness occurs in pain cries but their findings regarding

* Pain accompanying diagnostic (e.g., venipunctures) or treatment (e.g., intravenous therapy) procedures is referenced as procedural pain throughout this chapter. It is not considered a subset of acute pain.

pitch differed from the Wasz-Hockert et al and Fuller et al studies. Thus Johnston and Strada[78] and Johnston and O'Shaughnessy[77] concluded that a pain signature to a cry is not yet evident. Clearly, more research is needed to determine the reliability and validity of a pain cry for infants.

Little research has focused on cry for older children. Young children undergoing bone marrow aspirations and lumbar punctures exhibited more crying behavior than did older children.[41,85] Further, hospitalized postsurgical children older than 3 years did not cry in conjunction with pain experiences.[21,63,66] Therefore cry as a measure of pain for older children has questionable validity.

Interestingly, some studies suggest that vocalizations decrease as verbal facility increases. Craig et al[24] reported that of children from birth to 24 months, younger children vocalized more than the older children during immunizations. Similarly, Mills,[101,102] in examining acute pain behavior of infants and toddlers by developmental level, reported a decrease in crying behavior as verbal facility improved. However, Hester's[57,58] findings concerning vocalizations and verbalizations during immunizations suggested that preschool children tended to be quiet. Slightly more than half (54.5%) were quiet during the procedure and only 30% were either crying or screaming. Most (63.6%) children did not respond verbally; of those who did, all but one exhibited complaining behavior (e.g., "that hurts").

Verbalizations in relationship to pain have received little attention. Fuller and Hester[44] are currently studying acoustic parameters of verbalizations for the older (4 through 13 years) child. They are exploring whether the acoustic characteristics, such as pitch, shimmer, or jitter, are related to either the child's report or nurse's report of hospitalized children's pain. Support for these relationships would yield a new direction for measuring pain through acoustic indicators inherent in verbalizations of older children.

Facial expression. Facial expression is commonly assessed in studies on children's pain. Negative facial expression has occurred in response to painful care and pin pricks in preterms,[28,112] heel lances in infants,[42] and prolonged acute pain in infants and toddlers.[101,102] Negative facial behavior in response to immunizations, however, was evident in only about 25% of preschool children,[58,59] thus raising questions about this behavioral response as a valid measure of pain in older children.

Other researchers have analyzed facial expressions more minutely.[49,69,78] Grunau and Craig,[50] studying neonates undergoing heel lances, found a characteristic pain expression to include eye squeeze, brow contraction, nasolabial furrow, taut tongue, and open mouth. Johnston and Strada[78] commented that the facial expression of infants receiving immunizations was the most stable indicator of pain, showing the least variability across infants when compared with cry, heart rate, and body movement. Although facial expression seems to be a promising behavioral indicator of pain for infants, this parameter needs more clinical testing.

Motor behavior. Several researchers studying pain-related behaviors focus on large motor movements. For infants, movement of extremities occurs with pin pricks[112] and heel lances.[42] For preterms through toddlers, more generalized body movements occurred in response to arterial venipunctures,[43] painful care such as needle sticks, suctioning, or tape removal,[28] and tissue damage from surgery, burns, or fractures.[101,102] In preschool children receiving immunizations, movement was minimal: 61% of the children were quiet; 23% twisted or wriggled; 9% jerked their arms; and 7% jerked their bodies. Interestingly, exaggerated movements were associated with lower self-reports of pain rather than with higher pain levels.[58,59]

Inhibition of motor responses has been noted by Beyer et al[21] in children aged 3 to 7 postsurgically. Their findings substantiate the earlier work of Taylor,[134] who observed that as children "became more awake and alert, they seemed to realize that movements increased their pain" (p. 40).

These studies raise provocative questions about body movements in older children: Are motor behaviors indicators of pain, responses to pain, or ways of coping with pain? Possibly, motor behaviors are all of these and therefore lack specificity as a measure of pain.

Behavioral Measures

Tools for behaviors are designed to measure either a single behavior, such as cry or facial expression, or multiple behaviors. Most of these tools are in the early stages of development and may not be applicable for use in clinical practice settings. Additionally, most of these tools have been used to measure behavior associated with procedure-induced pain. The clinical use of these tools in situations of acute or chronic pain is inadvisable. Studies suggest that children in acute pain respond with *less exaggerated* and *fewer motor behaviors* than do children experiencing pain from procedures.[21,63] In addition, behaviors such as crying, negative facial expression, and large motor movement have yet to be documented as valid indicators of acute and chronic pain or of pain in older children.

Measures of single behaviors. Cry, facial expression, and motor behaviors have been measured independently from other behaviors. Some of these measures are simple focusing on the presence or absence of a behavior, but others are more sophisticated, incorporating the use of equipment or detailed analysis.

Measurement of cry in infants focuses on the presence or absence of crying[42,108,150] or spectrographic or acoustic analysis.[45,46,50,76-78] Presence or absence of crying is easily assessed in the clinical setting; however, although the presence of crying may indicate pain, the absence of crying should not be construed to mean there is no pain. Useful in research, spectrographic or acoustic analysis of vocalizations or verbalizations is not yet a practical method of clinical assessment of pain. Future research should demonstrate whether pain cries are different from other cries and whether pain cries can be identified in the practice setting without the aid of complicated equipment. Similarly, further research should reveal whether acoustic aspects of verbalizations have specific parameters associated with pain.

Simple measures of facial expressions focus on the identification by an observer of a negative facial expression, a cry face or a frown with or without crying.[28] Although practical for clinical use, the reliability and validity of such methods have yet to be established. Sophisticated tools include the Maximally Discriminative Facial Movement Coding System,[69,78] the Facial Action Coding Scales,[32] and the Neonatal Facial Coding System.[49,50] Although interrater reliability estimates are high (.83 to .98) for these coding scales, the use of these tools is limited to analyzing videotapes of infants undergoing procedures. Therefore the clinical application of these tools cannot yet be advocated nor may it be practical.

Few tools have been developed to measure only motor behaviors. Typically, researchers have examined single behaviors dichotomously, i.e., the motor behavior either occurred or it did not. For example, Davis and Calhoon[28] defined large movement as "a movement involving the extremities and the trunk" (p. 39). More large movements occurred when preterms received painful care than with routine care ($p < .001$). Froese-Fretz,[43] using an infant mattress for electronically recording movement,[84] found that body movement increased during arterial venipunctures. Through photogrammetry, Franck[42] demonstrated immediate withdrawal of both legs after a heel lance.

Multidimensional tools for measuring behavior. Most tools that measure behavior are multidimensional. The only behavior scale for infants (2 to 24 months of age), the Infant Pain Behavior Rating Scale,[24] was tested on infants receiving immunizations. Categories on the scale include infant vocal actions (crying, pain vocal, pain/fear verbal, and other), nonvocal-face (distortion of face, and eye orientation), nonvocal-torso (rigid and withdrawing), and nonvocal-limbs (protect/touch and kick/thrash). Interrater reliabilities were satisfactory only for behaviors that occurred most frequently; e.g., the reliability for crying was .98. Most interrater reliabilities were below .70. More psychometric work is needed on this tool before it can be used clinically with confidence.

The Children's Hospital of Eastern Ontario Pain Scale (CHEOPS),[94] a scale for young, 1-year-old to 7-year-old children, focuses on six behaviors: cry, facial, verbal, torso, touch, and legs. Although research has indicated high interrater reliability (greater than .80) and promising estimates of validity, recent evidence brings the scale into question for use with postoperative children. Beyer et al[21] reported a pattern of flat scores indicating few behavioral responses for children 3 to 7 years old, in the first 36 postoperative hours. Although observed to have no pain on the CHEOPS, the children reported pain on two different self-report scales.

The Behavioral Observation Tool[58,59], the first behavioral tool to be developed, was used with preschool children receiving immunizations. Interrater reliability estimates for measure of vocalizations, facial expression, and motor responses were high (greater than .75) but moderate for verbalizations (.50). Interestingly, the use of vocalizations and verbalizations was associated with higher self-reports of pain, and negative facial expression and exaggerated motor responses with lower self-reports of pain.

Abu-Saad and Holzemer[6] used a behavioral checklist to assess vocal, facial, and body movement behavior for 10 post-surgical children and adolescents, ages 9 through 15. Inter-rater reliability for the scale was estimated to be .98, and content validity of the categories was assumed since the categories were derived from the previous work of Johnson[75] and McCaffery.[90] Indicators for each of the three categories, vocal, facial, and body movement, were identified but the scoring of observations was unclear.

Katz, Kellerman, and Siegel[83] developed the procedure behavioral rating scale (PBRS) to measure pain and anxiety in children undergoing bone marrow aspirations. In the scale, 13 behaviors are scored dichotomously, thus providing data on occurrence but not intensity. This tool had an interrater reliabilty estimate of .85 but lacked information on validity. In fact, Katz et al[83] had difficulty determining which behaviors indicated pain, anxiety, or both, suggesting that the validity of the tool is problematic.

Jay and Elliott[70,71] developed the observation scales for behavioral distress (OSBD) by refining the PBRS. As with the PBRS, the OSBD was used in conjunction with bone marrow aspirations. Reliability estimates based on percent agreement between raters ranged from .80 to .91. Validity was substantiated by correlating the OSBD scores with nurse ratings of the child's distress, child's rating of anticipated and actual pain, and pulse rates at three times during the procedure. Although correlations were statistically significant, the magnitudes of correlation coefficients of the OSBD with the child's rating of pain and pulse rates were moderate, thus explaining little variance. These findings raise questions about the accuracy of the following statement by Jay and Elliot[71]: "Results of validity analyses indicated that the OSBD is a highly valid instrument" (p. 13).

LeBaron and Zeltzer[85] developed the procedure behavior check list (PBCL) from interviews with and observations of children and adolescents, through 18 years, undergoing bone marrow aspirations. This tool comprises eight behavioral categories similar to those in the PBRS. Interrater reliability ranged from .64 to .86. Evidence for concurrent validity between the PBCL and ratings of anxiety was stronger than between the PBCL and ratings of pain. In fact, the correlations between the PBCL and ratings of pain were low to moderate.

As with the OSBD, little variance is explained, thus raising questions about the validity of the PBCL.

Recently, Gauvain-Piquard, Rodary, Rezvani, and Lemerle[48] reported on a promising observational rating scale for acute and chronic pain in children 2 to 6 years of age. Used with children experiencing pain from cancer, the scale includes items related to pain, anxiety, and depression. Pain items include the child's rest position, protection of painful areas, protective behavior during movement, somatic complaints, control exerted by child when moved, and reactions to medical examination of painful regions. Preliminary evidence for sensitivity, reproducibility, and validity is promising.

Another promising scale is in the early formative stage of development. Through observations of infants and toddlers with surgical wounds, burns, or fractures, Mills[101,102] identified age-specific pain behaviors. Interrater agreement in the identification of these behaviors was a strong 91% to 94%. A measurement tool needs to be constructed with these behavioral indicators so that it can be tested for reliability, validity, and clinical applicability. Like the tool by Gauvain-Piquard et al, Mills' work is promising in that it focuses on pain from causes other than procedures.

Summary of Behavioral Methods

The methods used to assess behavioral indicators of pain are essentially immature. Many of the tools or indicators have been developed or tested in conjunction with procedures. Although potentially valid for procedure-related pain, these tools should not be used for acute or chronic pain. Behaviors consistent with the "spirited" child response[62] generally do not occur with pain from other etiologies except perhaps initially with traumatic injury. Behavioral inhibition, as identified by Beyer et al (1990), was common in postsurgical children although self-reports indicated pain was present. Few researchers have studied behaviors across time, that is, observed pain at more than one point in time. Thus it is unknown how the pattern of behavior might change during the course of a pain episode. More work is needed similar to that of Mills[101,102] and Gauvain-Piquard et al[48] to identify reliable and valid age-appropriate behavioral indicators of acute and chronic pain. Thus nurses should be cautious when applying the currently available behavioral measures clinically.

Physiological Methods

Physiological responses consistent with stress arousal often occur with pain episodes. The problem lies in the interpretation of these physiological responses as indicators of pain. For example, does an increase in heart rate indicate the presence of pain and a stable heart rate mean the absence of pain? Physiological responses most likely lack validity as specific indicators of pain. Researchers have studied the following physiological responses in association with pain: hormonal-metabolic levels, endorphins, heart rate/pulse, respiration, blood pressure, pallor, $TCpo_2$, and diaphoresis. As with the study of behavioral responses, much of the research is associated with procedure-related pain.

Hormonal-Metabolic Changes

Perhaps some of the most exciting research demonstrating the occurrence of physiological responses to pain is the work of Anand and colleagues. Anand, Brown, Bloom, and Aynsley-Green[8] concluded that both preterm and full-term neonates are "capable of mounting an endocrine and metabolic stress response to surgical trauma" (p. 125). Hormonal-metabolic changes have been observed with procedures such as venipunctures and circumcisions. For example, increases in plasma renin activity have been associated with venipunctures in neonates,[40] and increased plasma cortisol levels have been noted during and after circumcision.[51,133] Anand and Hickey,[9] in a critical review of several hormonal studies, noted that "preterm and full term neonates who underwent surgery under minimal anesthesia . . . (experienced) a marked release of catecholamines, growth hormone, glucagon, cortisol, aldosterone, and other corticosteroids as well as suppression of insulin secretion" (p. 1324). Although these findings are important in documenting that preterm and full-term neonates physiologically respond to pain, determining hormone/metabolic changes is not a practical method for assessing pain in the clinical setting.

Endorphins

Studies about endorphins and pain are conflicting. Olness, Wain, and Ng[107] reported the lack of detectable endorphin levels in children before and after they used self-hypnosis for pain control. Katz and colleagues[82] examined endorphin levels in cerebrospinal fluid obtained through lumbar punctures in children with leukemia. They found positive, but nonsignificant, associations between endorphin levels and nurses' ratings of anxiety, and between endorphin levels and behaviors measured on the PBRS. In contrast, Szyfelbein, Osgood, and Carr[132] reported that endorphin levels and self-reports of pain were inversely related in a sample of children with burns. Clearly, the research on endorphin levels is insufficient to provide any conclusive evidence. Several issues may have contributed to the discrepancy in findings:

1. The validity of the PBRS, nurses' rating of anxiety, and self-report measures used as criteria for the interpretation of endorphin levels as a pain indicator
2. The condition of the child, leukemia versus burn
3. A single measure[82] versus repeated measures[132]

As with hormonal-metabolic changes, the method for obtaining endorphin levels (i.e., invasive procedure) severely limits its clinical usefulness as an indicator of pain.

Heart/Pulse Rate, Respiration Rate, and Blood Pressure

Heart/pulse and respiration rates and blood pressure are enticing indicators since they are extremely objective and they are part of the nurse's usual routine. However, research on heart and/or pulse and respiration rates suggest the lack of a predictable response to pain. Although heart rates increase in response to heel lances and arterial venipunctures,[43,108] Johnston and Strada[78] described a general pattern of bradycardia during injection followed by a dramatic increase in heart rate after the injection. Important, however, is the finding that the responses of some infants were distinctly different from this general pattern. Studies by Dale[26] and by Field and Goldson[39] supported individual or variable heart rate responses in infants undergoing immunizations and heel lances, respectively. Field and Goldson[39] found no change in respiratory rate during heel lances. Froese-Fretz[43] found that patterns of respiration varied across infants undergoing arterial venipunctures; the majority of infants, however, experienced a decrease in respiratory rate at the time of venipuncture, which Froese-Fretz attributed to either crying or breath-holding.

Research on the use of heart rate in older children as an indicator of pain is extremely limited. Mischel, Fuhr, and McDonald[103] showed heart rates increasing consistently with behavioral measures of pain/distress in children undergoing orthodontic work. Jay and Elliott[70] measured pulse rate of children on arrival at the clinic and just before and after bone marrow aspirations. They found moderate relationships between pulse rates and OSBD scores for distress across time, with the highest coefficient occurring just before the procedure, indicating that pulse rate may be associated with anxiety. Additionally, Jay, Elliott, Katz, and Siegel[72] found similar relationships for blood pressure. Because these pulse rates and blood pressures were not taken during the actual procedure, any conclusions regarding the relationship between pulse rate or blood pressure and pain would be tentative.

Only a few studies have addressed heart and/or pulse rate in children in pain not related to procedures. Mills[101,102] found the heart and respiration rates of hospitalized infants and toddlers who had experienced surgery, burns, or fractures were at times higher than average but were within age-appropriate norms. Abu-Saad and Holzemer[6] examined pulse and respiration rates and blood pressure eight times for each of the 10 hospitalized school-age children and adolescents observed. The pulse and respiration rates and blood pressure parameters for both groups were near the expected age-appropriate means. Abu-Saad and Holzemer[6] categorized 80 observations according to the presence or absence of three types of behaviors, vocal, facial, and body. Pulse and respiration rates and blood pressure parameters for the group in which the behaviors were displayed were similar to or slightly higher than those for the group without the behaviors. Higher ratings of pain were reported for this group as well. Apparently, however, the researchers reported associations among these variables by visually inspecting the pattern of means for the two groups. Although they did not determine if there were statistical differences between the presence and absence groups of any of the physiological measures or in the pain ratings, Abu-Saad[1] later reported the absence of a relationship of physiological parameters with either behavioral responses or pain level.

Most of the studies have been conducted with children experiencing procedural pain. Even with relatively similar types of procedures, heart/pulse and respiration rates do not respond systematically, suggesting that autonomic stress arousal responses differ across children. Little research has addressed children who experience other than procedural pain. Thus heart/pulse and respiration rates and blood pressure may be sensitive indicators of stress arousal, but they are not specific as indicators of pain.

TCpo$_2$

Findings regarding TCpo$_2$ are inconsistent. Norris, Campbell, and Brenkert[106] found that TCpo$_2$ levels did not significantly change during heel lances. Mean TCpo$_2$ levels dropped during injection and dissection phases of the circumcision procedure[150] but increased for arterial punctures.[43]

Diaphoresis

Diaphoresis can occur as a physiological indicator of stress. A few researchers have studied palmar sweat as a potential indicator of pain associated with heel lances,[53] but these findings were not supported in studies on bone marrow aspirations[72] and acute pain.[101,102] Others have reported the occurrence of palmar sweating with anxiety rather than pain per se.[98,99] The inconsistent findings suggest that, as with vital signs, this indicator may be sensitive for stress arousal but may not be specific for pain.

Summary of Physiological Methods

Physiological methods are fraught with problems as indicators of pain in children. As with behavioral methods, most research has been conducted with infants undergoing procedures. The generalizability of these findings to situations of acute and chronic pain is unlikely. Determination of hormonal-metabolic changes and endorphin levels requires invasive procedures and is therefore inappropriate. Diaphoresis has been studied too infrequently to consider its value for pain. Unfortunately, these heart/pulse and respiratory rates and blood pressure lack specificity as measures of pain. In regard to physiological measures, P. A. McGrath[91] concluded:

> "Evidence suggests that physiological responses mirror the state of the infant or child in a stressful and painful situation. Thus, phys-

iological responses are often positively correlated with behavioral indices of overt distress and occasionally correlated with self-support indices of pain. However, there is insufficient evidence to conclude that physiological responses correlate directly with pain experience" (pp. 159-160).

Self-Report Methods

Researchers have approached the study of children's pain using a variety of self-report methods. McGrath and Unruh,[95] P. A. McGrath,[92] and Ross and Ross[117] identified the following types: verbal reports, interviews, questionnaires, diaries, projective tests, pain drawings, pain maps, and self-report rating scales.

Verbal Reports

Verbal reports of pain refer to a child's spontaneous statement denoting pain or a child's response to a question regarding hurt. Children's interpretation of their pain experiences may not always be conveyed in ways adults understand. An example from the study by Hester et al[61] vividly describes this issue:

> A preoperational child reported hurt like a "lion's roar." Puzzled, Hester and colleagues concluded that this response was uninterpretable. Several years later Rochelle, an adolescent, overheard her mother discussing how difficult this response was to interpret. Rochelle casually stated a plausible interpretation: "Oh, that's easy. It's the lion who roared when he had a thorn in his paw."

Rochelle's response was based on the familiar Aesop fable, *Androcles and the Lion.*[130] Inherent in her response was Rochelle's belief that the thorn had caused the lion to suffer from hurt.

In this scenario, the preoperational child's mode of verbal expression was consistent with her age and cognitive development but posed a barrier for adult understanding. Situations such as this may lead to the belief that children cannot accurately express or interpret their pain.[60]

In contrast, the mode of verbal expression can also provide a vivid picture of the child's pain. Ross and Ross[117] found that children tended to use descriptors unlike those of adults:

> It feels like my head is puffing up and shrinking down, then pushing against one side, then letting go (Boy, age 9, headache).

It feels like there's a big bomb in my stomach, it feels like it's going to explode or burst (Girl, age 7, stomachache) (p. 74).

Not all verbal children have the ability to be as expressive as these quotes might suggest.

Verbal responsiveness may be limited by a number of factors. Shyness may inhibit a child's verbal expressiveness, especially in the hospital situation. Fear of injections may inhibit a child's acknowledgment of pain.[37] A child may believe that denying pain will lead to discharge from the hospital (McCarthy, 1972, cited in Ross and Ross, 1988, p. 117).[117] Factors such as these must be considered in the interpretation of a child's verbal response.

Interviews

Interviews solicit information from children about their past and current pain experiences. Ross and Ross[116] discussed two types of questions that can be used in interviews: generate (open-ended) and supplied (forced-choice). Open-ended questions require children to generate the answers while forced-choice questions require either a yes or no response or a selection from provided alternatives. Examples of these types of questions are:

Generate: Tell me about the hurt you're having.

Supplied: Is your head hurting?

Supplied: Does your head hurt a little or a lot?

Generate questions will provide child interpretations of pain but supplied questions are apt to be laden with adult terminology or adult expectations. Generate questions, however, are more time-consuming and may not always be feasible in a hospital setting. Interestingly, Hester[57] found that generate questions tended to work well with adolescents but not with younger children.

In using the interview format (structured, semistructured, or unstructured), Ross and Ross[117] and Hester[57] found it important to clarify the meaning of pain terms. Hester,[57] in semistructured interviews, included a set of questions termed concept clarification. These questions focused on the meaning of the word *pain* and other pain words. If a child did not understand the word *pain,* the meaning of hurt was explored with the child. After determination of the child's understanding of the words, Hester proceeded to interview children about their pain experiences, tailoring the questions to use the appropriate pain word.

Hester and Barcus[60] designed interviews that nurses could use in their clinical practice. The set of interviews includes a pain experience history (elicited from parents and from verbal children) and a pain interview. See the three accompanying boxes. The use of these interviews has not been examined systematically through research, thus the reliability, validity, clinical feasibility, and subsequent value are yet to be determined.

Diaries

Pain diaries have been used infrequently with children. Diaries may include information such as the occurrence and duration of each pain episode, the potential triggers for each episode, the treatment, and the effectiveness of the treatment.

◆ PAIN EXPERIENCE HISTORY: CHILD INFORMANT

Name of child: ____________ Informant: ____________

Age: ____________ Sex: _____ Ethnicity: ____________

Tell me what pain is.

Tell me about the hurt you have had before.

Do you tell others when you hurt?

What do you want others to do for you when you hurt?

What don't you want others to do for you when you hurt?

What helps the most to take away your hurt?

Is there anything special that you want me to know about you when you hurt? (If yes, have child describe.)

From Hester NO and Barcus CS. (1986). Assessment and management of pain in children. *Pediatr Nurs Update, 1*(14), pp. 2-8. Used by permission.

Diaries have been used with children and adolescents with headaches[10,92,113] and with cancer and arthritis.

The limited use of pain diaries with children means that little is known about their reliability and validity. Conceivably, the information in the diary would assist clinicians in under-

◆ PAIN EXPERIENCE HISTORY: PARENT INFORMANT

Describe any pain your child has had before.

How does your child usually react to pain?

Does your child tell you or others when he or she is hurting?

What does your child do for himself or herself when he or she is hurting?

Which of these actions work best to decrease or take away your child's pain?

Is there anything special that you would like me to know about your child and pain? (If yes, please describe.)

From Hester NO and Barcus CS. (1986). Assessment and management of pain in children. *Pediatr Nurs Update, 1*(14), pp. 2-8. Used with permission.

◆ PAIN MEASUREMENT AND INTERVIEW

1. How much hurt are you having? (Use reliable and valid tool.)
2. Tell me about the hurt you're having now. (Elicit descriptors, location, cause.)
3. What would you like me to do? (e.g., give medication, be with you.)

From Hester NO and Barcus CS. (1986). Assessment and management of pain in children. *Pediatr Nurs Update, 1*(14), pp. 2-8. Used with permission.

standing the patterns of pain and the relative effectiveness of treatment regimes in children with chronic pain. The significance of diaries for acute pain situations has yet to be shown. A potential problem with diaries is the commitment needed from children and adolescents to maintain the data base as requested.

Projective Tests

Projective tools are strategies that indirectly elicit children's perception of pain. The Eland projective tool[33] consists of a dog cartoon character in five situations: one pain-free, three in common childhood pain experiences, and one in a situation similar to the preschool child's medical condition. The child rank-orders four black-and-white pictures from no hurt to the most hurt and then inserts the cartoon like the child's condition into the sequence of pictures to indicate the child's pain level. Eland[33] provided preliminary evidence for the reliability and validity of the tool.

Subsequently, in a study with hospitalized preschool children, Ward[145] used a similar tool but with six colored pictures. The sixth picture depicted the child's medical condition and was equated with one of the five pictures the child had previously ranked. Ward claimed to have established reliability and validity with this version of the tool.

Hester[58,59] used black-and-white cartoon pictures of a rabbit depicted in the same situations Eland[33] described. The fifth picture was standard for all children: a rabbit receiving an injection. Hester found that well preschool children had difficulty ranking pictures from no hurt to the most hurt; she questioned the appropriateness of this task for preschoolers. She did not arrive at the same conclusions about the reliability and validity of the tool as did Eland[33] and Ward.[145]

Scott[125] used two cartoon sequences, one depicting a child accidentally inflicting pain on himself with a hammer, and one with pain being inflicted upon a child in the form of an injection, to study color, shape, texture, pattern, and time sequences in the child's perception of pain. Reliability and validity of the cartoon sequences for measuring pain were not discussed and findings should be considered tentative, as they could have occurred by chance.

Lollar, Smits, and Patterson[87] developed the Pediatric Pain Inventory, consisting of 24 pictures representing medical, recreational, psychosocial, and common daily activities. The purpose of the tool is to assess how children perceive pain in regard to intensity and duration. Internal consistency estimates for intensity and duration were adequate ($\alpha > .70$) for the recreational and psychosocial pictures, but questionable ($\alpha = .41$ to $.62$) for the medical common daily activities pictures. Preliminary work suggested evidence for validity. The tool, however, has yet to be used with hospitalized children.

Projective tools involving cartoons are very appealing to use with children. Even with established psychometric properties, however, the tools may not be clinically applicable, especially in the hospital setting, because of the time required for administration. They may be more efficient as research tools than as clinical tools.

Pain Drawings

Researchers have had children portray their pain through drawings. Findings across studies reveal differences according to specific factors. Sturner, Rothbaum, Visintainer, and Wolfer[131] showed differences in the drawings of children who were prepared for needle procedures and those who were not, and Villamira and Occhiuto[142] reported differences between children with acute pain and with chronic pain. Developmental but not gender differences were found by Jeans and Gordon.[73] Unruh, McGrath, Cunningham, and Humphreys[137] categorized by content the drawings of children with migraine headaches or musculoskeletal pain. Children with musculoskeletal pain drew fewer pictures of helping themselves with the pain than did children with migraine headaches.

The most frequently used colors in the drawings were black and red.[73,137] Unruh et al[137] cautioned that "the significance of this finding is unclear" because red and black are preferred colors in any drawings (p. 391).

Pain drawings often reveal children's innermost perceptions of pain. Drawings may be of particular value in the clinical setting when the nurse suspects a child has pain but the child won't discuss it. Unruh et al[137] recommended the use of drawings as images for therapeutic modalities such as imagery and relaxation. However, the use of drawings is limited for severely ill or debilitated children. The reliability and validity of pain drawings is not easily documented. Expertise in evaluating drawings is important if the drawings are to be of clinical value.

Pain Maps

Pain maps are used to determine location of pain. Generally, researchers use clothed or unclothed, with or without genitals, child and adolescent, front and back body outlines as pain maps.* Generally, all researchers concluded that children can accurately and reliably represent the location of their pain on a body outline.

Pain maps can be useful for tracking the progression of pain across time. This strategy can be a useful adjunct in diagnosing a disease/illness or in determining its progression. A particular benefit of a pain map is evidenced in the following anecdote[66]:

> A seven-year-old girl, a subject in a study on pain, had experienced surgery for a cranio-facial disorder. When asked to rate the intensity of her pain, she responded: "Does it have to be on my head?" When the researcher said "No," the child proceeded to discuss her stomach pain.

When asked about pain, this child assumed the pain needed to be associated with her surgical site. If this young girl had not been assertive, the stomach pain may have been overlooked. A pain map would have provided this child an avenue to communicate pain other than that related to a surgical procedure.

Pain Words

Pain words are descriptors of the quality of pain experienced by a child or adolescent. Developed for adults, the McGill pain questionnaire[100] includes words that describe sensory, affective, and evaluative qualities of the pain experience; however, this tool is inappropriate for children. Thus researchers have attempted to develop a similar word list for children. Recently, Tesler, Savedra, Ward, Holzemer, and Wilkie[135] compiled a list of 129 words obtained from children[118,136,123] and determined that 43 of the words were appropriate for children in grades three through 12. These 43 words have undergone initial testing.[122] This child-generated

* References 34, 36, 61, 119, 121, 136, 140.

and research-tested list of words is incorporated in a pain questionnaire for children and adolescents with space to write in other words. Results from a series of studies support the test-retest reliability of the word list and its content, concurrent, and construct validity. Additionally, the list of words seems to be "relatively free of gender, ethnic, and developmental biases" (Wilkie, Holzemer, Tesler, et al, 1990, p. 8).[149]

Varni, Thompson, and Hanson[140] included a list of 31 words in their pediatric pain questionnaire that were generated from the McGill pain questionnaire (J. Varni, personal communication, April 18, 1990). This word list needs further psychometric work before the adequacy and appropriateness of the words can be determined for use with children.

Abu-Saad is one of the few researchers who has focused on examining cultural components of pain. She has studied pain descriptors from Arab-American children,[2,4] Asian-American children,[3,4] Latin-American children,[4] and Dutch children.[5] Differences in the selection of words were noted: Arab-American, Latin-American, and Dutch children tended to use sensory words to describe their pain, and Asian-American children used more affective and evaluative words. The findings from these studies are preliminary, and further study is warranted to determine how cultural differences should be included in pain assessment procedures.

Jerrett and Evans[74] studied the pain vocabulary of children attending a clinic for ear problems. Interestingly, some of the words reported by Jerrett and Evans are quite different from those in the studies by Savedra, Tesler, and colleagues and Abu-Saad. Examples are "lots of banging, buzzing, cymbals clapping, and mosquitos buzzing." These words potentially are descriptors specific to the ear problems experienced by the children in this study, suggesting that different words may be associated with different types of medical conditions.

Self-Report Scales

Self-report scales are methods that seek to quantify the amount of pain a child has. Scales generally fall within three categories: color-matching, visual analogue, and graphic rating. Five of the self-report scales are listed in Table 10-1. The criteria for inclusion in the table was that the scale has been cited frequently in the literature and/or is one of the best developed tools.

Text continued on p. 270.

◆ **Table 10-1**
Self-report methods and questionnaires

Tool	Description	Psychometric properties	Considerations for use
Eland color tool (ECT) Eland, 1975	Measures pain location and intensity. Child outline (front and back) is marked with crayon(s) chosen by the child from set of eight crayons to represent different amounts of hurt.	*Reliability:* No published information *Validity:* No research to support that choice of colors actually correlates with pain intensity. However, validity of use of body outline supported when 168 of 172 children, ages 4-10, located pain in keeping with their illness by placing an X on the body outline (Eland and Anderson, 1977; Hester et al, 1978).	Useful with children as young as 4 as an indicator of pain location(s). May help to elicit the child's perception of which body parts hurt most. Responses must be validated with the child. Children may make left/right and front/back mistakes when reporting pain on body outlines (Hester et al, 1978). Meaning of the colors used must also be validated with the child.
Eland color assessment tool (CAT) Eland, 1981	Measures pain intensity. Children select four of eight colors of felt squares to represent most hurt, not quite as much hurt, just a little hurt, and no hurt at all.	*Reliability:* No published information *Validity:* Expected reduction in pain evidenced by CAT when 20 of 22 children who rated an IM DPT injection as severe hurt indicated reduced pain by the time they left the office (Eland, 1981)	Limited evidence that children's color choices actually correspond to the amount of pain they feel. Clinical use necessitates careful validation of children's responses.

Eland color tool Eland, personal communication, 1983	Measures pain location and intensity. Child outline (front and back) is marked with four of eight crayons to represent different amounts of hurt as in the CAT.	*Reliability:* No published information *Validity:* Falco (1985) unable to demonstrate convergent validity for ECT and 10-point pain intensity scale	All versions available from the author: Dr. Joann Eland, 316 Nursing, University of Iowa, Iowa City, IA 52242.
Poker chip tool (PCT) Hester, 1976, 1979	Measures amount of pain. *Original version:* Four white poker chips in a horizontal line represent "pieces of hurt" on a 0 (none of the chips) to 4 (all of the chips) scale.	*Reliability:* Not established *Validity:* Significant and positive relationships among children's ratings of pain on the PCT and: (1) verbal and vocal responses during immunization (Hester, 1979), (2) children's pain ratings on the pain ladder and VAS (Hay and O'Brien, 1986). Pattern of pain intensity associated with immunizations (Alyea, 1978) similar to pattern in Hester (1979) study.	Useful with children 4-13 years to help determine the amount of pain present. Responses should be validated with words such as, "Tell me about the hurt." Clinical applicability rated high (Datz, 1989; Jordan-Marsh, 1990). Spanish version available (Jordan-Marsh et al, 1990a, 1990b). Chips are inexpensive, readily available, and easy to carry and disinfect.

Continued.

◆ **Table 10-1**
Self-report methods and questionnaires—cont'd

Tool	Description	Psychometric properties	Considerations for use
	Modified version: FIve poker chips (one white, four red) represent "pieces of hurt" on a 0 (white chip) to 4 (red chips) scale (Molsberry, 1979).	*Reliability:* Not established *Validity:* Children's ratings of pain on the MPCT significantly related to ratings: (1) on the hurt thermometer (Molsberry, 1979), (2) on the Oucher and vertical VAS (Aradine, Beyer, and Tomkins, 1988; Beyer and Aradine, 1987, 1988). Children and parents rated pain very similarly on MPCT, Oucher, and vertical VAS (Datz, 1989). Children's ratings on MPCT distinguished between more and less extensive procedures (Beyer and Aradine, 1987). Hurt decreased with analgesics (Aradine, Beyer, and Tomkins, 1988; Datz, 1989; Molsberry, 1979).	Manual and tool available from the author: Dr. Nancy Hester, School of Nursing, C288, University of Colorado Health Sciences Center, 4200 E. Ninth Ave., Denver, CO 80262.

Recommended version: Four red poker chips represent "pieces of hurt" on a 0 (none of the chips) to 4 (all of the chips) scale.	*Generalizability* (a property similar to reliability): In a study of 87 child-nurse-parent triads, children (4-13), nurses, and parents rated the child's pain similarly across measures taken at four different times (Hester et al, 1990) *Validity:* Ratings from child-nurse-parent triads were very similar at each pain measure (strong convergent validity), but significantly different from one measure to the next (strong discriminant validity) (Hester and Foster, 1989; Hester et al, 1990). Pain rated on the PCT significantly lower for children who received a topical skin coolant before an injection than for the control group (hypothesis testing) (Hagedorn, 1990).

Continued.

◆ **Table 10-1**
Self-report methods and questionnaires—cont'd

Tool	Description	Psychometric properties	Considerations for use
		Sensitivity: Pain ratings by 29 child-nurse-parent triads on the first postoperative day showed the PCT was moderately sensitive to the effects of analgesics (Hester, Foster, and Kristensen, 1989).	
Visual analogue scale (VAS) Scott et al, 1977; McGrath et al, 1985*	Measures amount of pain on a line that is typically 10 cm long. Usually positioned horizontally, but may be vertical. Line anchored by descriptors of the extremes of pain, e.g., "no hurt," "worst hurt." A true VAS contains no markings between the anchors (Huskisson, 1974).	*Horizontal VAS:* *Reliability:* No published information *Validity:* Pain scores of 33 and 40 children (respectively) on the VAS were very similar to scores on a simple descriptive pain scale (Scott et al, 1977) and to scores on a brightness scale (McGrath et al, 1985). Significant and positive relationships among children's ratings of pain on the original PCT, the	Needs additional testing to determine whether children (especially preschoolers) understand the concept of magnitude on a horizontal line. Of five scales, children and adolescents in a large study ($n = 896$) least preferred the horizontal VAS and found it hard to use (Savedra and Tesler, 1989).

pain ladder, and the VAS (Hay and O'Brien, 1986).

Vertical VAS:
Reliability: No published information
Validity: Pain scores of 23 mother-child pairs on the VAS significantly related to their scores on Oucher and MPCT (Datz, 1989). Pain scores among Oucher, MPCT, and vertical VAS highly correlated for children 3-12 years (Beyer and Aradine, 1988).

If either horizontal or vertical VAS used clinically, validate children's responses with additional questioning. Keep in mind that a 10 cm visual scale is different from the abstract thinking required to answer, "How much pain do you have on a 1-to-10 scale?"

No copyright; can easily be drawn for use. However, xeroxing may shorten or lengthen line slightly (Lorig, 1984). Whereas problematic for research, alterations in length may be acceptable for clinical purposes. No consensus about which anchor words should mark the extremes

*Abu-Saad and Holzemer (1981) also studied the psychometric properties of a 10 cm line. However, their use of 10 cross hatches along the line technically makes their tool a graphic rating scale (Huskisson, 1974).

Continued.

◆ **Table 10-1**
Self-report methods and questionnaires—cont'd

Tool	Description	Psychometric properties	Considerations for use
			of a pain scale. Length of line between zero point and child's mark must be measured to determine pain score.
Oucher Beyer, 1984	*Original version:* Measures amount of pain. Numerical (10-100 in tens) vertical scale for children who can count to 100; photographic vertical scale (6 faces of same white child with expressions from no hurt to the biggest hurt you could ever have) used with children who cannot count to 100 by ones.	*Reliability:* When 2-year-old to 6-year-old children were tested in two sessions 1 week apart, their scores on the Oucher were similar at both measures for hypothetical pain situations involving cartoon characters (Belter, McIntosh, Finch, and Saylor, 1988) *Validity:* As a group, 78 3-year-old to 7-year-old white children verified the ordering of the photographs from "no hurt" to "the biggest hurt you could ever have" for the original Oucher (Beyer and Aradine,	Useful with children as young as 4 to assess amount of pain. All children first asked to count from 1 to 100. Child who can count uses numerical Oucher. Child who cannot count is given Piagetian seriation test to determine ability to rank order by size. Child who can do seriation test uses photographic Oucher. Child who cannot do seriation is developmentally unable to use Oucher. Validation of children's responses important with either

1986). Pain scores among Oucher, MPCT, and VAS highly correlated for children 3-12 years. Oucher ratings conformed to expected patterns for pain before and after surgery (Aradine, Beyer, and Tomkins, 1988; Beyer, 1984; Beyer and Aradine, 1987, 1988). Significant relationship among pain scores on vertical VAS and MPCT and: (1) parents' scores on numerical Oucher, (2) children's scores on numerical and photographic Oucher (Datz, 1989). With 74 perioperative children, Oucher discriminated fear from pain (Beyer and Aradine, 1988). Pain scores decreased with analgesics (Aradine, Beyer, and Tompkins, 1988).

faces or numerical scale. Tool plasticized for disinfection.

Available from author:
Dr. Judith Beyer, School of Nursing, C288, University of Colorado Health Sciences Center, 4200 E. Ninth Ave., Denver, CO 80262.

Continued.

◆ **Table 10-1**
Self-report methods and questionnaires—cont'd

Tool	Description	Psychometric properties	Considerations for use
	African-American and Hispanic versions: Use faces of African-American or Hispanic child.	*Reliability:* No published information *Validity:* African-American and Hispanic children selected photographs and their relative rank order for two new ethnic versions of the Oucher (Denyes, 1990; Denyes and Villarruel, 1988a, 1988b; Neuman, Denyes, Stettner, and Villarruel, 1990; Villarruel and Denyes, 1989).	
Varni-Thompson pediatric pain questionnaire (Varni and Thompson, 1985)	Measures pain intensity, location, quality, and sensory affective and evaluative aspects using child, adolescent, and parent forms. Designed to assess chronic, recurrent pain. Uses: (1) VAS anchored with pain descriptors;	*Reliability:* No published information *Validity:* Pain descriptors chosen by children with juvenile rheumatoid arthritis (JRA) were very similar to those chosen by hospitalized and nonhospitalized children in a previous study by Savedra et al (1982) (Varni et al, 1987). Pain intensity rated on VAS by child and mother	Published results address only children with JRA, but results of studies in progress may validate the use of this tool for other populations. Length of the tool may preclude its use in some clinical situations, but the structured inter-

	(2) color-coded scale: body outline to be marked with four of eight crayons; (3) list of pain descriptors to circle; (4) questions about child/family social environment and background	increased as MD-rated disease increased (Varni et al, 1987). Studies in progress with children with acute, chronic, and recurrent pain (J. W. Varni, personal communication, April 18, 1990)	view for parents and children may be helpful in obtaining a detailed pain history. Available from the author: Dr. James W. Varni, Behavioral Pediatrics Program, Orthopaedic Hospital, 2400 S. Flower St., Los Angeles, CA 90007
Adolescent pediatric pain tool (APPT) Savedra, Tesler, Holzemer, and Ward, 1989	Multidimensional tool to measure pain location, intensity, and quality: (1) school age/adolescent body outline (front and back) to record pain sites; (2) word graphic horizontal rating scale (no pain, little, medium, large, worst possible); (3) list of 56	*Reliability:* Body outline judged to have adequate "alternate forms" validity when location, number, and surface area of sites marked by 175 children correlated 94%, 91%, and 83% of the time (respectively) with where children pointed to pain (Savedra et al, 1989). In test-retest situations, 16 children whose pain did not change across 10	Although the tool is relatively new, it has been developed with exceptional rigor and is ready for clinical use with children 8-17 years. As with other tools, careful validation of children's responses is encouraged. Available from author: Dr. Marilyn Savedra, University of

Continued.

◆ **Table 10-1**
Self-report methods and questionnaires—cont'd

Tool	Description	Psychometric properties	Considerations for use
	words to circle that describe pain, with opportunity to add words	measures in 5 days used similar words at each measure to describe their pain (Wilkie et al, 1990). *Validity:* Use of body outline by 175 children (8-17 years) validated when chart evidence supported most pain locations marked (Savedra et al, 1989). Word list shown free of ethnic and gender bias when used by a multiethnic sample of 958 nonhospitalized and 35 hospitalized boys and girls 8-17 years. Number of words circled tended to increase with increased pain scores. Moderate support for use of three categories of words (Wilkie et al, 1990). Patterns of pain scores decreased over the 5-day postoperative period (Savedra, Tesler, Holzmer, Wilkie, and Ward, 1990).	California, San Francisco, School of Nursing, San Francisco, CA 94143-0606

Children's pain inventory McGrath PA, 1990	Measures pain intensity (visual analogue scales) and pain affect (facial scale)	A series of reliability and validity studies were conducted from 1982 to 1990, assessing different types of pain for children ages 4-17. Only preliminary results have been published (McGrath et al, 1985) but manuscripts of final results are in progress (McGrath PA, personal communication, April 16, 1990).	Designed to be used in the home or hospital. Pain affect scale (facial scale) not intended for uses without accompanying pain intensity scales (visual analogue scales) (P.A. McGrath, personal communication, April 2, 1990). Available from author: Dr. Patricia A. McGrath, Department of Paediatrics, Children's Hospital of Western Ontario, London, Ontario, Canada, N6C 2V5

From Foster RL. (1990). A multi-method approach to the description of factors influencing nurses' pharmacologic management of children's pain. Unpublished doctoral dissertation, University of Colorado Health Sciences Center, Denver.

Color-matching. Many researchers have explored the use of color to measure the intensity of pain. The Eland color tool[34] measures pain location and intensity. Three versions of the tool exist (See Table 10-1). In the first version, children selected a color(s) from a set of eight color crayons to mark the location(s) of the pain on the body outline; the color represents the amount of hurt experienced in that location (see Figure 10-2). Although the location of pain was determined to be valid according to the child's history, the reliability and validity of the color use has been questioned. Hester et al[61] were unable to demonstrate convergent validity between the first version of the Eland color tool and the poker chip tool. They questioned whether colors actually represented amount of pain or whether they represented some other quality of pain.

The second version, the Eland color assessment tool, focused on the development of a child-generated intensity scale using colors but without using a pain map.[35] This tool uses eight colored squares of felt from which children select four colors, each representing a designated amount of hurt: most hurt, not quite as much, just a little hurt, and no hurt at all. Subsequently, J. Eland (personal communication, 1983) ap-

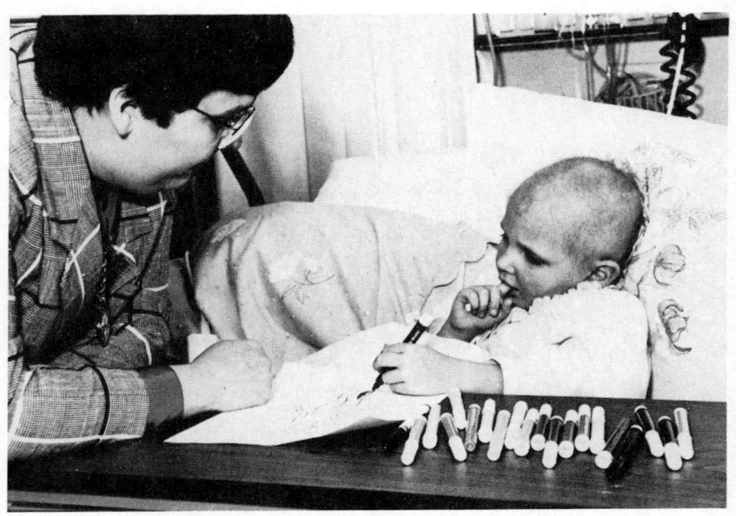

FIGURE 10-2. Administration of the Eland Color Tool. (Courtesy University of Colorado Health Sciences Center, Denver.)

plied the idea of the child-generated color scale to the Eland color tool such that children colored the location of pain, i.e., the third version. Although Eland[35] found some evidence for construct validity and sensitivity of the child-generated scale using the felt squares, Falco[38] was unable to demonstrate convergent validity for the third version of the Eland color tool and a 10-point pain intensity scale. Varni and colleagues[140] used a tool similar to the adapted Eland color tool in the pediatric pain questionnaire, but they have yet to provide evidence of its reliability and validity.

Savedra and Tesler[119] developed a horizontal color scale with red representing the most hurt and yellow no hurt. In a study comparing different types of horizontal scales: color, visual analogue, graphic rating, word-anchored rating, and magnitude estimation, they found that nonhospitalized children preferred the color scale whereas hospitalized children selected the word-anchored rating scale.

The interest in color scales is based on the assumption that colors represent quantity of pain. However, research has yet to establish the reliability and validity of this claim. As with pain drawings, red tended to be selected more frequently than other colors.[34,61,89,140] More work is needed on color tools to establish their clinical value in measuring children's pain.

Visual analogue scales. A visual analogue scale (described in Chapter 4) is used to measure a single attribute of pain, its intensity. The visual analogue scale can be positioned either vertically or horizontally, as the correlation between pain scores on the two forms was highly significant ($r = .99$, $p < .001$).[128] The validity of the visual analogue scale for children has been questioned by Beyer and Knapp.[20] The works of Scott, Ansell, and Huskisson[126] and Beales, Keen, and Holt[12] showed that younger children reported less pain on the visual analogue than adults and adolescents. Beyer and Knapp[20] did not accept their conclusion that younger children must experience less pain; rather they noted the serious disregard for the validity of the scale for children and adolescents: "Validity was assumed but not tested. Evaluation of the instrument was apparently based solely on whether or not each child could draw a mark across the 10 cm line" (p. 236).

Maunuksela, Olkkola, and Korpela[96] examined the validity of an adapted form of the visual analogue scale using an increased amount of red coloration for increasing pain, and

Beyer and Aradine[19] tested the validity of a vertical visual analogue scale. The scale with the red coloration was strongly correlated with a faces scale and verbal self-report of pain intensity but only moderately associated with a behavioral assessment. The vertical scale was strongly correlated with the numerical and photographic oucher (γ = .888 and .732, respectively) and the poker chip tool (γ = .881 and .732*), but the correlation coefficients were of a lesser magnitude than were the correlation coefficients between the poker chip tool and the numerical and photographic scales on the oucher (γ = .946 and .981, respectively). These findings provide some evidence for the convergent validity of these two forms of the visual analogue scale. In addition, P. A. McGrath[92] demonstrated that children did understand the concept of the horizontal visual analogue scale. Children and adolescents, however, ranked the visual analogue scale as the least preferred and the most difficult to use in comparison with four other horizontal scales: a color scale, a word graphic rating scale, a graded graphic rating scale, and a magnitude estimation scale.[119]

Although the visual analogue scale has been used satisfactorily in a few studies with children, its appropriateness for use with children is questionable. This type of scale may be confusing for children and adolescents who lack cognitive ability to understand its abstractness. An inherent difficulty with the visual analogue is an increase or decrease in length that occurs during photocopying.[88,119] Clinical or research use of the visual analogue scale with young children to document patterns of pain or effects of interventions should proceed cautiously until the psychometric issues related to the visual analogue scale have been cogently addressed.

Graphic rating scales. As with the visual analogue scale, graphic rating scales measure one attribute, intensity, of the pain experience. They differ from the visual analogue scale in that they have markers indicating levels of pain. Several types of graphic rating scales prevail in the literature: numerical rating scales,† word graphic rating scales,[119] pain thermometers,[104,132] and facial scales.[15,16,85,93,152]

* The first correlation coefficient represents the relationship between the PCT and the VAS for children who rated their pain with the numerical oucher. The second coefficient represents the relationship between the PCT and the VAS for children in the photographic oucher group.

† References 6, 15, 16, 54, 58, 59, 95, 115, 119.

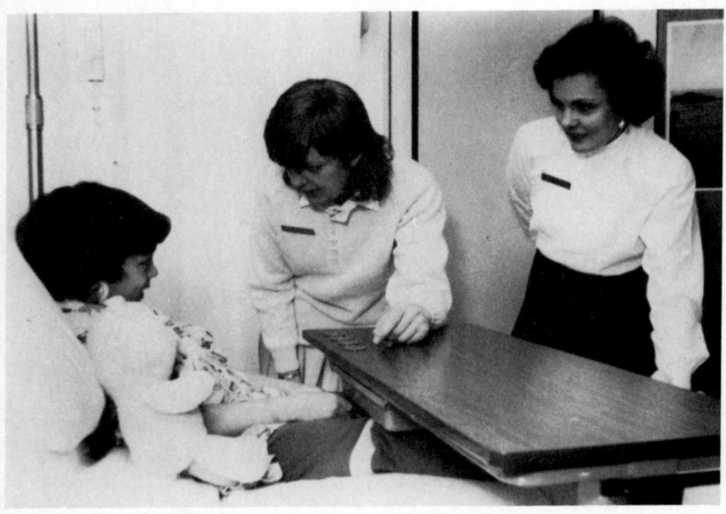

FIGURE 10-3. Administration of the Poker Chip Tool. (Courtesy Pain Topics, Vol 3, (3), 1990, New York.)

NUMERICAL RATING SCALES. Numerical rating scales involve scoring of pain with a numerical value. (See Chapter 4.) Tools vary in their range of scores, e.g., zero to four, zero to five, one to five, zero to 10, and zero to 100. The scales are arranged either vertically or horizontally; neither arrangement has been documented as superior.

The first numerical rating scale to be developed was the poker chip tool.[58,59] It consists of four poker chips with one chip representing a little bit of hurt and four chips, the most hurt possible (see Figure 10-3). Originally, the tool consisted of four white chips; later, it was revised by Molsberry[104] to include one white chip for no hurt and four red chips for various levels of hurt. The current version consists of four red chips; this version has been tested with both hospitalized and well children. Evidence for the psychometric properties of the poker chip tool is strong for generalizability,* strong for convergent and discriminant validity, and moderate for sensitivity

* Generalizability[25] is a psychometric property that is similar to reliability but is generally considered superior to reliability. For a brief discussion of the generalizability of the poker chip tool, see Hester N, Foster R, and Kristensen K. (1990). Measurement of pain in children: generalizability and validity of the pain ladder and the poker chip tool. In Tyler D and Krane E (eds). *Advances in pain research and therapy: vol 15. Pediatric pain,* (pp. 79-84). New York: Raven Press.

(see Table 10-1). The instructions are also available in Spanish.[80,81] Datz[27] rated the poker chip tool high on criteria for clinical applicability.

The pain ladder[54] is a drawing of a nine-rung ladder on which the child marks or points to the amount of pain. Although purported to be a 10-point scale, it is actually a 20-point scale (counting the rungs and the spaces between, above, and below the rungs) with an ambiguous zero point.[66] Hospitalized children 4 through 13 years of age were often perplexed when presented with this tool. The pain ladder has evidence for marginally adequate generalizability, partial to strong support for convergent validity, partial support for discriminant validity, and a moderate degree of sensitivity.[54,64,65] Because of problems with administration and limited research on the psychometric properties, this tool is not recommended for use with children and young adolescents.

Abu-Saad and Holzemer,[6]* Abu-Saad,[1] Ross and Ross,[115] and Savedra and Tesler[119] all developed and tested numerical rating scales, 10 centimeters long, positioned horizontally. Ross and Ross[117] reported that children had no difficulty using a 10-centimeter numerical rating scale but evidence for test-retest reliability was weak. Although Abu-Saad and Holzemer[6] conjectured through inspection that pain scores were positively related to the occurrence of vocalizations, facial expressions, body movements, and physiological parameters, a later report by Abu-Saad[1] did not substantiate the earlier claim that the tool had evidence for construct validity. Savedra and Tesler[119] used a graded graphic rating scale in their comparison of five self-report scales. Although the tool functioned similarly to the others, children did not prefer to use it.

Beyer[15,16] imbedded a vertical, zero-to-100, numerical rating scale on the Oucher. The scale numbers increase by 10s. Children who can count to 100 by ones purportedly can use this tool. Colleagues questioned this assumption, and recently Beyer revised her instructions to include questions on children's understanding of larger and smaller numbers. To use this scale, children must be able to count and demonstrate a conceptual understanding of numbers. A series of small studies suggest strong evidence for construct validity.[11,18,19] Pain

* Abu-Saad and Holzemer (1981) referred to this scale as a visual analogue scale, but the scale had 10 hash marks on the 10-centimeter line. Thus, by definition, it is a rating scale rather than a visual analogue scale.

scores from this scale were highly correlated with the poker chip tool and a vertical visual analogue scale. Pain scores also decreased, as expected, after administration of analgesics (see Table 10-1).

McGrath and Unruh[95] developed a six-point, zero-to-five, numerical-verbal pain scale for use in the clinic. To assist children in selecting the appropriate pain level, a verbal description of pain severity accompanied a numerical value. Children used the scale without difficulty. The only psychometric property discussed by McGrath and Unruh[95] was interrater reliability based on the relationship between child and parent ratings. Consistent ratings between parents and children, however, provide support for convergent validity in that child and parent ratings represent two different ways of measuring pain.

WORD GRAPHIC RATING SCALES. Scott and Huskisson[127] and Savedra and Tesler[119] used word graphic rating scales in studies comparing different types of self-report measures. Both teams of investigators found that words distributed across the length of the line were satisfactory. In fact, a large sample of hospitalized children in the Savedra-Tesler study preferred the word graphic scale over four other scales. In using this type of scale, ascertaining children's understanding of the words is imperative.

PAIN THERMOMETERS. Pain thermometers are based on the principles of a temperature thermometer. They are vertical, numerically-graded scales anchored at the bottom with no hurt and at the top with the most or worst hurt. Molsberry's hurt thermometer[104] was positively correlated with the poker chip tool, suggesting evidence for convergent validity. Szyfelbein et al[132] found their pain thermometer adequate to assess rapid fluctuations of pain intensity in children undergoing burn dressing changes. Although intriguing, the use of the pain/hurt thermometer in the clinical setting is not advised because of the limited information available on reliability, validity, and sensitivity.

FACIAL SCALES. Facial scales use an arrangement of faces with expressions that indicate various levels of pain from no pain to severe pain. The Oucher[15,16] uses photographs of an androgenous-appearing male child experiencing various postsurgical levels of pain (see Figure 10-4 and Table 10-1). Beyer and Aradine[17] tested the order of the pictures by determining the percentage of 3-year-old to 7-year-old children who could

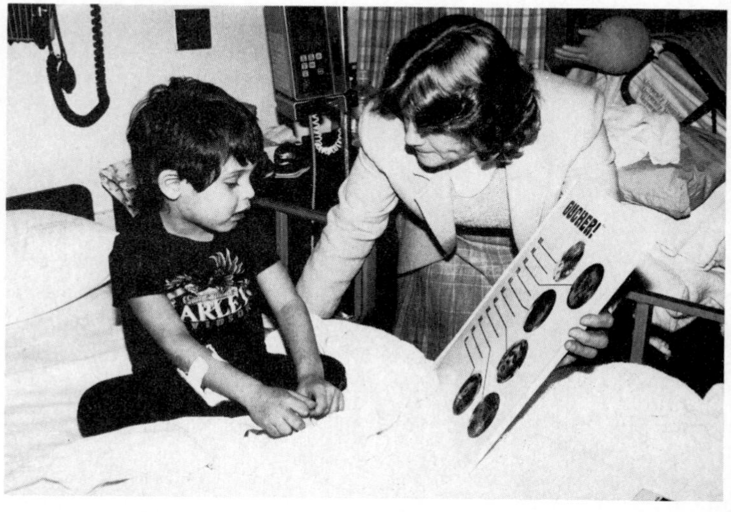

FIGURE 10-4. Administration of the Oucher. (Courtesy University of Colorado Health Sciences Center, Denver.)

correctly sequence the photographs. The success rate for properly sequencing the photographs was lowest for 3-year-olds. Content validity was considered adequate because the majority of children properly sequenced most of the photographs. Pain scores obtained on the photographic scale were highly correlated with those on the poker chip tool and a visual analogue scale, suggesting convergent validity.[11,18,19] In addition, discriminant validity was supported by weak correlations between scores on the Oucher and two fear scales.[19] On a small sample of hospitalized children, mean and median scores at preanalgesic times were higher than those at postanalgesic times, thus supporting construct validity.[11] The culture-specificity of the Oucher, which uses photographs of a white child, is a major concern. Currently, Denyes and Villarruel[30,31,105,144] are developing Hispanic and African-American photographic tools.

Other facial scales include five caricatures of a human face with increasing levels of distress,[85] a series of nine cartoon faces with various emotional expressions,[93] five faces ranging from smiling to crying,[96] and a faces rating scale with six facial expressions.[148,152] Research on the psychometric properties of these scales is extremely limited; therefore the clinical application of these scales is not advised.[23]

Questionnaires. Questionnaires are structured formats focusing on issues such as pain history and the child's understanding of pain (see Table 10-1). They can be administered to children in interview format or children can respond to the questions by themselves. The format of the questionnaires varies and may include supplied and/or generate questions. Often other self-report methods are imbedded in a questionnaire; examples include rating scales, pain maps, and pain drawings. Some questionnaires include both parent and child/adolescent sections. Length can be a problem for clinical application, particularly in the hospital.

Based on Schultz's work,[124] Tesler et al[136] developed the pediatric pain questionnaire, which focused on topics such as causes, descriptors, feelings, coping strategies, and location. Continued efforts by Savedra, Tesler, and colleagues[119,120,122,135] resulted in the development of the adolescent pediatric pain tool (APPT). This tool, similar in format to the McGill pain questionnaire,[100] includes a pain map, a rating scale, and a list of pain words (see Figure 10-5). Rigorous development and testing of the tool in various settings provide strong evidence for reliability, validity, sensitivity, and clinical applicability.

The Varni-Thompson pediatric pain questionnaire,[139] also similar to the McGill pain questionnaire, was developed for use with chronic pain[141] (see Table 10-1). The tool includes separate forms for children, adolescents, and parents. It includes a visual analogue scale, a body outline, a list of pain descriptors that assess sensory, affective, and evaluative pain qualities, and a socioenvironmental history. Content validity of the pain descriptors and concurrent validity of the visual analogue scale were addressed in an early study of children with juvenile rheumatoid arthritis.[140] Recognition of the lack of psychometric evidence has resulted in new studies, currently in progress, with children experiencing acute, chronic, and recurrent types of pain. These studies should provide additional information on the psychometric properties of this tool (J. Varni, personal communication, April 18, 1990).

The children's comprehensive pain questionnaire[92] was designed for use with children experiencing recurrent and chronic pain (see Table 10-1). It includes generate and supplied questions, a visual analogue scale, and an affective facial scale. The questionnaire consists of a pain history obtained from the parent(s) and a subjective pain experience obtained

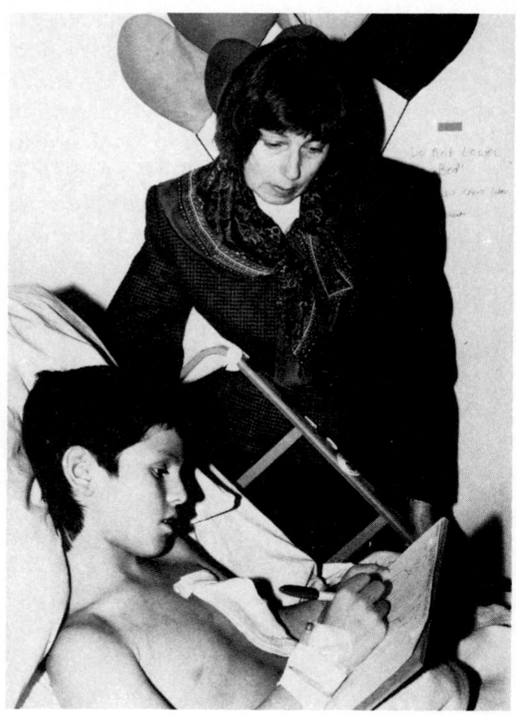

FIGURE 10-5. Administration of the APPT. (Courtesy University of Colorado Health Sciences Center, Denver.)

from the child. It is a versatile questionnaire that can be used for specific pain problems simply by substituting the appropriate pain problem. For example, the request, "Describe one of your usual headaches" (P. A. McGrath[92] p. 393) could be easily adapted to other acute or chronic pain problems such as stomachaches, leg aches, or sore throats. The questionnaire, which is extremely long, is to be administered by a trained interviewer. Results of studies on the psychometric properties of the questionnaire have yet to be published (P. A. McGrath, personal communication, April 2, 1990).

Of these questionnaires, the adolescent pediatric pain tool is the most reliable and valid. It is the only questionnaire to be tested with hospitalized children. Savedra et al[122] cautioned, however, that "for practical use in clinical settings, the length of time required to complete the tool must be determined" (pp. 92-93).

Summary of Self-Report Methods

Researchers have developed several different methods to assist children and adolescents in reporting pain. Some methods focus on one dimension of pain (e.g., measure only intensity) but others are multidimensional (e.g., measure intensity, location, and quality). Some tools are in the preliminary stages of development and others are, comparatively, quite well developed. To date, however, most tools have been examined only by the developer, which potentiates the threat of investigator bias. Additionally, conclusions about the psychometric adequacy of the scales often are drawn from the results of one study. *Cumulative evidence is important in determining the psychometric properties of any tool.*

A recurrent problem particularly evident in the psychometric research related to self-report scales is memory lag, the phenomenon of marking pain intensity similarly on successive scales. Many studies have been conducted using two or more tools. Memory lag, especially when the tools are similar, may create a misleading interdependence between or among the tools. "This potential interdependence threatens conclusions drawn about validity; thus, results from the studies using two or more tools must be regarded as tentative" (Hester et al,[64] p. 81).

◆ CUES NURSES USE IN ASSESSING CHILDREN'S PAIN

Research on the cues nurses use in assessing children's pain is in its infancy. Three of the earliest studies[89,111,138] and one of the more recent studies[114] are unpublished. Only three studies[22,63,110] have been published; one is in abstract form and another is in a newsletter with limited distribution.

Primm[111] stated that a nurse's assessment of pain in children was based on four criteria:

1. The child's behavior
2. The child's verbalizations
3. The child's emotional state
4. The pain expected according to the child's diagnosis or operative date

Lukens[89] used Primm's[111] data collection form to obtain data on the importance of each criterion in assessing a specific child's pain and the child's behavior postoperatively. Verbalization was the only criterion of the four that received a ranking of "not important" by some of the nurses. It is not known whether this ranking reflected a characteristic of the child or a nurse bias. As a characteristic of the child, it would suggest the importance of viewing the child as an individual and pain as a human experience. As a nurse bias, it would exemplify a point articulated by Hester and Barcus[60]: children's interpretation of their body cues may be considered suspect because of the assumption that children cannot accurately interpret their body cues. Changes in the nurses' use of criteria on different assessments suggest that nurses may not use a static set of criteria across time.

Varchol[138] implemented a study similar to that of Lukens.[89] She used Primm's data collection form and examined the importance of the four criteria for nurses on day and evening shifts in assessing chronic and acute pain. Rating the importance of the four criteria revealed different patterns of importance for day and evening nurses in assessing chronic and acute pain. Interestingly, for children with acute pain, regardless of the nurses' shift, behavior was rated as very important more than 85% of the time and verbalization as very important only about 50% of the time. Distinct patterns for day and evening nurses evolved for children with chronic pain. The most frequently observed child behaviors at the time of assessment for both chronic and acute pain were how the child was occupied, degree or description of body activity, and verbalization or vocalizations. Nurses identified physical signs least often for both chronic and acute pain.

Bradshaw and Zeanah[22], using an open-ended question, elicited nine categories of criteria used by nurses in assessing children's pain. They were ranked in the following descending order: body language, oral expression, physiological changes, affect, verbal communication, facial expression, nurse's judgment, relief action, and parent's assessment. Rank ordering of the criteria revealed differences according to the years of experience in pediatric nursing. Both experienced and inexperienced nurses tended to use body language, physiological measures, and oral expressions. Experienced nurses also used facial expressions and verbal requests but inexperienced nurses used affect. Surprisingly, the least experienced nurses also relied on nursing judgment. As did Varchol,[138] Bradshaw and Zeanah found differences in the rank-ordering of criteria by acute care and chronic care nurses. Regardless of the acute and chronic care orientation, the majority of nurses used physiological measures, affect, oral expressions, and body language. In addition, chronic care nurses frequently used verbal requests and facial expressions.

Pomietto[110] and Ritchie[114] used Bradshaw and Zeanah's criteria to determine the use of the criteria by nurses in other settings. Pomietto[110] reported findings similar to those in the Bradshaw-Zeanah study. Frequently used criteria included body language and facial expression,* verbal expression and verbal requests, affect, and physiological changes. Nursing judgment, relief action, and parental assessment were least used.

Ritchie[114] approached analyses differently from Bradshaw and Zeanah[22] and Pomietto.[110] She determined that age of the child affected the criteria nurses used to assess pain. For example, oral expressions and responses to relief actions were highly ranked criteria for infants; oral expression and affect for the preschool age child; verbal communication for the school age child; and verbal requests and body language for adolescents. Identified criteria were more similar for children in juxtaposed age groups. Ritchie's study suggests that development was an important influence on the use of criteria by nurses to assess pain. One criterion, physiological measures, was ranked as an important criterion despite the age of the child.

Hester, Foster, Kristensen, and Bergstrom[66] and Hester and Foster[63] elicited cues nurses used when they rated pain in hospitalized children, using either the pain ladder or the poker chip tool. Analysis of the cues led to eight categories of cues: appearance, physiology, temperament, activity, interaction, verbalization, vocalization, and body language. Collection of cue data over time, up to four times within the nurse's shift, resulted in another important category, change.

Congruency exists across these studies. Six of the Hester-Foster categories are similar to six criteria described by Bradshaw and Zeanah,[22] and seven are similar to the categories described by Primm.[111] Four of Bradshaw and Zeanah's criteria are similar to three of Primm's categories. Three criteria from Bradshaw and Zeanah (nursing judgment, response to relief measures, and parental assessment) were not evident in the other two sets of categories. Interestingly, these three categories were the least used by nurses in studies by Bradshaw and Zeanah,[22] Pomietto,[110] and Ritchie.[114] The category

* It is unclear from Pomietto's article whether these criteria were combined before collecting data or after analyzing it.

"change"[63] was not present in the other categorical schemes, although change could be inferred from Lukens'[89] findings. A rationale for this finding is that the Hester-Foster study involved nurse-generated cues for each child on repeated occasions, whereas the other studies involved data collection at one point in time.

The studies using Primm's and Bradshaw and Zeanah's criteria serve to demonstrate potential influences on the selection and use of cues. The shift nurses' work[138] may indirectly influence the cues nurses use. It could be postulated that:

1. Variation in work responsibilities for different shifts affects the attention nurses give pain cues
2. Nurses who work different shifts vary in personal characteristics that influence cue usage
3. Pain manifests differently according to time of day
4. Parents are present more often on the evening shift, and their presence alters children's expression of pain.

Cues for children with chronic pain may be different from those with acute pain.[22,138] Children with chronic pain may suppress or inhibit certain responses to pain and may learn to function as though pain-free even during pain episodes. Nurses may expect children with chronic pain to be different from those with acute pain.

Years of experience in pediatric nursing may alter cue selection and usage. Longevity should affect the degree of nurse expertise. Novice nurses may lack experience in working with children in pain, and therefore may be less sensitive to pain cues. Age of the child influences the types of cues nurses use in assessing pain.[114] Expert nurses may note more subtle pain cues. However, continued exposure to children in pain may desensitize the nurse's response to pain such that pain becomes a normal expectation for some conditions.

These few studies provide a beginning framework for understanding how nurses assess pain in children. None of the studies indicated that nurses used measurement tools in conjunction with the cues they identified.

◆ CRITICAL APPRAISAL OF RESEARCH ON CHILDREN'S PAIN

Critical appraisal of the research related to assessing and measuring children's pain suggests that pain is an individualized experience. Pain as an individual experience may be affected by the child's physical/psychological condition, developmental level, gender, personal concerns, background meanings, family issues, culture, emotions, reflective thoughts, and environment. The individual nature of the experience is evident in the cues nurses used when they assessed pain. Although they reported using information such as children's verbalizations, temperament or affect, appearance, activity, and body language, indicators for these categories varied across children. Change in these indicators was a primary process through which nurses knew a child had pain. Judgments of pain were influenced by factors such as the child's age, developmental level, and type of pain. However, research failed to show that nurses strongly considered factors such as psychological aspects, gender, background meanings, culture, and family issues.

The research on pain measurement has focused on behavior, physiological parameters, and subjective reports. An assumption underlying measurement research is that a common pain response exists, particularly for behavioral and physiological parameters. Research findings suggest that, *although some behavioral and physiological responses may be similar, a common pain response among children does not exist or, at least, has yet to be documented.* The inability to document a common pain response among children lends credibility to viewing pain as an individual experience and to the importance of obtaining a subjective report whenever possible.

Several self-report tools yield reliable, generalizable, and valid information about pain. Although nurses used child verbalizations in their assessment of pain, they did not document the validity of the child's report through the use of psychometrically-sound self-report methods.

Research concerning vocalizations is less clear. Many of the behavioral measures of pain include vocalizations as a parameter. Although nurses reported vocalizations as a cue, they did not use the cue frequently. The use of vocalizations, such as crying, whining, and groaning, as indicators of pain poses some problems. First, these types of behaviors may be linked to development; infants and toddlers may use vocalizations to communicate pain and other types of distress but older children may use verbalizations. Second, vocalizations may signal only the sudden onset of pain that accompanies procedures. Third, during periods of acute or chronic pain, children may limit vocalizations that exacerbate pain. Fourth, vocalizations may represent the occurrence of a stress arousal but not necessarily pain. Fifth, the absence of vocalization does not mean the absence of pain even though some behavioral tools so suggest.

In consideration of these issues, the finding that nurses use vocalizations sparingly in assessing pain is not surprising. The nurses who were studied focused on the hospitalized child from infancy through adolescence, suffering primarily from acute or chronic pain. If the nurses had worked primarily with infants or with painful procedures, vocalizations might have been used more frequently as pain indicators.

Most of the measurement research on motor behaviors has been conducted in conjunction with procedures (e.g., injections, venipunctures, and circumcision) in which behaviors such as body movement or movement of extremities may be exaggerated. In contrast, measurement research on children suffering from postoperative pain suggests that behavioral responses are often limited or inhibited. The findings from postoperative research are congruent with the cues nurses report using. Nurses reported cues, such as, "the child is lying quietly, is guarding his side, or doesn't want to move."

The research on physiological parameters and pain suggests an inconsistency between their value from a measurement perspective and their value from a clinical perspective. The measurement research has yet to identify physiological indicators (e.g., heart rate, respiratory rate, and blood pressure) as reliable, valid, and sensitive methods for assessing pain. Interestingly, however, nurses often report heart rate, respiratory rate, and blood pressure as important indicators of pain.

◆ GUIDELINES FOR CLINICAL JUDGMENT IN ASSESSING CHILDREN'S PAIN

Guidelines for clinical judgment in assessing children's pain are based on viewing pain as an individualized experience and on the knowledge generated through research on pain measurement and on nurse cues or criteria for pain. The implementation of these guidelines depends on the *nurse's recognition of pain as a priority for each child.*

- "Recognize that ill children are *likely* to experience pain" (Stevens, 1989, p. 877).[129]
- Assume responsibility for pain assessment.
- Know the child and how pain might affect him or her. The interviews in the boxes beginning on p. 252 may yield important information about the child and previous painful experiences. Through interviews such as these,

the nurse may identify the most salient factors for a child.

- Develop a plan for pain assessment with the child, family, physician, and other health care providers.[129]
- Assess pain routinely in *every* child, regardless of diagnosis. The nurse may individualize a schedule for pain assessments based on factors such as the child's medical history, previous pain experiences, current condition, and anticipated pain episodes.
- Use reliable, generalizable, valid, and sensitive methods to measure pain. To select appropriate tools, the nurse should consider the following about specific tools:
  - The characteristics of the population on which the tool has been tested
  - The setting in which the testing occurred
  - The evidence available attesting to the tool's reliability, generalizability, validity, and sensitivity in measuring pain
  - The appropriateness of the content of the tool for the developmental level of the child, the setting, and the type of pain the child is experiencing
  - The training to learn to use the tool
  - The time to administer the tool
- Assess pain from a multidimensional perspective. The nurse should combine several ways of determining a child's pain level, for example:
  - Ask the child about his pain but also measure the amount of pain using a valid self-report scale.
  - Observe the child for signs of pain but also measure the pain using a valid observation scale.
  - Use physiological indicators, but not alone.
- Observe pain-related changes in the child, particularly the subtle cues.
- Document conclusions about pain on a flow sheet or in the chart. The nurse should routinely record the intensity of pain, the tool used, and other supporting evidence.
- Review the documentation to discern patterns of pain and pain relief for an individual child.

The assessment of pain must be prioritized as an important aspect of care for children. Research on the assessment of children's pain has provided a number of significant assessment and measurement strategies that can improve the clinical judgment of nurses in assessing pain. Good clinical judgment in assessing children's pain forms the foundation for adequate treatment that should yield the desired patient-centered outcome of *adequate pain relief.*

REFERENCES

1. Abu-Saad H. (1984a). Assessing children's responses to pain. *Pain, 19,* 163-171.
2. Abu-Saad H. (1984b). Cultural components of pain: the Arab-American child. *Iss Comp Pediatr Nurs, 7,* 91-99.
3. Abu-Saad H. (1984c). Cultural components of pain: the Asian-American child. *Child Health Care, 13*(1), 11-14.
4. Abu-Saad H. (1984d). Cultural group indicators of pain in children. *Mat Child Nurs J, 13,* 187-196.
5. Abu-Saad H. (1990). Toward the development of pain in children: Dutch study. In Tyler D and Krane E (eds), *Advances in pain research and therapy, vol 15: pediatric pain* (pp. 101-106), New York: Raven Press.
6. Abu-Saad H and Holzemer WL. (1981). Measuring children's self-assessment of pain. *Iss Comp Pediatr Nurs, 5,* 337-349.
7. Alyea B. (1978). *Child pain rating after injection preparation.* Unpublished master's thesis, University of Missouri, Columbia.
8. Anand KJS, Brown R, Bloom S, and Aynsley-Green A. (1985). Studies on the hormonal regulation of fuel metabolism in the human newborn infant undergoing anesthesia and surgery. *Horm Res, 22,* 115-128.
9. Anand KJS and Hickey P. (1987). Pain and its effects in the human neonate and fetus. *N Engl J Med, 317,* 1321-1329.
10. Andrasik F, Burke E, Attanasio V, and Rosenblum E. (1985). Child, parent, and physician reports of a child's headache: relationships prior to and following treatment. *Headache, 25,* 421-425.
11. Aradine C, Beyer J, and Tompkins J. (1988). Children's perceptions before and after analgesia: a study of instrument construct validity. *J Pediatr Nurs, 3,* 11-23.
12. Beales JG, Keen JH, and Holt PJL. (1983). The child's perception of the disease and the experience of pain in juvenile chronic arthritis. *J Rheumatol, 10,* 61-65.
13. Belter R, McIntosh J, Finch A, and Saylor C. (1988). Measurement of pain in preschool children: three self-report methods. *Clin J Child Psychol, 17,* 327-335.
14. Benner P and Wrubel J. (1989). *The primacy of caring: stress and coping in health and illness.* Menlo Park, Calif: Addison-Wesley Publishing.
15. Beyer JE. (1984). *The oucher: a user's manual and technical report.* Charlottsville, Va: University of Virginia Alumni Patent Foundation.
16. Beyer JE. (1988). *The oucher: a user's manual and technical report.* Denver: University of Colorado Health Sciences Center.
17. Beyer JE and Aradine CR. (1986). Content validity of an instrument to measure young children's perceptions of the intensity of their pain. *J Pediatr Nurs, 1*(6), 386-395.
18. Beyer J and Aradine C. (1987). Patterns of pediatric pain intensity: a methodological investigation of a self-report scale. *Clin J Pain, 3,* 130-141.
19. Beyer JE and Aradine CR. (1988). Convergent and discriminant validity

of a self-report measure of pain intensity for children. *Child Health Care, 16*(4), 274-282.

20. Beyer JE and Knapp TR. (1986). Methodological issues in the measurement of children's pain. *Child Health Care, 14,* 233-241.
21. Beyer JE, McGrath PJ, and Berde CB. (1990). Discordance between self-report and behavioral measures in 3-7 year old children following surgery. *J Pain Sympt Manage, 5*(6), 350-356.
22. Bradshaw C and Zeanah PD. (1986). Pediatric nurses' assessments of pain in children. *J Pediatr Nurs, 1*(5), 314-322.
23. Carpenter P (1990). New method for measuring young children's self-report of fear and pain. *J Pain Sympt Manage, 5*(4), 233-240.
24. Craig KD, McMahon RJ, Morison JD, and Zaskow C. (1984). Developmental changes in infant pain expression during immunization injections. *Soc Sci Med, 19*(12), 1331-1337.
25. Cronbach L, Gleser G, Wanda H, and Rajaratnam N. (1972). *The dependability of behavioral measurements theory of generalizability for scores and profiles.* New York: Wiley.
26. Dale JC. (1986). A multidimensional study of infants' responses to painful stimuli. *Pediatr Nurs, 12*(1), 27-31.
27. Datz L. (1989). *Comparison of mother's and children's ratings of children's tonsillectomy pain intensity.* Unpublished master's thesis, University of California, Los Angeles.
28. Davis DH and Calhoon M. (1989). Do preterm infants show behavioral responses to painful procedures? In Funk SG, Tornquist FM, Champagne MT, Copp LA, and Wiese RA (eds), *Key aspects of comfort: management of pain, fatigue, and nausea,* (pp. 35-45) New York: Springer Publishing.
29. Denyes M. (1990). Effect of nursing actions to alleviate pain in children. Grant funded by NIH, National Center for Nursing Research.
30. Denyes M and Villarruel A. (1988a). *Content validity of a self-report pain intensity instrument with young black children.* Unpublished manuscript, Wayne State University, Detroit.
31. Denyes M and Villarruel A. (July 1988b). *Development of culturally sensitive measures of pain in young children.* Paper presented at the First International Symposium on Pediatric Pain, Seattle.
32. Ekman P and Friesen WV. (1978). *Facial action coding system: a technique for the measurement of facial movement.* Palo Alto, Calif: Consulting Psychologists Press.
33. Eland JM. (1974). *Children's communication of pain.* Unpublished master's thesis, University of Iowa, Iowa City.
34. Eland JM. (1975). *Assessment and management of pain in children.* Paper presented at The Children's Hospital, Denver.
35. Eland JM. (1981). Minimizing pain associated with prekindergarten intramuscular injections. *Iss Comp Pediatr Nurs, 5,* 361-372.
36. Eland JM. (1983). Children's pain: developmentally appropriate efforts to improve identification of source, intensity and relevant intervening variables. In Felton G and Albert M (eds), *Nursing research: a monograph for non-nurse researchers* (pp. 64-79). Iowa City: University of Iowa Press.
37. Eland JM and Anderson JE. (1977). The experience of pain in children. In Jacox AK (ed), *Pain: a sourcebook for nurses and other health professionals* (pp. 453-473). Boston: Little Brown.

38. Falco J. (1985). Pain experienced by children with juvenile rheumatoid arthritis. Unpublished raw data.
39. Field T and Goldson E. (1984). Pacifying effects of nonnutritive sucking on term and preterm neonates during heelstick procedures. *Pediatrics, 74,* 1012-1015.
40. Fiselier T, Monnens L, Moerman E, et al. Influence of the stress of venipuncture on basal levels of plasma renin activity in infants and children. *Int J Pediatr Nephrol, 4,* 181-185.
40a. Foster RL. (1990). *A multi-method approach to the description of factors influencing nurses' pharmacologic management of children's pain.* Unpublished doctoral dissertation, University of Colorado Health Sciences Center, Denver.
41. Foster RL. (1981). *Coping strategies of the child with leukemia: the stress of invasive procedures.* Unpublished master's thesis, University of Colorado Health Sciences Center, Denver.
42. Franck LS. (1986). A new method to quantitatively describe pain behavior in infants. *Nurs Res, 35,* 28-31.
43. Froese-Fretz A. (1986). *The use of transcutaneous electrical nerve stimulators (TENS) during radial arterial blood sampling in newborn infants.* Unpublished master's thesis, University of Colorado Health Sciences Center, Denver.
44. Fuller B and Hester N. (1990). Concurrent validity of acoustic, self-report, and caretaker's measures for assessing children's pain. Unpublished raw data.
45. Fuller B, Connor D, and Horii Y. (1990). Potential acoustic measures of infant pain and arousal. In Tyler D and Krane E (eds), *Advances in pain research and therapy, vol 15: pediatric pain* (pp. 137-145), New York: Raven Press.
46. Fuller B, Horii Y, and Connor D. (1989). Vocal measures of infant pain. In Funk SG, Tornquist EM, Champagne MT, Lopp LA, and Wiese RA (eds), *Key aspects of comfort: management of pain, fatigue and nausea* (pp. 46-51). New York: Springer Publishing.
47. Gaffney A and Dunne E. (1986). Developmental aspects of children's definitions of pain. *Pain, 26,* 105-117.
48. Gauvain-Piquard A, Rodary C, Rezvani A, and Lemerie J. (1987). Pain in children aged 2-6 years: a new observational rating scale elaborated in a pediatric oncology unit—preliminary report. *Pain, 31,* 177-188.
49. Grunau R and Craig K. (1990). Facial activity as a measure of neonatal pain expression. In Tyler D and Krane E (eds), *Advances in pain research and therapy, vol 15: pediatric pain* (pp. 147-155), New York: Raven Press.
50. Grunau RVE and Craig KD. (1987). Pain expression in neonates: facial action and cry. *Pain, 28,* 395-410.
51. Gunnar MR, Fisch RO, Korsvik S, and Donhowe JM. (1981). The effects of circumcision on serum cortisol and behavior. *Psychoneuroendocrinology, 6,* 269-275.
52. Hagedorn M. (1990). *Does a topical skin cooling agent alter a child's pain perception during a D.P.T. injection?* Unpublished master's thesis, University of Colorado Health Sciences Center, Denver.
53. Harpin VA and Rutter N. (1982). Development of emotional sweating in the newborn infant. *Arch Dis Child, 57,* 691-695.
54. Hay H. (1984). *The measurement of pain intensity in children and*

adults—a methodological approach. Unpublished master's research report, McGill University, Montreal, Canada.

55. Hay H and O'Brien C. (1986). The measurements of pain intensity in children and adults . . . a methodological approach. *Proceedings of the International Nursing Research Conference,* University of Alberta: Edmonton, Alberta, Canada.
56. Hester NO. (1989). Comforting the child in pain. In Funk SG, Tornquist EM, Champagne MT, Copp LA, and Wiese RA (eds), *Key aspects of comfort: management of pain, fatigue, and nausea* (pp. 290-298). New York: Springer Publishing.
57. Hester NO. (1986). The human experience of pain for children. Unpublished raw data.
58. Hester NO. (1976). *The preoperational child's reaction to immunizations.* Unpublished master's thesis, University of Kansas Medical Center, Kansas City, Kan.
59. Hester NO. (1979). The preoperational child's reaction to immunization. *Nurs Res, 28*(4), 250-254.
60. Hester N and Barcus C. (1986). Assessment and management of pain in children. *Pediatr: Nurs Update, 1*(14), 1-8.
61. Hester NO, Davis RC, Hanson SH, and Hassanein RS. (1978). *The hospitalized child's subjective rating of painful experiences.* Unpublished manuscript, University of Kansas Medical Center, Kansas City, Kan.
62. Hester NO and Foster RL. (October 1988). *Assessment of pain in children: the state of the art.* Paper presented at The Art of Caring and the Pediatric Oncology Nurse, Association of Pediatric Oncology Nurses, Denver.
63. Hester NO and Foster RL. (1990). Cues nurses and parents use in making judgments about children's pain. *Pain,* Supplement 5, S31.
64. Hester NO, Foster RL, and Kristensen K. (1990). Measurement of pain in children: generalizability and validity of the pain ladder and the poker chip tool. In Tyler DC and Krane EJ (eds), *Advances in pain research and therapy, vol 15: pediatric pain.* New York: Raven Press.
65. Hester NO, Foster RL, and Kristensen K. (March 1989). *Sensitivity, convergent and discriminant validity of the pain ladder and the poker chip tool.* Paper presented at Third International Nursing Research Symposium, Clinical Care of the Child and Family, Montreal, Canada.
66. Hester NO, Foster R, Kristensen K, and Bergstrom L. (1989). *Measurement of children's pain by children, parents, and nurses: psychometric and clinical issues related to the poker chip tool and the pain ladder.* Final report for study entitled *Generalizability of procedures assessing pain in children.* Research funded by NIH, National Center for Nursing Research under grant number NRO1382.
67. Holve R, Bromberger P, Groveman H, et al. (1983). Regional anesthesia during newborn circumcision. *Clin Pediatr, 22*(12), 813-818.
68. Huskisson EC. (1974). Measurement of pain. *Lancet, 2,* 1127-1131.
69. Izard CE, Huebner RR, Risser D, McGiness GC, and Dougherty LM. (1980). The infant's ability to produce discrete emotional expressions. *Dev Psychol, 16,* 132-140.
70. Jay SM and Elliot C. (1984). Behavioral observation scales for measuring children's distress: the effects of increased methodological rigor. *J Consult Clin Psychol, 52,* 1106-1107.
71. Jay SM and Elliott C. (1986). *Observation scale of behavioral distress: information, scoring procedures, definitions of behaviors, OSBD inter-*

val coding form (revised manual). Los Angeles: Children's Hospital of Los Angeles.

72. Jay SM, Elliott CH, Katz E, and Siegel SE. (1987). Cognitive-behavioral and pharmacologic interventions for children's distress during painful medical procedures. *J Consult Clin Psychol, 55,* 860-865.
73. Jeans ME and Gordon DJ. (1981). An investigation of the developmental characteristics of the concept of pain. *Pain* (Suppl 1), S11.
74. Jerrett MD and Evans K. (1986). Children's pain vocabulary. *J Adv Nurs, 11,* 403-408.
75. Johnson M. (1977). Assessment of clinical pain. In Jacox A (ed), *Pain: a sourcebook for nurses and other health professionals* (pp. 139-166). Boston: Little, Brown.
76. Johnston CC. (1989). Pain assessment and management in infants. *Pediatrician, 16,* 16-23.
77. Johnston CC and O'Shaughnessy D. (1988). Acoustical attributes of infant pain cries: discriminating features. In Dubner R, Gebhart GF, and Bond MR (eds), *Pain research and clinical management, 3* (pp. 336-340). Amsterdam: Elsevier.
78. Johnston CC and Strada ME. (1986). Acute pain response in infants: a multidimensional description. *Pain, 24,* 373-382.
79. Jordan-Marsh M. (October 1990). *Criteria for selecting pain assessment tools.* Paper presented at the Ninth Annual Scientific Meeting, American Pain Society, St. Louis.
80. Jordan-Marsh M, Brown R, Watson R, and Duncan L. (1990a). *The Harbor-UCLA Medical Center humor for pain in children project* (funded by the Research and Education Institute, Inc.). Los Angeles: Harbor-UCLA Medical Center.
81. Jordan-Marsh M, Brown R, Watson R, and Duncan L. (1990b). *Pediatric pain assessment research: application challenges in multicultural acute care setting.* Unpublished manuscript, Harbor-UCLA Medical Center, Los Angeles.
82. Katz ER, Sharp B, Kellerman V. (1982). Beta-endorphin immunoreactivity and acute behavioral distress in children with leukemia. *J Nerv Ment Dis, 170,* 72-77.
83. Katz ER, Kellerman J, and Siegel SE. (1980). Behavioral distress in children with cancer undergoing medical procedures: developmental considerations. *J Consult Clin Psychol, 48,* 356-365.
84. Keefe M. (1984). *The effect of the hospital environment on infant state behavior and maternal sleep.* Unpublished doctoral dissertation, University of Colorado, Denver.
85. LeBaron S and Zeltzer L. (1984). Assessment of acute pain and anxiety in children and adolescents by self-reports, observer reports, and a behavior checklist. *J Consult Clin Psychol, 52*(5), 729-738.
86. Levy DM. (1960). The infant's earliest memory of innoculation: a contribution to public health procedures. *J Genet Psychol, 96,* 3-46.
87. Lollar DJ, Smits SJ, and Patterson DL. (1982). Assessment of pediatric pain: an empirical perspective. *J Pediatr Psychol,* 7(3), 267-276.
88. Lorig K. (1984). Measurement of pain. (Letter to the editor). *Nurs Res, 33,* 367.
89. Lukens M. (1982). *The identification of criteria used by nurses in the assessment of pain in children.* Unpublished master's thesis, University of Cincinnati, Cincinnati.

90. McCaffery M. (1972). *Nursing management of the patient with pain.* Philadelphia: JB Lippincott.
91. McGrath PA. (1987). An assessment of children's pain: a review of behavioral, physiological and direct scaling techniques. *Pain, 31,* 147-176.
92. McGrath PA. (1990). *Pain in children: nature, assessment, and treatment.* New York: Guilford Publications.
93. McGrath PA, deVeber LL, and Hearn MT. (1985). Multidimensional pain assessment in children. *Adv Pain Res Ther, 9,* 387-393.
94. McGrath PJ, Johnson G, Goodman JT, et al. (1985). The CHEOPS: a behavioral scale to measure post operative pain in children. In Fields HL, Dubner R, and Cervero F (eds), *Advances in pain research and therapy* (pp. 395-402). New York: Raven Press.
95. McGrath PJ and Unruh AM. (1987). *Pain in children and adolescents.* New York: Elsevier.
96. Maunuksela E, Olkkola K, and Korpela R. (1987). Measurement of pain in children with self-reporting and behavioral assessment. *Clin Pharmacol Ther, 42,* 137-141.
97. Maxwell L, Yaster M, Wetzel R, and Niebyl J. (1987). Penile nerve block for newborn circumcision. *Obstet Gynecol, 70*(3), 415-419.
98. Melamed BG and Siegel LJ. (1975). Reduction of anxiety in children facing hospitalization and surgery by use of filmed modeling. *J Consult Clin Psychol, 43,* 511-521.
99. Melamed BG, Yurcheson R, Fleece EL, Hutcherson S, and Hawes R. (1978). Effects of film modeling on the reduction of anxiety-related behaviors in individuals varying in level of previous experience in the stress situation. *J Consult Clin Psychol, 46,* 1357-1367.
100. Melzack R. (1975). The McGill pain questionnaire: major properties and scoring methods. *Pain, 1,* 277-299.
101. Mills N. (1989a). Acute pain behavior in infants and toddlers. In Funk S, Tournquist E, Champagne M, Copp L, and Wiese R (eds), *Key aspects of comfort: management of pain, fatigue, and nausea* (pp. 52-59). New York: Springer Publishing.
102. Mills N. (1989b). Pain behaviors in infants and toddlers. *J Pain Sympt Manage, 4*(4), 184-190.
103. Mischel H, Fuhr R, and McDonald M. (1986). Children's dental pain: the effects of cognitive coping training in a clinical setting. *Clin J Pain, 1,* 235-242.
104. Molsberry D. (1979). *Young children's subjective quantification of pain following surgery.* Unpublished master's thesis, University of Iowa, Iowa City.
105. Neuman BM, Denyes MJ, Stettner L, and Villarruel AM. (1990). Facial expression as an emotional response to pain: a study of instrument content validity. *Pain,* Suppl 5, S25.
106. Norris S, Campbell L, and Brenkert S. (1982). Nursing procedures and alterations in transcutaneous oxygen tension in premature infants. *Nurs Res, 31*(6), 330-336.
107. Olness K, Wain HJ, and Ng L. (1980). A pilot study of blood endorphins in children using self-hypnosis. *J Dev Behav Pediatr, 1,* 187-188.
108. Owens M and Todt EH. (1984). Pain in infancy: reaction to a heel lance. *Pain, 20,* 77-86.
109. Piaget J and Inhelder B. (1969). *The psychology of the child.* New York: Basic Books.

110. Pomietto M. (1988, Spring). Pain management at Children's Hospital: results of 1987 survey. *Express 88* 1, 8.
111. Primm P. (1971). *Identification of criteria used by nurses in the assessment of pain in children.* Unpublished master's thesis, University of Iowa, Ames.
112. Rich E, Marshall R, Volpe J. (1974). The normal neonatal response to pinprick. *Dev Med Child Neurol, 16,* 132-140.
113. Richardson GM, McGrath PJ, Cunningham SJ, and Humphreys P. (1983). Validity of the headache diary for children, *Headache, 23,* 184-187.
114. Ritchie J. (1989, May). *Nurses' assessments and management strategies for children's pain.* Paper presented at Research in Pain, the annual meeting of the Association for the Care of Children's Health, Anaheim, Calif.
115. Ross DM and Ross SA. (1982). *A study of the pain experience in children* (final report, ref. no. 1 R01 HD13672-01). Bethesda, Md: National Institute of Child Health and Human Development.
116. Ross DM and Ross SA. (1984). The importance of type of question, psychological climate, and subject set in interviewing children about pain. *Pain, 19,* 71-79.
117. Ross DM and Ross SA. (1988). *Childhood pain: current issues, research, and management.* Baltimore: Urban & Schwartzenberg.
118. Savedra M, Gibbons P, Tessler M, Ward J, and Wegner C. (1982). How do children describe pain? A tentative assessment. *Pain, 14,* 95-104.
119. Savedra MC and Tesler MD. (1989). Assessing children's and adolescents' pain. *Pediatrician, 16,* 24-29.
120. Savedra MC, Tesler MD, Holzemer WL, and Ward JA. (1989). *Adolescent pediatric pain tool (APPT) preliminary user's manual.* San Francisco: University of California.
121. Savedra MC, Tesler MD, Holzemer WL, Wilkie DJ, and Ward JA. (1989). Pain location: validity and reliability of body outline markings by hospitalized children and adolescents. *Res Nurs Health, 12,* 307-314.
122. Savedra M, Tesler M, Holzemer W, Wilkie D, and Ward J. (1990). Testing a tool to assess postoperative pediatric and adolescent pain. In Tyler DC and Krane EJ (eds), *Advances in pain research and therapy, vol 15: pediatric pain* (pp. 85-93). New York: Raven Press.
123. Savedra M, Tesler M, Ward J, and Wegner C. (1988). How do adolescents describe pain? *J Adoles Health Care, 9,* 315-320.
124. Schultz NV. (1971). How children perceive pain. *Nurs Outlook, 19,* 670-673.
125. Scott R. (1978). "It hurts red": a preliminary study of children's perception of pain. *Percep Motor Skills, 47,* 787-791.
126. Scott PJ, Ansell BM, and Huskisson EC. (1977). Measurement of pain in juvenile chronic polyarthritis. *Ann Rheum Dis, 36,* 186-187.
127. Scott J and Huskisson EC. (1976). Graphic representation of pain. *Pain, 2,* 175-184.
128. Scott J and Huskisson EC. (1979). Vertical or horizontal visual analogue scales. *Ann Rheum Dis, 38,* 560.
129. Stevens B. (1989). Nursing management of pain in children. In Foster R, Hunsberger M, and Anderson J (eds). *Family-centered nursing care of children,* Philadelphia: WB Saunders.
130. Stevens J. (1989). *Androcies and the lion* (an adapted Aesop fable). New York: Holiday House.

131. Sturner R, Rothbaum F, Visintainer M, and Wolfer J. (1980). The effects of stress on children's human figure drawings. *J Clin Psychol, 36,* 324-331.
132. Szyfelbein SK, Osgood PF, and Carr DB. (1985). The assessment of pain and plasma B-endorphin immunoactivity in burned children. *Pain, 22,* 173-182.
133. Talbert LM, Kraybill EH, and Potter HD. (1976). Adrenal cortical response to circumcision in the neonate. *Obstet Gynecol, 48,* 208-210.
134. Taylor P. (1983). Post-operative pain in toddler and pre-school age children. *Mat Child Nurs J, 12,* 35-50.
135. Tesler MD, Savedra MC, Ward JA, Holzemer WL, and Wilkie DJ. (1989). Children's words for pain. In Funk SG, Tornquist EM, Champagne MT, Copp LA, and Wiese RA (eds), *Key aspects of comfort: management of pain, fatigue, and nausea* (pp. 60-65). New York: Springer Publishing.
136. Tesler M, Ward J, Savedra M, Wegner C, and Gibbons P. (1983). Developing an instrument for eliciting children's description of pain. *Percept Motor Skills, 56,* 315-321.
137. Unruh A, McGrath P, Cunningham SJ, and Humphreys P. (1983). Children's drawings of their pain. *Pain, 17,* 385-392.
138. Varchol D. (1983). *The relationship between nurses' and children's perception of pain in the acute and chronic pain experiences of children.* Unpublished master's thesis, University of Cincinnati.
139. Varni JW and Thompson KL. (1985). *The Varni/Thompson pediatric pain questionnaire.* Unpublished manuscript.
140. Varni J, Thompson K, and Hanson V. (1987). The Varni/Thompson pediatric pain questionnaire. I. Chronic musculoskeletal pain in juvenile rheumatoid arthritis. *Pain, 28,* 27-38.
141. Varni J, Walco G, and Katz E. (1989). Assessment and management of chronic and recurrent pain in children with chronic diseases. *Pediatrician, 16,* 56-63.
142. Villamira M and Occhiuto M. (1984). Psychological aspects of pain in children, particularly relating to their family and school environment. In Rizzi R, Visentin M (eds), *Pain* (285-289). Padua, Italy: Piccin/Butterworths.
143. Villarruel A and Denyes M. (May 1989). Cultural considerations in the assessment of pain in children. Paper presented at the 24th Annual Conference of the Association for the Care of Children's Health, Anaheim, Calif.
144. Villarruel A and Denyes M. (1990). *Content validity of a self-report pain intensity instrument for Hispanic children.* Unpublished manuscript, University of Michigan, Detroit.
145. Ward B. (1975). *Externally observed pain—associated behavior and internally perceived pain intensity in the four through eight year old child.* Unpublished master's thesis, University of Kansas Medical Center, Kansas City.
146. Wasz-Hockert O, Michelson K, and Lind J. (1985). Twenty-five years of Scandinavian cry research. In Lester BM, Boukydis CFZ (eds), *Infant crying: theoretical and research perspectives* (83-104). New York: Plenum.
147. Watson J. (1985). *Nursing: human science and human care.* Norwalk, Conn: Appleton-Century-Crofts.
148. Whaley L and Wong D. (1987). *Nursing care of infants and children* (ed 3). St. Louis: CV Mosby.

149. Wilkie DJ, Holzemer WL, Tesler MD, et al. (1990). Measuring pain quality: validity and reliability of children's and adolescents' pain language. *Pain, 41*(2), 151-159.
150. Williamson PS and Williamson ML. (1983). Physiologic stress reduction by a local anesthetic during newborn circumcision. *Pediatrics, 71,* 36-40.
151. Wolff PH. (1969). The natural history of crying and other vocalizations in early infancy. In Foss BM (ed), *Determinants of infant behavior, vol 4.* London: Methuen.
152. Wong D and Baker C. (1988). Pain in children: comparison of assessment scales. *Pediatr Nurs, 14,* 9-17.

11

Clinical Judgment in Managing the Crisis of Children's Pain

Judith E. Beyer
Susan A. Clegg
Roxie L. Foster
Nancy O. Hester

THE CLINICAL MANAGEMENT of children's pain is a complex and challenging responsibility that rests primarily on pediatric nurses. The process requires expert knowledge of developmental principles and skill in implementing assessment (Chapters 3, 4, and 9) and intervention strategies. This chapter begins with evidence showing that the treatment for pain in children is inadequate. A framework follows that develops the notion that unrelieved pain may precipitate a state of crisis in children. Reasons that treatment may be inadequate are suggested, and an overview of common pediatric pain experiences and an explanation of new pain management techniques are then presented. Finally, suggestions are provided for reducing or relieving pain in children.

◆ INADEQUACY OF PAIN MANAGEMENT

Numerous studies in recent literature present evidence to suggest that children are seriously undertreated for pain.* Most of this evidence comes from research relating to postoperative analgesic use. According to Schechter,[98] the pain of

* References 15, 24, 31, 34, 69, 100.

burn injuries and invasive medical procedures is also undertreated in children. In addition, Schechter, Berrien, and Katz[101] reported that the pain of sickle cell crisis is probably undertreated in children and adolescents. Few studies have focused on the efficacy of nonpharmacological techniques in pediatric patients with painful conditions. More research is necessary to thoroughly investigate the quality of pain management practices with children.

A review of the results of available studies indicates that children receive fewer and less frequent doses of medication than adults postoperatively.[15,31,100] The details of the findings of these studies are reported in Chapter 12. Several additional studies also raise questions about the appropriate pharmacological management of children's pain experiences. Mather and Mackie[69] found that nonnarcotics were often used instead of narcotics in a group of 170 postoperative Australian children. Burokas[24] found subtherapeutic dosage ranges and intervals among a group of 40 children after abdominal or thoracic surgery. Foster and Hester[34] found that in a sample of 150 4- to 13-year-old hospitalized children, analgesics were administered only 39% of the time when subjects were eligible for them. For this sample, there was no relationship between the children's pain scores and the nurses' decisions to medicate. A number of the studies showed that significant proportions of postoperative pediatric samples did not receive any analgesics: 24%;[15] 52%;[31] and 16%.[69] Two studies reported proportions of samples not given narcotics after major injuries or surgeries: 13%[24] and 13%.[100] One subject in the study by Burokas[24] was a 2-day-old infant who had a repair of a tracheoesophageal fistula and who received a total of 22 doses of Pavulon (muscle paralyzer) but no narcotics. Clearly, the process of pain management in children requires more attention from the nursing community to sort out and solve the many issues and problems.

◆ PAIN AS A CRISIS FOR CHILDREN

Unrelieved pain, regardless of the origin, may represent a crisis to children experiencing it. As noted by Brownell,[21] crisis is a concept that nurses confront daily, yet the term itself lacks clarity. Caplan[25] described crisis as an upset in a steady state and indicated that crisis occurs when an individual faces a problem or obstacle in life that he or she cannot manage by using customary methods of problem-solving. Pain would qualify as a "situational crisis," defined by Geissler[44] as "one which results from unexpected or sudden externally imposed stress or trauma" (p. 2). Through an extensive review of literature, Geissler concluded that crisis is neither positive nor negative and that several assumptions about crisis are widely accepted:

- Crisis occurs in healthy individuals and is not equated with psychopathology.
- Crises are temporary and acute, not chronic.
- The seriousness of an obstacle or event must be defined by the experiencing individual, not by the magnitude of the event itself.
- A crisis situation contains the potential for psychological growth or deterioration. (p. 2)

In addition, Geissler[44] said that four provisional criteria are common in addressing the concept of crisis:

- An impediment to the desired goal
- A decisive point requiring action
- The inability to act constructively
- A period of psychological instability (p. 3)

In crisis, an individual attempts to maintain a state of equilibrium by employing a variety of adaptive and problem-solving techniques.[91] The inability to cope with a situation or problem disrupts normal equilibrium, and a state of disequilibrium occurs.[25]

Pain may create a state of disequilibrium in children.[95] Children are more vulnerable to disequilibrium because they have limited coping strategies. Children attempt to cope with noxious stimuli by using the limited resources at their disposal. Younger children are even more limited than older children in effectively mobilizing coping strategies.[19,93] Young children typically use more motor and emotional coping strategies, such as physical resistance and crying. Cognitive strategies, such as verbal expression of anxiety and verbal stalling, are increasingly incorporated as children get older, thus enhancing their repertoire of coping mechanisms.[33,78] It follows that younger children, who have fewer coping strategies, may be especially vulnerable to disequilibrium when experiencing pain.

Children are also more vulnerable to disequilibrium when pain is severe, continuous, or recurrent. Coping with pain requires a great deal of energy, and pain that is intense or prolonged may leave a child physically and emotionally exhausted. Fatigue, in turn, further reduces coping abilities, predisposing the child to crisis. This situation is potentiated when caregivers (1) fail to recognize the child is in pain, (2) fail to treat the pain, and/or (3) fail to evaluate the effectiveness of treatment.

When children perceive that they cannot change, stop, or escape their pain,[95,103] a crisis may ensue. If adult caregivers fail or are unable to provide pain relief, children may feel helpless, frustrated, and angry. Children interviewed by Hester[49] expressed feelings of anger and frustration in relation to the pain they had experienced during hospitalization. A 10-year-old girl explained:

> I don't like it when people ignore me when I'm in pain, like if I buzz the nurse and she says "Can I help you?" and I ask for a pain pill and she says "Well I don't think we should give you one because you're a child." I've had them (pain pills) all the time . . . I can take them. It makes me mad because (she) should have been informed that I am able to take up to two pain pills at one time and I can take them up to three times a day (p. 292).

A 13-year-old boy told Hester that when he was in pain he felt "like screaming. I get mad, I mean, I have a bad temper anyway and when I hurt, I want to get revenge . . . I want to grab my doctor's neck" (p. 293).

Crisis precipitated by unrelieved pain may know no developmental boundaries. Mills[78] reported that two infants in her study of pain behaviors pinched or bit their own arms. She speculated that this behavior may have related, in part, to the infants' frustration with their pain.

In addition to the moral issues associated with needless suffering, there may be other reasons to avoid crises precipitated by unrelieved pain. Citing Lazarus and Folkman's[65] theory of coping, Caty, Ritchie, and Ellerton[26] suggest that children's ability to cope with the stresses of hospitalization may influence overall somatic health, morale, and social functioning. Lazarus and Folkman assert, "The question should not be whether stress is good or bad, but rather how much, what kinds, at which times during the life course, and under what social and personal conditions it is harmful or helpful" (p. 182). Pain can be counted among the stresses many, if not most, hospitalized children face that, when unrelieved, may precipitate a state of crisis.

◆ REASONS PAIN MANAGEMENT IS PROBLEMATIC

Decision-making in pain management is influenced by many factors. These contributing factors probably include the existing knowledge base about pain and pain relief, the inaccurate beliefs about pediatric pain, the attitudes of nurses and physicians regarding children in pain, and the complexity of the nursing role in pediatric pain assessment and management. Erroneous beliefs or misbeliefs are discussed in Chapter 3. Few studies have explored systematically the factors that contribute to decisions about pain management in children. A major funded study of decision-making among nurses in regard to children's pain should clarify some of the issues in pain management.[50]

The Knowledge Base

Eland and Anderson[31] were the first to systematically review the content on pediatric pain in medical and nursing journals and textbooks. Their analysis showed that major nursing and medical texts severely lacked content about pediatric pain. Rana[90] supported this finding in medical texts and provided a detailed table showing how many pages in each volume were devoted to pain. For the majority of pediatric medical texts, pain content was nonexistent. This void is being addressed by the fact that entire books are now being written on pediatric pain.[1,71,76,95] In addition, the proceedings of the First International Conference on Pediatric Pain held in Seattle, Wash., in July of 1988 have also been published in book form.[112] Further, chapters specific to children are now being included in textbooks on pain (e.g., Wall and Melzack[117]). Certain current nursing references also devote entire chapters to pediatric pain.[36,42,70] Information on pain in nursing and medical texts should alert students and professors alike that pain is "essential content" in curricula and must be addressed more emphatically in educational programs.

Just a decade ago, journal articles related to pediatric pain were rare. Eland and Anderson[31] conducted a search of the journal literature between 1970 and 1975 and found a total of 33 articles on pediatric pain. Most were medically oriented and related to chronic pain conditions, such as recurrent abdominal pain or headache. They found little information related to assessment of intensity, children's pain responses, or appropriate management.

Over the past 5 years, the number of articles on children's pain in the journal literature has increased dramatically. Part or all of an issue was devoted to this topic in *Pediatric Clinics of North America* (1984 and 1989), *Nursing Clinics of North America* (1987), *Issues of Comprehensive Pediatric Nursing* (1981 and 1988), *Pediatrician* (1989), and *Journal of Pain and Symptom Management* (1989).

Despite the accumulating findings from many studies, little is certain about children's pain.[14] A list of corroborated research findings related to pain in children is provided (see box). These issues are addressed later in this chapter or in Chapter 10.

◆ KNOWLEDGE BASE ABOUT PAIN IN CHILDREN

1. Children receive fewer doses of analgesics for pain than adults with similar conditions.[15,31,100]
2. Pain management with analgesics often is not sufficient to relieve children's pain.*
3. Several validated pain self-report assessment tools for children 3 years and older could, if used correctly, provide more accurate assessment of children's pain experiences than is traditionally practiced.[18,54,96]
4. Infants respond behaviorally and physiologically to presumably pain-producing stimuli.†
5. Children respond behaviorally to pain, but the nature of this response varies. The details of, and the meaning of, these behavioral responses as they relate to the amount of pain have not been thoroughly explored or elucidated.[16,51,52,53]
6. Children seem to benefit from a variety of pharmacological and nonpharmacological pain management techniques used in clinical settings, although these techniques are just beginning to be tested through research for their efficacy.‡
7. Inaccurate beliefs about pain and personal biases and experiences of health care providers influence their pain assessment and management practices with children.[24,46,99] Many of these beliefs and biases may result in the provision of inadequate pain relief.

*References 29, 31, 34, 50, 69, 97.
†References 3, 38, 39, 40, 47.
‡References 8, 10, 11, 29, 30, 71, 76, 102, 118.

Inaccurate Beliefs about Children's Pain

The notion of inaccurate beliefs about children's pain is considered in more depth in Chapter 3. However, the undertreatment of pain in children is strongly related to these inaccurate beliefs, and they are still prevalent among health care providers despite research and practice findings to the contrary. For this reason, it seems important to address these beliefs here too. Some of the most common "myths" about pain[31,70,98] include the following:

1. Children do not feel pain as adults do
2. Since children cannot verbalize the nature of their pain, they are not in pain
3. Narcotics depress respirations and cause addiction in children more readily than in adults
4. Children require fewer narcotics because their metabolism of these drugs is different from adults

Those who hold these inaccurate beliefs would not be able to assess or manage the pain experience of children accurately.

Recent literature and research on the physiological[2,3,4,92] and behavioral[47,48,111] responses of infants and young children strongly suggest that they do indeed feel pain meaningfully. Owens[86,86a] argued that pain is one of the very first emotions to appear because it is a response to tissue damage and is of utmost importance to the survival of the neonate.

Children's inabilities to discuss or describe pain has nothing to do with their abilities to feel pain. They may even hide expressions of pain altogether,[20,31,103] such as by playing or sleeping. Hester and Barcus[52] reported that children may sleep as a means of coping with the severity of pain. Hiding pain may also be related to children's fears of additional pain, as from injections.[31]

Infants over a month old and children are not more prone than adults to respiratory depression and addiction resulting from the use of opioid analgesics.[98] Doses of narcotics that are appropriately calculated are generally no more dangerous than any other drug.[31,77] Ross and Ross[95] assert that respiratory depression is a rare complication that should not deter the use of narcotics for pain control. Further, the duration of pain, for example, postoperative pain, is too short to allow addiction to occur.[31,95] Although pharmacokinetic differences exist, no firm evidence shows that children require less analgesia than adults because of differences in the rate of drug metabolism and excretion.[95,99]

Researchers and clinicians alike are working to sort out the differences between fact and fiction on the topic of children's pain. Inaccurate beliefs, at least in part, account for some inappropriate and inaccurate pain management practices.

Attitudes/Beliefs

Along with knowledge and skill, nurses bring their own belief systems and attitudes to the work environment, which are interwoven into the way they practice nursing. Nurses' attitudes, values, and beliefs are bound to affect how they manage the patient in pain. Burke and Jerrett[23] studied BSN students' pain management strategies for patients in acute pain across all age groups. Findings did not consistently correspond with what the students were taught in an extensive learning module on pain. Burke and Jerrett concluded that attitudes and beliefs of the nursing students had a stronger influence on their ideas of pain management than did the curriculum content. Burokas[24] also provided evidence to suggest that attitudes and beliefs affected nurses' decisions to medicate for pain. Nurses whose offspring had experienced a severe painful episode medicated their postoperative pediatric patients significantly more frequently. In a vignette study by Holm and colleagues,[57] nurses who had experienced more intense pain in their own lives seemed more sympathetic in their assessment of patients in pain, regardless of age, race, or sex of the patient.

In the study by Burokas,[24] nurses' goals for pain relief seemed to have the most influence on their decisions to use medications with children. When 84 nurses were asked about their goals for pain relief postoperatively, only 12% indicated their goal was complete pain relief. Gadish, Gonzalez, and Hayes[43] reported similar findings, in regard to pediatric patients. Cohen's[28] study of adults also reported similar findings: Only 3% believed that the goal was complete pain relief. Essentially, complete pain relief seems to be a low priority among nurses.

Physicians' attitudes and beliefs about pain in children can also affect pain management practices. A recent study by Schechter and Allen[99] surveyed pediatricians, family practitioners, and surgeons about their attitudes on children's pain and its treatment. Only 59% of the surgeons, 91% of the pediatricians, and 77% of the family practitioners believed that children experience adult-like pain by the age of 2. Also, 49% of the surgeons, 80% of the pediatricians, and 64% of the family practitioners stated that they would use narcotics on children by the time they were 2. Further, 25% of the surgeons and 6% of the pediatricians perceived that children experienced less pain than adults with similar injury. The study determined that many physicians fear addiction, despite numerous sources that report its infrequent occurrence. Overall, surgeons were the most conservative of all physicians surveyed about children's pain. Clearly, these attitudes have the potential to influence how physicians prescribe analgesics for children's pain. However, a study by Foster and Hester[35] reported that even when orders were available, nurses often chose not to administer analgesics.

Schechter[98] noted the general societal beliefs that complaints about pain are considered a sign of weakness, that denial of pain is a sign of strength, and that drug use is generally frowned on. Health care providers believe that a "correct" amount of pain exists for particular conditions. Thus nurses and physicians may believe a patient is "entitled to" only a certain amount of pain; if they have more than the "correct" amount, their credibility and honesty are questioned. These beliefs can seriously hamper a health care provider's ability to be objective and sensitive in the pain assessment/management process.

The Complexity of Pediatric Pain Management

The process of using problem-solving skills to relieve children's pain is both complex and time-consuming. Decision-making centers on two questions: Are interventions necessary for pain relief? If so, what strategies should be used with this particular child?

The first question involves several factors. Is the pain causing the child distress, is it hindering the child's recovery in any way, what are the parents' and child's wishes for treatment, what has the physician made available to the child in terms of analgesia, and what is the cause of the pain? From the answers to these questions, the nurse can determine if pain relief strategies can be instituted.

The second question requires a decision about the type of treatment that will best relieve the pain for each individual child. Many factors are involved here as well. Are there cultural, religious, or personal factors that will influence the kind of care offered? Are there any constraints to using analgesics (cultural, religious, physiological)? Does the age of the child allow or prohibit certain strategies? Are there any physical comfort measures that can be employed (e.g., positioning, therapeutic touch, holding, rocking)? What psychosocial or cognitive-behavioral measures need to be employed (such as relaxation exercises, imagery)? Are safety measures necessary with certain analgesic regimens (such as assessment of respirations every hour, apnea monitoring, availability of naloxone, frequent observation)? The actual management of pain should be a tailor-made, multidimensional attempt to alleviate the discomfort of each individual child. Decision-making involves answering the above questions and then using safe, appropriate, and effective methods for the particular child.

This process requires careful data gathering, testing of a variety of techniques, and then evaluating the effects on the child. This complex individualized process requires much time and attention. A shortage of nurses on clinical units threatens the time nurses have to carry out this decision-making process fully. The nursing shortage, in addition to recent budget cuts, has placed increasing demands on nurses who are caring for patients with increasingly acute conditions. The combination of the time needed to effectively assess and manage pediatric pain, the time shortage caused by inadequate staffing, and the increased difficulty of care greatly increases the possibility of inadequate pain management for the child. Treatment of pain must be a priority if it is to occur.

◆ COMMON PAIN EXPERIENCES IN CHILDREN

Addressing all painful conditions that occur in children would be impossible here. Like adults, children experience acute, chronic, recurrent, and cancer-related pain of varying intensities, locations, qualities, and durations.[17,73] According to a study of 994 subjects,[95] children themselves reported that the most common pain events for them were lacerations, infections, insect bites, burns, sprains, sore throats, stomachaches, headaches, and earaches.

The most common pain experiences in children discussed in this section are acute pain (postoperative, procedural), chronic pain (juvenile rheumatoid arthritis, hemophilia, and sickle cell disease), recurrent pain (abdominal pain and headache), and cancer pain.

Acute Pain

Postoperative Pain

One of the most common types of acute pain in children is postoperative pain. Much of the research on postoperative pain focuses on the undertreatment of children with analgesics and on the variety of treatment modalities. Postoperative pain can result from the manipulation and retraction of organs and tissues, tissue damage from the surgical procedure, including irritation of tissues from intubation and intravenous therapy, and the position of the patient during surgery. Damaged tissues release chemical substances, such as seratonin, histamine, bradykinen, and potassium ions, that stimulate the transmission of pain impulses along A-delta fibers.[27,110]

Although acute pain usually serves to warn an individual of tissue damage, postoperative pain "serves no useful function" (Chapman and Bonica,[27] p. 20). Physiological, emotional, and behavioral responses to postoperative pain may actually increase morbidity and mortality if not relieved. For example, some restriction of activity is necessary after surgery to protect the suture line until healing occurs. However, greatly reduced mobility resulting from pain can lead to complications associated with inadequate lung aeration and compromised circulation. Thus postoperative pain should be and can be reduced or abolished with a variety of pharmacological and nonpharmacological nursing interventions (see New Pain Management Techniques in this chapter and recommendations in Chapter 12).

Previously, research examining the effects of postoperative pain relief techniques was hindered by the lack of validated research instruments to measure pain in children. Measurement of pain in infants remains a problem.[60] However, the measurement of pain in 3-year-old children and older children has been clarified[18,54,96] and studies are providing empirical data with which to make practice decisions.

Procedural Pain

Other common types of acute pain in children include that resulting from traumatic injuries, burns, and invasive medical procedures (such as bone marrow aspirations, lumbar punctures, circumcisions, injections, venipunctures, and skin-testing). Some of these pain conditions are recurrent episodes of acute pain, such as the bone marrow aspirations required with cancer or the dressing changes required with burns. Some researchers argue that procedural pain is distinct from other forms of acute pain. Each of these distressful sources of pain and relief measures are being explored.

Chronic Pain

Chronic pain in children is usually related to diseases, such as arthritis, hemophilia, or sickle cell anemia. Chronic pain is complex, and multidimensional assessment, including somatic, affective, and behavioral components, is required.[73]

Juvenile Rheumatoid Arthritis

The most prevalent arthritic condition in children is juvenile rheumatoid arthritis (JRA).[73] Children with this condition experience joint stiffness and pain, night pain, limitation of mobility and activities of daily living, irritability, and fatigue. JRA varies in severity, and the course of the condition is unpredictable. Several forms of the disease exist, characterized by the degree of systemic involvement and number of joints affected. JRA has a substantial effect on school performance, psychological adaptation, and vocation. It continues into adulthood for most of the children affected.[68]

Most of the research on JRA has been conducted by psychologists who have developed sophisticated cognitive-behavioral programs to assist children in coping with their chronic pain by encouraging regulation of their pain perceptions and more self-control over their pain behaviors.[68,113] Nonsteroidal antiinflammatory drugs in conjunction with cognitive-behavioral therapy, such as relaxation and imagery, seem to be the pharmacological treatment of choice. Varni[113] has reported that the child's disease and psychological adjustment to it, and the family's psychosocial environment play important roles in the amount of pain the child experiences. As such, the pain of JRA is a complex and multidimensional phenomenon.

Early studies about children with JRA suggested that the level of pain experienced by children was low in comparison with that of adults.[104] However, these studies predated the development of psychometrically sound and developmentally appropriate pain measures for children. Findings from these earlier studies are now being questioned, and the pain associated with JRA is being reexamined in terms of its patterns, severity, and effects on the child and family. As with other forms of pain, the pain of arthritis and its effects on children are most likely misunderstood. Guidelines for the use of analgesics are only beginning to evolve. Treatment has focused on the amelioration of the disease rather than on pain control.[68]

Hemophilia

The pain of hemophilia results from the characteristic bleeding into the soft tissues, muscles, and joint capsules. Frequent bleeding into joints results in degenerative and painful arthropathy[73] similar to that of osteoarthritis.[113] Varni, Walco, and Katz[114] and Varni[113] noted that in hemophilia, two types of pain exist: the acute recurring pain of active bleeding into the tissues and the potentially debilitating chronic arthritic pain resulting from recurrent bleeding into the joints. Treatment of pain incorporates the use of opioid and nonopioid analgesics and a comprehensive and systematic program of cognitive-behavioral strategies, such as relaxation, imagery, and meditation.

With the exception of the work of the psychologist Varni and his associates, little has been written about the pain associated with hemophilia. Nurses could play an important role in helping to describe the patterns of pain experienced by these children and in documenting the effectiveness of pain relief techniques.

Sickle Cell Disease

Sickle cell anemia is the most common hemoglobinopathy in North America, causing significant morbidity and mortality in children.[97] Although sickle cell anemia is most often included under the categories of conditions causing chronic pain, it might more correctly be termed a recurrent form of acute pain. The pain of sickle cell disease is associated with vasoocclusive crisis (VOC), which results in repeated episodes of mild to severe pain over the individual's lifetime. This pain occurs when sickle-shaped red blood cells occlude arterioles.

The ischemia, tissue hypoxia, infarction, and necrosis that can result produce pain of varying intensity.[66] Interestingly, pain associated with hypoxia of myocardial tissues (angina pectoris and myocardial infarction) is widely accepted, whereas pain resulting from tissue hypoxia in VOC is often regarded with suspicion.

Despite the intense pain of VOC, pain medications are often withheld or administered in inadequate doses. Schechter and colleagues acknowledged that children with sickle cell anemia have been labeled unfairly as "manipulative" in their attempts to obtain pain relieving medication during crises.[101] Burghardt-Fitzgerald,[22] a nurse, acknowledged the frequent conflicts that arise between health care providers and patients over narcotic dosages, activities of daily living, compliance with fluid intake, breathing exercises, and activity requirements in in-patient settings. Varni and colleagues[114] noted that the pain complaints of children in sickle cell crises are often questioned or dismissed by health care providers because of their biases about sickle cell patients.

The latest thinking is that during vasoocclusive crises, children should be treated aggressively with opioid analgesics, such as morphine.[97,105,106,76] Withholding pain-relieving medications only serves to increase patients' drug-seeking behaviors and the chance of needless suffering, and decrease trust in health care providers. Unrelieved pain, as noted by Shapiro,[105,106] may contribute significantly to the development of psychopathology. Although addiction is a widespread fear in relation to sickle cell anemia, it probably occurs infrequently.[97,115] Schechter warned that the fear of addiction should not be considered a justification for withholding narcotics needed by children in sickle cell crisis.

One reason for the reluctance to provide adequate analgesia to children in VOC may relate to a lack of understanding about the variability of the pain experienced. Within the same individual, pain crises can vary greatly in intensity and duration.[83,115] Ranging from mild to severe, the pain of VOC is usually sudden in onset. In infants and toddlers VOC frequently presents as dactylitis, soft tissue swelling, and pain in the hands and feet. In children over 2 years, the pain often begins in the long bones of an extremity and then spreads throughout the body.[83,115] However, pain can occur anywhere in the body and may remain localized.[106] The pain of VOC has been described as deep, gnawing, and throbbing in the acute stage but may linger as a dull ache.[83] Although it can subside in a matter of minutes, pain may also persist for weeks.[106]

For reasons poorly understood, vasoocclusive crises also vary in frequency of occurrence. Shapiro and colleagues[106] stated that about 20% of the patients with sickle cell anemia experience about 70% of all VOC episodes. Similarly, Walco and Dampier[116] reported that of 260 pediatric patients, 95% experienced infrequent crises and were hospitalized no more than once per year. The other 5% had more severe and more frequent crises and were hospitalized up to 12 times per year for periods of 10 to 12 days.

Additionally, individual differences in metabolism of narcotics add to the complexity of pain assessment for children with VOC.[115] A given milligram per kilogram dose of narcotic that relieves pain in one child may be totally ineffective for another. Vichinsky and Lubin[115] suggested that drug dosage and administration should be individualized for each child and limited only by drug toxicity.

The human propensity to compare patients' reactions to disease in the process of drawing conclusions about their suffering[62] can only lead to confusion and suspicion when applied to children with VOC. Caregivers who recognize that the manifestation of and response to VOC vary will be better prepared to individualize care to the child and each episode.

Caregivers' attitudes about the child's and family's health behaviors constitute another potential reason for inadequate treatment. According to Parson's[88] classic sick role model, persons are generally not held responsible for their illness. As long as they accept the responsibility to get well, they enjoy certain social exemptions. Taken one step further, persons considered the unwitting victims of disease usually garnish a good measure of sympathy from their caregivers. But what if a child or family is considered responsible for the illness? Could caregiver attitudes lead to punitive treatment?

Commonly, discussions of sickle cell anemia list factors that predispose to VOC. These factors are associated with decreased oxygen concentration and include exposure to cold, dehydration, high altitude, vigorous exercise, infection, smoking, and consumption of alcohol.[83,97] Viewing this list, one might conclude that prevention of VOC is a matter of child and family education and that a painful crisis is evidence of noncompliance. A fact less known, however, is that VOC is unpredictable, and it often occurs in the absence of precipitating factors.[83,106] The uncertainty of when the next crisis will occur and its intensity, and the patient's helplessness to prevent it, have been termed some of the most disabling aspects of sickle cell anemia.[106] Sensitivity to this issue will improve the effectiveness of care.

The cure for sickle cell anemia is unknown, and care is based on judicious use of blood transfusions, aggressive treatment for infection, and analgesics for pain relief.[107] Recent advances in therapy, at least for adolescents with sickle cell anemia, may include patient-controlled analgesia (PCA) and behavioral contracting. In a small pilot study, PCA was shown to be effective as a treatment strategy for pain associated with sickle cell anemia.[101] Behavioral contracting involves detailed individual treatment plans on which the patient and health team agree as written behavioral objectives. The treatment plans are designed to provide the patient more control over his or her care and greater resources for coping with the sickle cell crisis.[22,116] According to the work of Shapiro[105,106] and Walco and Dampier,[116] psychotherapy may also be required to assist patients to deal with the consequences of sickle cell anemia in the long term.

Shapiro[105,106] indicated that psychopathology and psychosocial dysfunction characteristically appear in adolescents and adults with sickle cell anemia. She suggested that this dysfunction may be the cumulative effect of the unpredictability and intensity of the recurrent pain, and the lack of control over the disease. Sickle cell anemia can be very disruptive to the child's activities of daily living, normal development, and school performance and attendance, and can significantly affect the quality of life for the child and family.

A better understanding of the intensity of pain associated with tissue hypoxia, the biases and inappropriate care practices of health care providers, and the "lived experience" of a child with sickle cell anemia would help nurses to provide more empathetic and effective care to children affected by this condition.

Recurrent Pain

The two most common forms of recurrent pain in children are recurrent abdominal pain and headache. Children with these conditions are often seen by nurses in the private offices and pain clinics of physicians and psychologists or in the hospital during diagnostic work-ups.

Recurrent Abdominal Pain (RAP)

According to Rappaport,[89] RAP occurs in approximately 15% of the school age population and most characteristically presents as periumbilical pain lasting 1 to 3 hours. This condition has received a bad name, and children so afflicted have previously been unfairly accused of malingering. In the past, many cases of RAP were labeled psychogenic in origin. McGrath and colleagues[74,72] severely criticized the indiscriminant use of the term "psychogenic" when an organic cause for the pain could not be found. In the recent past, 90% of all children with RAP were classified as having "psychogenic" pain.[89]

New evidence suggests that only about 10% of the children with RAP have psychogenic pain.[89] Another 10% have pathological conditions causing the pain, for example, diabetes, Hirschsprung's disease, or giardiasis. A third category may account for the large group of children (80%) in which RAP may occur as the result of an imbalance between normal physiological processes and stressors. An example of the third category is the discovery that children with lactose and sorbital intolerance develop RAP with excessive ingestion of these substances. Other examples are irritable bowel syndrome and pain associated with constipation. Although these are not pathological conditions, they can result in severe pain.

Levine and Rappaport[67] shed further light on the cause of RAP with the creation of a multidimensional model. Factors hypothesized to influence the recurrence of episodes of abdominal pain include: a somatic predisposition, dysfunction, or disorder; the milieu and critical events; temperament and learned response patterns; and lifestyle and habits. These factors interact and cause pain of different types and varying intensities.

Rappaport[89] reported that pain for one third of the children with RAP is resolved within 5 years. For another one third, the pain persists at 5 years. For the final one third of RAP cases in children, the pain continues but changes to a new and different pain problem. Thus, for most of the children with RAP, the pain persists over a long time.

Rappaport[89] and McGrath and Unruh[76] recommend careful diagnostic tests sufficient to rule out serious problems, but they discourage the use of aggressive, invasive, and continuous testing if a cause cannot be found. Rappaport cautions that the children and their families need to be protected from iatrogenic trauma and that a "fishing expedition" is not appropriate. Important to the treatment of these children is the use of cognitive-behavioral strategies to help children cope with their pain and control the onset, duration, and intensity of the pain episodes. Although still experimental, Feldman and colleagues[32] reported positive results of the inclusion of over-the-counter fiber cookies in the daily diet of a sample of children with RAP. Analgesics are not usually used in this recurrent pain condition. Opiates further decrease gastrointestinal motility, and aspirin irritates the gastric tissue.

Headache

According to statistics reported by McGrath and Humphreys,[75] recurrent headaches are a frequent problem in children and adolescents, particularly in older children and girls. Headaches in children have several causes. They are most frequently the result of vascular dilation (migraine) or muscle contraction of the scalp or neck (tension headache).[87] Few actually are the result of serious pathology, such as brain tumors. Sinus congestion is another common cause of headaches; these are usually treated with medical and surgical interventions to relieve the congestion.

After serious pathology for vascular and tension headaches is ruled out, the child and family need to be reassured. The recurrent nature, the intensity, and the disruption the pain causes can be extremely troublesome to children and their families. They need to be helped to identify the "triggers," the situations that precipitate the headaches, and avoidance strategies should be explored. Some postulated "triggers" are: tests at school, lack of sleep, noise, being upset, activity, arguing, and the consumption of chocolate. Adequate rest and sleep, stress management, and cognitive-behavioral techniques (such as biobeedback, imagery, and relaxation) may help to prevent these recurrent pain episodes or to alleviate the pain.[75,109] "Cognitive restructuring" has shown positive results in decreasing pain frequency, duration, and intensity. This strategy teaches the child to think differently about the pain and the accompanying stress that triggers it. McGrath and co-workers[75] have called this "thinking straight," and Ross and Ross[95] have called it "thought-stopping."

According to McGrath and Humphreys,[75] ergotamine preparations may help prevent migraine headaches in some adolescents if taken early enough in the attack. Although there are no published studies of the use of tricyclic antidepressants (such as amitriptyline) with children, McGrath and Humphreys[75] suggest they may be useful in preventing pediatric migraine, based on the unpublished findings of one of their own studies. Although frequently ordered for reducing headache activity in children and adolescents with severe migraine, propranolol (a beta adrenergic blocker) has not been shown to be consistently effective in experimental studies.[71,75,76] Once headaches occur, drug therapy usually involves nonopioid analgesics, although meperidine may be used for severe migraine pain.

Cancer Pain

Pain associated with cancer in children has been categorized into four major etiologic groups: cancer-related, therapy-related, procedure-related, and debilitation.[79] Cancer-related pain includes bone metastases and other physiological manifestations of the disease. This type of pain is frequently present at diagnosis and usually subsides soon after the onset of therapy.[80] Pain associated with the tumor itself may recur later, in the event of relapse and metastasis. Miser and colleagues,[80] in monitoring patterns of cancer pain, reported that, of 92 young adults and children with cancer, 50% of the inpatients and 25% of the outpatients experienced pain. Miser and Miser[82] suggested that cancer-related pain can be severe and persistent, and that it generally is undertreated with analgesics. Intermittent caudal epidural administration of narcotic analgesics has been shown effective in one case study for relieving terminal cancer pain.[6]

Therapy-related pain is associated with side effects of chemotherapy and radiation therapy (e.g., mucositis, infection, neuropathic pain, abdominal pain from intractable vomiting, radiation dermatitis). Procedure-related pain includes invasive diagnostic procedures (e.g., lumbar puncture, bone marrow aspiration, and surgical insertion of an indwelling catheter). Children have reported that treatments related to cancer were worse than the cancer itself.[58,63] Eight adolescent survivors of cancer interviewed by Fowler-Kerry[37] said lumbar punctures, bone marrow aspirations, and surgery were the most painful aspects of cancer. Interestingly, however, the adolescents reported that recurrent venipunctures and the infusion of chemotherapeutic agents were the most difficult types of pain to handle. They perceived the chemotherapy treatment rooms as cold and the persons present as "just watching and not doing anything to help me" (p. 368). Adjectives used by these adolescents to describe their procedure-related pain were shooting, ripping, stabbing, cutting, burning, and aching.

Describing what she believed her young son experienced before his death from leukemia, Offsay,[84] a nurse, invoked a scene not unlike the recollections of Fowler-Kerry's[37] adolescent informants:

> For a moment, I would ask you to play a childhood game of imagining . . . You are in a room and your mom is holding you tightly curled up and someone is shooting needles in your back. You can't see anything and it goes on and on. People tell you to stay still but you are screaming to be let go since you hate to be restrained in any way, and you feel you are being attacked . . . You want to escape this torture chamber now before anyone thinks of anything else to do to you (p. 174).

The pain of debilitation includes bed sores, infections, and other conditions associated with the terminal, bedridden stages of cancer.

Many psychological techniques have been developed to assist children in dealing with procedures. Strategies such as breathing and bubble blowing, behavioral distraction, and hypnotic techniques have proven effective with children as young as 2 and a half and as old as 15.[63,64] Other successful strategies include imagery, distraction, and relaxation[58,72] and hypnotic techniques.* The effective use of such techniques, however, depends on careful instruction of the child, adequate practice before the stressful event, and often the presence of the psychologist during the event.

Although discussions of cancer pain often focus on invasive diagnostic procedures and pain in the terminal stages, many stressful events for the child with cancer occur in the course of "usual" nursing care. For example, Offsay[84] related her son's aversions to recurrent finger sticks and the taste of prednisone. Stress of this nature can sometimes be avoided when caregivers are willing to employ common sense and innovation rather than relying solely on the established procedures. Offsay reasoned, "Because living with childhood cancer is itself a horrible burden, it becomes the responsibility of every caregiver to

* References 55, 56, 59, 61, 85, 120.

consider each action, down to the smallest detail" (p. 175).

In the future, cancer pain may be treated more effectively with alternate routes and techniques such as patient-controlled analgesia, transdermal delivery of opioids, enhanced transmucosal analgesics, and inhalation analgesia.[79] Caring and compassion, however, are the mainstay of pain management and supportive care for children with cancer and their families.

Two recent documents focus on the pain relief needs of the oncology population in revolutionary new ways. These include: (1) the Report of a Consensus Conference on the Management of Pain in Childhood Cancer held in 1988 by a multidisciplinary panel of experts[99a] and (2) the Oncology Nursing Society (ONS) Position Paper on Cancer Pain.[109a,b] These documents took aggressive stands on the alleviation/abolition of cancer pain, and both provided valuable guidance for the assessment and management of cancer pain in children. Nurses are encouraged to become familiar with the suggestions made in these sources, because they promise to make an impact on oncology nursing practice.

Summary

Children experience a variety of forms of pain: acute, chronic, recurrent, and cancer pain. Each form of pain raises special issues and problems. Recent research is showing an increase in the body of knowledge about children with each of these pain conditions, which will contribute to the nursing care given to these children.

◆ NEW PAIN MANAGEMENT TECHNIQUES

Pharmacological Methods

Several pharmacological measures for pain control have recently been used in ambulatory pediatric settings or in situations to reduce the pain of invasive medical procedures. Topical applications, such as Frigiderm (a skin coolant) or EMLA (Eutetic Mixture of Local Anesthetics; a new anesthetic cream) are useful for procedures, such as intramuscular injections, venipunctures, lumbar punctures, and wound cleaning.[29,119] Injections of local anesthetics, such as Nesacaine, can be used for short procedures such as suturing and burn dressing changes.[29,119]

For the treatment of mild to moderate postsurgical pain or chronic pain with an inflammatory origin, the use of nonsteroidal antiinflammatory drugs (NSAIDs) appears to be effective (Berde et al, 1989).[10,11,29] Few studies have focused on these medications for effectiveness and side and toxic effects in children under 12 years, but they appear to be safe and effective for short-term use.[10,11] Eland[29] recommended the use of morphine suppositories for children who do not have intravenous lines and who cannot tolerate oral forms of morphine because of the gastrointestinal effects. These suppositories may be uncomfortable for the few seconds it takes to insert them, but they are effective and relatively inexpensive, and can be made by the hospital pharmacist.

Several new techniques are being used for the management of more severe postsurgical pain in children. According to Berde et al,[8] peripheral nerve blocks are now being used in children having general anesthesia to allow them to be pain free for a prolonged period of time after surgery. Nerve blocks, in conjunction with general anesthesia, permit the use of smaller amounts of the general anesthetic agent, thus permitting faster recovery and emergence from general anesthesia. In addition to nerve blocks with surgery, continuous epidural and intrapleural infusions of local anesthetics are used postoperatively in patients on general nursing units as well as in intensive care units.[6,11] These epidural and intrapleural infusions are especially helpful for patients who have had thoracic or abdominal surgery or those with severe respiratory diseases, such as cystic fibrosis or bronchopulmonary dysplasia. These new methods of pain relief allow patients to turn, cough, and deep breathe more easily postoperatively.[11]

Berde[5] and Gilbert[45] advocated the use of continuous infusions of opioid analgesics as the preferred method of pain management in the postoperative pediatric patient. However, if intravenous boluses are used, they suggested that they should be given at intervals no greater than every 2 hours. Providing frequent intravenous infusions of analgesics to patients may, however, be a problem for the nurses if the unit is short staffed, because close monitoring is necessary.

Another recent alternative available for the management of pain in the pediatric patient is patient-controlled analgesia (PCA), in which patients can deliver their own opioid analgesics through an intravenous line, either central or peripheral. Although PCA has been used and studied extensively in adults, use has just begun with the pediatric population.[94,118] The youngest age at which it could or should be used is not documented, although some pain centers have used it with patients as young as 6 years.[5] The few studies with children using PCA have been confined to the adolescent and older school age group. In the younger age groups, *parent-controlled* analgesia may be a consideration.

Other pharmacological techniques that may prove to be useful with children include the use of methadone postoperatively[7,79] as well as sublingual and transdermal forms of fentanyl. Methadone has a half-life in children of almost 20 times that of the same dose of morphine.[9,79] Sublingual and transdermal forms of fentanyl offer potent analgesia via noninvasive routes. In a small pilot study, Schechter and colleagues[102] found fentanyl lollipops, the buccal route, to be effective in the relief of pain in five 7- to 18-year-olds after lumbar punctures or bone marrow aspirations. These techniques require more testing before full use with children.

With chronic forms of pain in adults, tricyclic antidepressants are an important part of the pain therapy. These medications are also now being used with success in children with chronic pain. The tricyclics help by allowing the patient to sleep, a factor that is essential for improving patients' abilities to cope with chronic pain.[10,82]

Nonpharmacological Methods

Nonpharmacological methods are helpful adjuncts to analgesics in the treatment of pain in children. Several techniques have been suggested in the literature, such as distraction/attention, imagery, art and play therapy, having parents present, relaxation exercises, holding or rocking the infant, hypnosis, physical therapy, use of cold or heat, positioning, massage, whirlpools, acupuncture, exercise, biofeedback, modeling, and music therapy. The three comprehensive books on children's pain[71,76,95] provide information about the details and the efficacy of these techniques. Nurses can use some of these techniques with reading and practice. Several of these methods, such as hypnosis, biofeedback, and play therapy, would take additional training. Acupuncture is performed by a physician.

A recent nonpharmacological technique that has gained considerable attention in the treatment of pain is transcutaneous electrical nerve stimulation (TENS). TENS is the delivery of a low-grade electrical stimulus through the skin at a site near the area of the pain. It is thought to work by blocking the transmission of pain impulses at the spinal cord level.[108] Smith et al.[108] found TENS helpful in patients with chronic pain as well as postoperative pain. Berde[5] reported that TENS can be used as an adjunct to postoperative analgesia. Eland[30] reported success with TENS in children undergoing painful injections, intravenous needle insertion, muscle spasms, burn graft donor site pain, abrasions, and bone metastasis from cancer.

◆ DECISION-MAKING IN PRACTICE

Pain problems in children can most successfully be identified and treated by multidisciplinary teams of health professionals, particularly nurses, physicians, and psychologists. Pharmacologists, physical and occupational therapists, and child life workers can add greatly to this team effort. Pain treatment services are just beginning to appear throughout the world, although they in no way match the proliferation of similar services for adults. It has been estimated that there are about 1500 pain clinics in North America for adults, whereas there are only 13 pain treatment services for children.[10] The services for adults are most often those that focus on patients experiencing chronic low back pain and headaches. For children, most of the pain centers are located in medical or health sciences centers in major metropolitan areas, treating a variety of forms of both acute and chronic pain. Pain is a multidisciplinary problem, and health providers need to work together to find solutions, each making his or her own unique contribution. Pain management in the past has created many adversarial situations among health providers. This is counterproductive, and the one who suffers most is the patient. Conflicts between nurses and physicians in regard to the route, type, or dose of a medication have been common in the past.

The characteristics and underpinnings of nurses' decisions about pain management are just beginning to be investigated.[24,50,57] Decision-making in pediatric pain management requires consideration of a variety of factors. Major suggestions can be made to improve the effectiveness of pain relief and thus to reduce or eliminate the chance of pain-related crises for children (see box).

◆ SUMMARY OF CLINICAL SUGGESTIONS: PAIN RELIEF IN CHILDREN

1. Make complete pain relief your goal.
2. Differentiate between children's needs for pain relief and apprehension control, and implement the appropriate nursing strategies.
3. Assess pain frequently and systematically, using valid pain assessment tools. Use this information, in part, to make decisions about the use of pain management techniques.
4. Use "noninvasive" pain management techniques whenever possible. Avoid injections.
5. Use analgesics to relieve pain appropriately, safely, and effectively.
6. Use nonpharmacological pain relief techniques appropriately and liberally.
7. Test new pain management techniques in practice settings.
8. Do not subscribe to the inaccurate beliefs, myths, and misconceptions about children's pain.

- Health providers need to become more liberal in their goals for pain relief in children. Although 100% pain relief may not be feasible, providers need to strive for this level, within safe and therapeutic parameters. Relieving only enough pain to allow the patient to function is not an adequate or appropriate goal. The patient is entitled to much higher quality of care.
- The safe but effective use of analgesics is addressed elsewhere in this volume (see Chapter 12). Eland provides some of the important details about pharmacological management that when used correctly will enhance the effectiveness of pain management. In many instances, such as in the postoperative situation, analgesics are the first line of defense against this acute, self-limited form of pain.[12] They should be used properly both to prevent and to relieve pain.
- Providers need to use nonpharmacological pain relief techniques more liberally. In many instances, these techniques may be all that is needed. In other instances, they serve to augment the effects of analgesic administration.
- Providers need to differentiate more clearly between

their interventions for pain relief and those for apprehension control. Although both types of interventions may be needed to adequately relieve a child's pain and distress, the actual strategies are different. It is not appropriate to use strategies to reduce apprehension without using analgesics when pain may be present. Health providers have been known, however, to use distraction, tranquilizers, and Pavulon with "fresh" postoperative children without administering analgesics. Similarly, cognitive-behavioral strategies are often used with painful medical procedures, such as burn dressing changes, without the help of analgesics. In addition, acetaminophen has been given to children as their only analgesic after major trauma "so as not to mask the symptoms." The best pain management, however, will incorporate both pharmacological and nonpharmacological techniques to treat pain as well as the apprehension, fear, and anxiety that often accompany it.

- One of the most important ways to improve pain management is to improve assessment procedures. Without thorough, accurate, and systematic assessment, management cannot be effective. To approach assessment more accurately, the child's self-report needs to be obtained whenever it is developmentally possible. The best way to ensure accuracy of this report is to use clinically validated pain measurement devices. Nurses should be knowledgeable about the psychometric properties of the tools they select for use. Pain measurement efforts will be wasted if the measuring tools do not yield valid data.

  Nurses have been heard to say that they will not use the measuring tools because they do not have time. This practice does not make good sense since accurate and thorough assessment form the foundation for all nursing care. Obtaining pain scores from children actually takes only a few seconds once the child has learned how to use the instruments. Orientation to the instruments can easily take place during the admission procedure.
- Providers, particularly nurses, need to be more systematic in their assessment of pain. Systematic means pain measures should be taken frequently and at regular intervals. Pain should be assessed at least as often as vital signs, preferably more often. It is more time-consuming to take a blood pressure than to obtain a child's self-report of pain intensity. Management of pain will not be

effective if the assessment procedures are sporadic, haphazard, or an afterthought. The pain scores obtained should be recorded as an aid to evaluating pain relief measures.

- In the management of children's pain, providers need to avoid injections. Numerous sources document the trauma and terror experienced by children confronted with the possibility or reality of receiving an injection. It is one of the unfortunate paradoxes of health care that painful procedures are necessary to relieve pain. In modern practice, a growing number of noninvasive pharmacological pain management techniques are available. These techniques should be used with children whenever possible. A major goal in the care of children should be to eliminate unnecessary iatrogenic suffering.
- Providers need to enhance their repertoires of pain management methods. Many new methods of pain control have appeared in just the last few years. These methods need to be tested for their safety and effectiveness.
- Providers need to avoid, at all costs, subscribing to the myths and unproven assumptions about children's pain. They have been harmful to children's health and well-being, and they need to be put to rest.

The field of pain management in children has advanced rapidly in the last several years. Health providers across disciplines are beginning to work together to alleviate and prevent pain in children. Nurses have played key roles in this effort, both in the clinical area and in research. In the hospital setting, no other health care provider is available to monitor and treat pain on a continuous 24-hour basis. In research, nurses have contributed most to identifying children's pain as a patient care problem in need of more attention; developing methods of pain measurement; identifying behavioral and physiological responses to pain in infants and children; examining the factors affecting nurses' abilities to manage pain and the cues nurses use to assess pain; and testing interventions designed to relieve pain. Nursing has been and will continue to be instrumental in advancing knowledge about and improving care for children in pain.

REFERENCES

1. Anand KJS and McGrath PJ. (In press). *Pain in infants.* The Netherlands: Elsevier.
2. Anand KJS and Aynsley-Green A. (1988). Does the newborn infant re-

quire potent anesthesia during surgery? Answers from a randomized trial of halothane anesthesia. In Dubner R, Gebhart G, and Bond M (eds), *Proceedings of the Vth World Congress on Pain.* The Netherlands: Elsevier, pp. 329-335.

3. Anand KJS and Hickey P. (1987). Pain and its effects in the human neonate and fetus. *N Engl J Med, 317,* 1321-1347.
4. Anand KJS, Sippell W, and Aynsley-Green A. (1987). Randomized trial of fentanyl anesthesia in preterm babies undergoing surgery: effects on the stress response. *Lancet, 1,* 243-248.
5. Berde C. (1989). Pediatric postoperative pain management. *Pediatr Clin North Am, 36,* 921-940.
6. Berde C, Fischel N, Filardi J, et al. (1989). Caudal epidural morphine analgesia for an infant with advanced neuroblastoma: report of a case. *Pain, 36,* 219-223.
7. Berde C, Holzman R, Sethna N, Dickerson R, and Brustowicz R. (1988). A comparison of methadone and morphine for postoperative anelgesia in children and adolescents. *Anesthesiology, 69,* A519.
8. Berde C, Sethna N, and Anand KJS. (In press). Pediatric pain management. In Gregory GA (ed). *Pediatric anesthesia.* New York: Churchill Livingstone.
9. Berde C, Sethna N, Holzman R, Reidy P, and Gondek E. (1987). Pharmacokinetics of methadone in children and adolescents in the perioperative period. *Anesthesiology, 67,* 519.
10. Berde C, Sethna N, Masek B, Fasburg M, and Rocklin S. (1989). Pediatric pain clinics: recommendations for their development. *Pediatrician, 16,* 94-102.
11. Berde C and Warfield C. (1988). Pediatric pain management. *Hosp Pract, 23,* 83-101.
12. Beyer J, Ashley L, Russell G, and DeGood D. (1984). Pediatric pain after cardiac surgery: pharmacologic management. *Dimen Crit Care Nurs, 3,* 326-334.
13. Beyer J and Bournaki M. (1989). Assessment and management of postoperative pain in children. *Pediatrician, 16,* 30-38.
14. Beyer J and Byers ML. (1985). Knowledge of pediatric pain: the state of the art. *Child Health Care, 13,* 233-241.
15. Beyer J, DeGood D, Ashley L, and Russell G. (1983). Patterns of postoperative analgesic use with adults and children following cardiac surgery. *Pain, 17,* 71-81.
16. Beyer J, McGrath P, and Berde C. (1990). Discordance between self-report and behavioral pain measures in children aged 3-7 after surgery. *J Pain Sympt Manage 5*, 350-356.
17. Beyer J and Levin C. (1987). Issues and advances in pain control in children. *Nurs Clin North Am.*
18. Beyer J and Wells N. (1989). The assessment of pain in children. *Pediatr Clin North Am, 36,* 837-854.
19. Brown J, O'Keefe J, Sanders S, and Baker B. (1986). Developmental changes in children's cognition to stressful and painful situations. *J Pediatr Psychol, 11,* 343-357.
20. Bradshaw C and Zeanah P. (1986). Pediatric nurses' assessments of pain in children. *J Pediatr Nurs, 1,* 314-322.
21. Brownell M. (1984). The concept of crisis: its utility for nursing. *Adv Nurs Sci, 6,* 10-21.

22. Burghardt-Fitzgerald D. (1989). Pain-behavior contracts: effective management of the adolescent in sickle-cell crisis. *J Pediatr Nurs, 4,* 320-324.
23. Burke S and Jerrett M. (1989). Pain management across age groups. *West J Nurs Res, 11,* 164-180.
24. Burokas L. (1985) Factors affecting nurses' decisions to medicate pediatric patients after surgery. *Heart Lung, 14,* 375-379.
25. Caplan G. (1964). *Principles of preventive psychiatry.* New York: Basic Books.
26. Caty S, Ritchie J, and Ellerton M. (1989). Mothers' perceptions of coping behaviors in hospitalized preschool children. *J Pediatr Nurs, 4,* 403-410.
27. Chapman C and Bonica J. (1983). *Acute pain. Current concepts.* Kalamazoo: Upjohn.
28. Cohen F. (1980). Postsurgical pain relief: patients' status and nurses' medication choices. *Pain, 9,* 265-274.
29. Eland J. (1988). Pharmacologic management of acute and chronic pediatric pain. *Iss Comp Pediatr Nurs, 11,* 93-111.
30. Eland J. (1989). The effectiveness of transcutaneous electrical nerve stimulation (TENS) with children experiencing cancer pain. In Funk S, Tornquist E, Champagne M, Copp L, and Wiese R. (eds) (1989). *Key aspects of comfort: pain, fatigue, and nausea.* New York: Springer.
31. Eland J and Anderson J. (1977). The experience of pain in children. In Jacox A. (ed) *Pain: a sourcebook for nurses and other health professionals,* pp. 453-473. Boston: Little, Brown.
32. Feldman W, McGrath P, Hodgson C, Ritter H, and Shipman R. (1985). The use of dietary fiber in the management of simple childhood idiopathic recurrent abdominal pain: results in a prospective double blind randomized controlled trial. *Am J Dis Child, 139,* 1216-1218.
33. Foster R. (1981). *Coping strategies of the child with leukemia: the stress of invasive procedures.* Unpublished master's thesis, The University of Colorado, Denver.
34. Foster R and Hester N. (1990). The relationship between pain ratings and pharmacologic interventions for children in pain. In Tyler DC and Krane EJ (eds) *Advances in pain research and therapy,* vol. 15, (pp. 31-36). New York: Raven Press.
35. Foster R and Hester N. (1989). Variations in analgesic administration by pain ratings and other personalogic or situational variables. Unpublished raw data.
36. Foster R, Husberger M, and Anderson J. (1989). *Family-centered nursing care of children.* Philadelphia: Saunders.
37. Fowler-Kerry S. (1990). Adolescent oncology survivors' recollection of pain. In Tyler DC and Krane EJ (eds) *Advances in pain research and therapy,* vol. 15, (pp. 365-371). New York: Raven Press.
38. Franck L. (1986). A new method to quantitatively describe pain behavior in infants. *Nurs Res, 35,* 28-31.
39. Fuller B, Conner D, and Horii Y. (1990). Potential acoustic measures of infant pain and arousal. In Tyler D and Krane E (eds), *Advances in pain research and therapy,* vol. 15 (137-146). New York: Raven Press.
40. Fuller B and Horii Y. (1986). Differences in fundamental frequency, jitter, and shimmer among four types of infant vocalizations. *J Comm Dis, 19,* 441-447.
41. Fuller B and Horii Y. (1988). Spectral energy distribution in four types of infant vocalizations. *J Comm Dis, 21,* 111-127.

42. Funk S, Tornquist E, Champagne M, Copp L, and Wiese R. (eds) (1989). *Key aspects of comfort: pain, fatigue, and nausea.* New York: Springer.
43. Gadish H, Gonzalez J, and Hayes J. (1988). Factors affecting nurses' decisions to administer pediatric pain medication postoperatively. *J Pediatr Nurs, 3,* 383-390.
44. Geissler E. (1984). Crisis: What it is and is not. *Adv Nurs Sci, 6,* 1-9.
45. Gilbert H. (1990). Pain relief methods in the postanesthesia care unit. *J Post Anesth Nurs, 15,* 6-15.
46. Gonzales J and Gadish H. (1990). Nurses' decisions in medicating children postoperatively. In Tyler DC and Krane EJ (eds), *Advances in pain research and therapy,* vol 15, (pp. 37-42). New York: Raven Press.
47. Grunau R and Craig K. (1987). Pain expression in neonates: facial action and cry. *Pain, 28,* 395-410.
48. Haslam D. (1969). Age and perception of pain. *Psychosom Sci, 15,* 86.
49. Hester N. (1989). Comforting the child in pain. In Funk S, Tornquist E, Champagne M, Copp L, and Wiese R (eds), *Key aspects of comfort: pain, fatigue, and nausea* (pp. 290-302). New York: Springer.
50. Hester N. (1988). *Nurse clinical decision-making: pain in children.* A 3-year grant supported by the National Institutes of Health, National Center for Nursing Research under grant number R23 NRO 1382.
51. Hester N. (1979). The preoperational child's reaction to immunizations. *Nurs Res, 28,* 250-254.
52. Hester N and Barcus C. (1986). Assessment and management of pain in children. *Pediatr Nurs Update, 1,* 1-8.
53. Hester N and Foster R. (In press). Cues nurses and parents use in making judgments about children's pain. *Pain research and clinical management.* New York: Elsevier.
54. Hester N, Foster R, and Beyer J. (1992). Clinical judgment in assessing children's pain. In Watt-Watson J and Donovan M (eds), *Pain management: nursing perspective.* St. Louis: Mosby–Year Book, Inc.
55. Hilgard J and LeBaron S. (1984). *Hypnotherapy of pain in children with cancer.* Los Altos, Calif: William Kaufmann.
56. Hilgard E and LeBaron S. (1982). Relief of anxiety and pain in children and adolescents with cancer: Quantitative measures and clinical observations. *Int J Clin Exp Hyp, 30,* 417-442.
57. Holm K, Cohen F, Dudas S, Medema P, and Allen B. (1989). Effect of personal pain experience on pain assessment. *Image, 21,* 72-75.
58. Jay S, Elliott C, Ozolins M, Olson R, and Pruitt S. (1985). Behavioral management of children's distress during painful medical procedures. *Behav Res Ther, 23,* 513-520.
59. Jay S, Elliott C, and Varni J. (1986). Acute and chronic pain in adults and children with cancer. *J Consult Clin Psychol, 54,* 601-607.
60. Johnston C. (1989). Pain assessment and management in infants. *Pediatrician, 16,* 16-23.
61. Kellerman J, Zeltzer L, Ellenberg L, and Dash J. (1983). Adolescents with cancer: hypnosis for the reduction of the acute pain and anxiety associated with medical procedures. *J Adolesc Health Care, 4,* 85-90.
62. Kreidler M. (1984). Meaning in suffering. *Int Nurs Rev, 31,* 174-176.
63. Kuttner L. (1989). Management of young children's acute pain and anxiety during invasive medical procedures. *Pediatrician, 16,* 39-44.
64. Kuttner L. (1990). No fears, no tears: children with cancer coping with

pain. In Tyler DC and Krane EJ (eds), *Advances in pain research and therapy,* vol 15 (p. 391). New York: Raven Press.
65. Lazarus R and Folkman S. (1984). *Stress, appraisal, and coping.* New York: Springer.
66. Leonard M. (1989). Nursing strategies: altered hematologic function. In Foster RL, Hunsberger M, and Anderson JJ (eds), *Family-centered nursing care of children* (pp. 1339-1374). Philadelphia: WB Saunders.
67. Levine M and Rappaport L. (1984). Recurrent abdominal pain in school children: the loneliness of the long-distance physician. *Pediatr Clin North Am, 31,* 969-992.
68. Lovell D and Walco G. (1989). Pain associated with juvenile rheumatoid arthritis. *Pediatr Clin North Am, 36,* 1015-1027.
69. Mather L and Mackie J. (1983). The incidence of postoperative pain in children. *Pain, 15,* 271-282.
70. McCaffery M and Beebe A. (1989). *Pain: clinical manual for nursing practice.* St. Louis: Mosby–Year Book, Inc.
71. McGrath PA. (1990). *Pain in children: nature, assessment, and treatment.* New York: The Guilford Press.
72. McGrath PA and deVeber L. (1986). The management of acute pain evoked by medical procedures in children with cancer. *J Pain Sympt Manage, 1,* 145-150.
73. McGrath PA and Hillier L. (1989). The enigma of pain in children: an overview. *Pediatrician, 16,* 6-15.
74. McGrath PJ, Goodman J, Firestone P, Shipman R, and Peters S. (1983). Recurrent abdominal pain: a psychogenic disorder? *Arch Dis Child, 58,* 888-890.
75. McGrath PJ and Humphreys P. (1989). Recurrent headaches in children and adolescents: diagnosis and treatment. *Pediatrician, 16,* 71-77.
76. McGrath PJ and Unruh A. (1987). *Pain in children and adolescents.* Amsterdam: Elsevier.
77. Melzack R. (1990). The tragedy of needless pain. *Sci Am, 262,* 27-33.
78. Mills N. (1989). Pain behaviors in infants and toddlers. *J Pain Sympt Manage, 4,* 184-190.
79. Miser A. (1990). Evaluation and management of pain in children with cancer. In Tyler D and Krane E (eds), *Advances in pain research and therapy,* vol 15 (pp. 345-364). New York: Raven Press.
80. Miser A, Dothage J, Wesley R, and Miser J. (1987). The prevalence of pain in a pediatric and young adult cancer population. *Pain, 29,* 73-83.
81. Miser A, McCalla J, Dothage J, Wesley M, and Miser S. (1987). Pain as a presenting symptom in children and young adults with newly diagnosed malignancy. *Pain, 29,* 85-90.
82. Miser A. and Miser S. (1989). The treatment of cancer pain in children. *Pediatr Clin North Am, 36,* 979-999.
83. Morrison R and Vedro D. (1989). Pain management in the child with sickle cell disease. *Pediatr Nurs, 14,* 595-599, 613.
84. Offsay JB. (1989). The pain of childhood leukemia: a parent's recollection. *J Pain Sympt Manage, 4,* 174-178.
85. Olness K and Gardner G. (1988). *Hypnosis and hypnotherapy with children,* ed 2. Philadelphia: Grune & Stratton.
86. Owens M. (1984). Pain in infancy: Conceptual and methodological issues. *Pain, 20,* 213-230.

86a. Owens, M. (1986). Assessment of infant pain in clinical settings. Pain Sympt Manage, *1,* 29-31.

87. Painter MJ and Bergman I. (1990). Neurology. In Behrman RE and Kliegman R (eds), *Nelson essentials of pediatrics* (pp. 622-669). Philadelphia: WB Saunders.

88. Parsons T. (1951). *The social system.* New York: Free Press.

89. Rappaport L. (1989). Recurrent abdominal pain: theories and pragmatics. *Pediatrician, 16,* 78-84.

90. Rana S. (1987). Pain—a subject ignored (letter to the editor). *Pediatrics, 79,* 309-310.

91. Rapoport L. (1965). The state of crisis: some theoretical considerations. In Parad JJ (ed) *Crisis intervention: selected readings.* New York: Family Service Association of America, pp. 22-31.

92. Rawlings D, Miller P, and Engel R. (1980). The effect of circumcision on transcutaneous po_2 in term infants. *Am J Dis Child, 134,* 676-678.

93. Reissland N. (1983). Cognitive maturity and the experience of fear and pain in the hospital. *Soc Sci Med, 17,* 1389-1395.

94. Rodgers B, Webb C, Stergios D, and Newman B. (1988). Patient controlled analgesia in pediatric surgery. *J Pediatr Surg, 23,* 259-262.

95. Ross D and Ross S. (1988). *Childhood pain: current issues, research, and management.* Baltimore: Urban & Schwarzenberg.

96. Savedra M and Tesler M. (1989). Assessing children's and adolescents' pain. *Pediatrician, 16,* 24-29.

97. Schechter N. (1985). Pain and pain control in children. *Curr Prob Pediatr, 15*(5), 1-67.

98. Schechter N. (1989). The undertreatment of pain in children. *Pediatr Clin North Am, 36,* 781-794.

99. Schechter N and Allen D. (1986). Physicians' attitudes toward pain in children. *Dev Behav Pediatr, 7,* 350-354.

99a. Schechter N, Altman A, and Weisman S, eds. Report of the consensus conference on the management of pain in childhood cancer. *Pediatr,* Suppl 5(part 2), 86:813-834.

100. Schechter N, Allen D, and Hanson K. (1986). Status of pediatric pain control: a comparison of hospital analgesic usage in children and adults. *Pediatrics, 17,* 11-15.

101. Schechter N, Berrien F, and Katz S. (1988). The use of patient-controlled analgesia in adolescents with sickle cell pain crisis: a preliminary report. *J Pain Sympt Manage, 3,* 109-113.

102. Schechter N, Weisman S, Rosenblum M, et al. (1990). Sedation for painful procedures in children with cancer using the fentanyl lollipop: a preliminary report. In Tyler DC and Krane EJ (eds) *Advances in pain research and therapy,* vol 15 (pp. 209-214). New York: Raven Press.

103. Schultz N. (1971). How children perceive pain. *Nurs Outlook, 19,* 670-673.

104. Scott J, Ansell B, and Huskisson E. (1977). Measurement of pain in juvenile polyarthritis. *Ann Rheum Dis, 36,* 186-187.

105. Shapiro B. (1989). The management of pain in sickle cell disease. *Pediatr Clin North Am, 36,* 1029-1045.

106. Shapiro B, Dinges D, Orne E, Ohene-Frempong K, and Orne M. (1990). Recording of crisis pain in sickle cell disease. In Tyler D and Krane E (eds), *Advances in pain research and therapy,* vol 15 (pp. 313-321). New York: Raven Press.

107. Shurin S. (1990). Hematology. In Behrman RE and Kliegman R (eds), *Essentials of pediatrics* (pp. 492-522). Philadelphia: WB Saunders.
108. Smith M, Tyler D, Womack W, and Chen A. (1989). Assessment and management of recurrent pain in adolescence. *Pediatrician, 16,* 85-93.
109. Smith M, Womack W, and Chen A. (1990). Intrinsic patient variables and outcome in the behavioral treatment of recurrent pediatric headache. In Tyler DC and Krane EJ (eds), *Advances in pain research and therapy,* vol 15 (pp. 305-311). New York: Raven Press.
109a. Spross J, McGuire D, and Schmitt R. (1990). Oncology Nursing Society position paper on cancer pain. *Oncol Nurs Forum Part I: 17(4)*:595-614.
109b. Spross J, McGuire D, and Schmitt R. (1990). Oncology Nursing Society position paper on cancer pain. *Oncol Nurs Forum Part II: 17(5)*:751-760.
110. Sweeney S. (1977). Pain associated with surgery. In Jacox A (ed), *Pain: a sourcebook for nurses and other health professionals.* Boston: Little Brown.
111. Taylor P. (1983). Postoperative pain in toddler and preschool age children. *Child Nurs J, 12,* 35-50.
112. Tyler D and Krane E (eds). (1990). *Advances in pain research and therapy: pediatric pain,* vol 15. New York: Raven Press.
113. Varni J. (1990). Behavioral management of pain in children. In Tyler D and Krane E (eds), *Advances in pain research and therapy,* vol 15. New York: Raven Press.
114. Varni J, Walco G, and Katz E. (1989). Assessment and management of chronic and recurrent pain in children with chronic disease. *Pediatrician, 16,* 56-63.
115. Vichinsky E and Lubin B. (1987). Suggested guidelines for the treatment of children with sickle cell anemia. *Hematol Oncol North Am, 1,* 493-501.
116. Walco G and Dampier C. (1987). Chronic pain in adolescent patients. *J Pediatr Psychol, 12,* 215-225.
117. Wall P and Melzack R (eds). (1989). *Textbook on pain,* ed 2. New York: Churchill Livingstone.
118. Webb C, Stergios D, and Rodgers B. (1989). Patient-controlled analgesia as postoperative pain treatment for children. *J Pediatr Nurs, 4,* 162-171.
119. Williams J. (1987). Managing pediatric pain. *Nurs Times, 83,* 36-39.
120. Zeltzer L and LeBaron S. (1982). Hypnosis and nonhypnotic techniques for reduction of pain and anxiety during painful procedures in children and adolescents with cancer. *J Pediatr, 101,* 1032-1035.

12

Pharmacological Management of Children's Pain

Joann M. Eland

◆ INTRODUCTION

Two separate research studies 10 years apart confirm the fact that, although administration of analgesics is a frequent nursing intervention for adults, analgesics are not given with the same frequency to children. In a study completed in 1975, Eland and Anderson[10] found that adults received *26 times* the amount of analgesics given children with the same surgical diagnosis. A decade later Beyer, Ashly, Russell, and DeGood[6] evaluated 50 adults and 50 children undergoing the exact same open heart surgery procedure and found that adults received 70% of the analgesic medications given. There are certainly many ways to treat people in pain besides pharmacologically, but one is hard pressed to identify a more prudent intervention for the specific postoperative situations these studies surveyed.

Eight-year-old Jessica wakes up one morning with a very sore throat and a headache. She cries when she swallows and refuses to drink anything because "it hurts too much!" Her mother takes her to the clinic where a diagnosis of strep thoat is made. The appropriate antibiotics are prescribed and Jessica's mother is told to have her daughter drink 2-3 liters of fluid per day, have her stay home from school, and give her some acetaminophen if she develops a fever. When her mother asks for something for the pain in her throat she is told to "wait until the antibiotics take effect."

Jessica's pain was what brought her to the clinic where the

diagnosis was made, but it is interesting to note that none of the treatments prescribed are specifically for pain. When the infection is under control the pain will diminish, but why do Jessica and her parents have to wait? Additionally Jessica is not going to be very cooperative in drinking 2 to 3 liters of fluid per day.

Danny is 10 years old and had his spleen removed today after an automobile accident. In change of shift nursing report, data are given about vital signs, intravenous fluids, his incision, intravenous antibiotics, and his persistent refusal to cough. The staff nurse giving report states that he has been uncooperative and she is concerned about the risk of him developing pneumonia. When a nurse from the oncoming shift asks about analgesics given since surgery, the day nurse replies, "I haven't given him anything. I don't think he needs any!"

Danny's refusal to cooperate, ambulate, and cough are seen as antecedents to pneumonia, but no connection is made between the behaviors and the likelihood that pain caused them. When the causes of pain from abdominal surgery are listed (see Table 12-1), his refusal to cough becomes even more understandable.

It is physiologically impossible for Danny to be pain free in the first 72 postoperative hours, yet it is highly unlikely he will receive the analgesia he requires. Ineffective pain management has many undesirable physiological consequences (see Table 12-1). If one looks only at the causes of pain, there is little question that Danny will require around-the-clock analgesia for at least 48 hours postoperatively so that he can be pain free, cooperate with his caregivers, and spend his energy getting well rather than fighting pain.

The purpose of this chapter will be to provide clinically relevant information for the practicing nurse in the area of pharmacological management of pediatric pain. It will proceed from the assumption that the reader is familiar with the previous chapters on pharmacology and misbeliefs regarding pain, and will focus on clinical roadblocks and recent discoveries that affect practice.

◆ CLINICAL ROADBLOCKS IN PEDIATRIC PAIN MANAGEMENT

There are many clinical roadblocks in pain management that are present in the day-to-day practice of pediatric nursing.

◆ **Table 12-1**
Causes and consequences of unrelieved pain

Cause	Consequences
The incision itself	Respiratory
Severing nerve fibers in the skin	Rapid shallow breathing; can lead to alkalosis
Cutting and stretching of muscle fibers from the surgery	Inadequate expansion of lungs; bronchiectasis, atelectasis
Manipulation of abdominal contents	Inadequate cough; retention of secretions
Chemical irritation from the cell breakage associated with the accident itself and the surgery	Cardiovascular Increased heart rate Tissue ischemia
Pain and stiffness from lying on the operating room table for hours in one position	Mobility Will not spontaneously move in bed Will not ambulate
Miscellaneous pains: NG tube, IV, lying in one position to minimize pain postoperatively	Fluid and electrolyte losses increased Rapid respiration and increased perspiration Increased metabolic rate
Other soft tissue injury from the trauma of the automobile accident	Psychological Will have nightmares about pain and surgery Will be less cooperative in the future for procedures Increased anxiety

This section will identify these concerns or roadblocks that prevent effective practice and result in unrelieved pain (see Table 12-1). Rationale for change based on current literature can be used to negotiate changes in practice.

Substance Abuse Versus Therapeutic Use

The use of illicit drugs for psychic effect has become a major problem on this continent. The current documentation of substance abuse has only encouraged the public to believe that taking opiates for pain will result in addiction. To combat this problem children and their families must be educated from the beginning of any illness in which opiates are likely to play a role. Children should be encouraged to reject street drugs but also to recognize that opiates given for pain have a therapeutic effect and do not cause addiction. They need to be taught that being pain free will help them get well by enabling them to move earlier and by preventing respiratory problems.

The practice world almost daily misuses the word *addiction* in conversation, and the author believes this is not going to change in the near future. Although it is *inappropriate* use of the word addiction, a statistic from a study by Porter and Jick[22] is useful in discussions with nurse and physician colleagues concerning the "fear of addiction." Only 4 out of 11,882 patients became "addicted" to their narcotic analgesics during their hospitalizations, and all four had a previous history of substance abuse. Comparing the risk of addiction to side effects of other drugs nurses administer frequently can serve as a reference point to eliminate unrealistic fears. Although 4 out of 11,882 people will become "addicted" to their narcotic analgesics, *15 out of 1,000 people* who take penicillin G will develop a *true* anaphylaxis.[17]

It is a clinical challenge when a physician is unwilling to prescribe or a nurse is unwilling to administer an opiate analgesic to a specific child who appears to be in pain. An appropriate response could be something similar to:

> You know, it was once thought that there was a significant risk in "addicting" someone to narcotics, and that for that reason they should not be administered very often. A couple of researchers named Porter and Jick found that only 4 out of 11,882 people became "addicted" to their narcotics, and all 4 had a history of substance abuse. When you compare that risk with the chance of a true anaphylaxis from antibiotics, it's not as scary. Did you know, for example, that 15 out of every 1,000 doses of potassium penicillin G we give will cause a true anaphylaxis? Also, people only become "addicted" when they are using drugs for nonmedical reasons.

Recognizing Tolerance in Children

Because analgesics are being administered more frequently to children with long-term pain, some children become tolerant to their narcotic analgesics. Tolerance means that a larger dose of analgesic is required to achieve the same analgesic effect and occurs most frequently when a disease process is progressing.

Children and parents will often have as their chief complaint the fact that the current analgesic "won't work" anymore. To ascertain whether a child is tolerant to the current narcotic analgesic, the child and family should be asked, "I believe that the current medicine isn't working for you anymore but I have one question, does the medicine work for a little while and then stop working?" If the answer to this question is "yes," then the child is tolerant and the dosage needs to be increased. It is important to include the first part of the question about believing they have pain in spite of analgesics. Children and parents often think it is their credibility that is being questioned when additional data are being asked of them.

Nurses and physicians may also need to be reminded that doses of other categories of drugs are increased as disease processes advance or body systems change. Insulin dosages are adjusted over time for diabetics, renal disease frequently requires an increase in dosage of antihypertensives and diuretics, and antibiotic doses are increased for children with chronic infections.

Respiratory Depression Concerns

Many nurses have been taught that the most common side effect of narcotic analgesics is respiratory depression. This is incorrect because the most common side effect of narcotic analgesics is constipation.[26] It is certainly true that analgesics can depress the respiratory center to the point of cessation of respiration in certain individuals, but it is also true that the only large study on the incidence of this found that 3 out of 3,263 patients developed respiratory depression and it was not dose related.[18] Health professionals need to use statistics to calm fears about the likelihood of such occurrences of respiratory depression and addiction and use the statistics to help change attitudes of those with whom they work to eliminate unrealistic fears in both nurses and physicians.

Recently a group of nurses approached the author and stated that they were opposed to intravenous analgesics because physicians were requiring vital signs to be taken every 15 minutes for the entire time a child was receiving a continuous intravenous morphine drip. Taking vital signs every 15 minutes for the duration of an intravenous drip is totally inappropriate and is a waste of valuable nursing time. The timing of peak respiratory depression of individual drugs being used should be ascertained so that vital signs can be monitored for the appropriate time. For example, the peak respiratory depression for morphine sulfate occurs at the following times[14]:

1. Intravenous, 7 minutes
2. Intramuscular, 30 minutes
3. Subcutaneous, 90 minutes

It is possible that an increase in the occurrence of respiratory depression may occur as health professionals unfamiliar with narcotics become more aggressive in pain management. The increase will occur because of the inexperience of practitioners increasing analgesic dosages more frequently than they should and omitting the essential ongoing assessment. The judgment that the current regimen is unsuccessful may be premature, because it takes 5 half lives of a narcotic analgesic to reach the maximum analgesic efficiency and incidence of side effects.[12] Dosages should not be changed before the maximum analgesic effect has been reached for the current dosage.

If the rare case of respiratory depression does occur, naloxone HCl (Narcan) .4 mg/cc should be diluted with 10 cc of saline, and .5 cc given by IV push every 2 minutes until the respiratory rate returns to an acceptable level. Administering naloxone in this manner will reverse the respiratory depression, the patient will retain analgesia, and the patient will not develop narcotic abstinence symptoms.[20]

Increase in Sleep Requirement

All too often children with advanced cancer enter the hospital because of unrelieved pain. When questioned they provide a description of severe pain accompanied by loss of morale, sleeplessness, fatigue, irritability, restlessness, and inability to be distracted. These children behave like a "wounded animal"—withdrawn, irritable, and striking out at almost everything.[26] When questioned further, they describe many weeks of sleeping only 3 to 4 hours per night, which explains why the child will sleep for long periods when pain is relieved. Unfortunately many nurses believe that sleeping is an undesirable side effect of opiates and refrain from giving the necessary doses. The questions that determine whether sleep is an undesirable side effect of opiates are: (1) What is the respiratory rate? (2) How appropriate is the child's speech when aroused? and (3) Is the child behaving like someone who wants to be left alone to sleep? Most children who have been in overwhelming pain sleep for a minimum of 3 to 4 days around the clock. When awakened for routine nursing care, meals, or medicines they behave like grouchy children who want to be left alone. Their respiratory rate rarely approaches the predetermined cutoff point, and their speech is completely articulate.

Misinterpreting Children's Behaviors

Previous chapters have thoroughly addressed the assessment of children's pain. However, there can be hundreds of reasons children behave as they do in the hospital: pain itself, fear of the unknown, social expectations, or even the fact that they may be missing an important school activity. If analgesics are being administered via the intramuscular route, children who have been hospitalized before often will modify their pain behavior and verbally deny pain to avoid an injection. This should not be confused with the presence or absence of pain but is an indication of how much children hate injections. In a young child's mind, admission of pain results in more pain—an injection, and the fact that they feel better later has nothing to do with the injection because they have a limited concept of time. The obvious solution to the problem is to change the route of administration to one that is acceptable.

Nurses have often been in the process of convincing a colleague that a specific child is experiencing unrelieved pain when the child appears at the doorway of his or her room and walks down the hall. The second caregiver sees the child and concludes that because the child is up and walking in the hall the child cannot be experiencing pain. This judgment is based on an adult model of pain. Adults have found by experience that activity often makes pain worse, whereas children do not know this.

Children may become more active as a way of coping with unrelieved pain. Children who have experienced multiple hospitalizations know that if they stay in their hospital "bedrooms" people will come there to poke, probe, and stick them, and take them places where they will be hurt. Many of these children believe that if they cannot be found in their "bedrooms" these events will not take place, so they leave their rooms.

Failure to Effectively Communicate Information About Pain

Questions asked of patients about their pain may be too general and therefore not effective. Nurses are frequently the professionals who know the most about a child's pain; however, the way in which the information is communicated to others can often be improved. Physicians and nurses ask children, "How are you?" believing the question is a pain question. Children and families perceive this as a social question and answer, "Fine" automatically. The caregivers assume that there is no pain problem.

Physicians need to ask specific *pain* questions, and until physicians begin doing this, nurses need to realize they may be dealing with a physician who perceives that he or she is receiving conflicting information about pain from the child and the nurse. It is helpful to complete the steps in the accompanying box before requesting a change in analgesics and to communicate the information about ineffective analgesia (see box) when talking with a physician about unrelieved pain.

Negative Physiological Consequences of Unrelieved Pain

For the first time the dangers associated with prolonged pain have begun to be demonstrated. Research on newborns undergoing surgery under minimal anesthesia has docu-

◆ **REQUESTING A CHANGE OF ANALGESIC ORDERS FROM A PHYSICIAN**

Before notifying the physician be certain the current analgesics have been given:

- At the prescribed interval
- Around the clock, with no doses omitted
- And remained in the body long enough to be effective (i.e., vomiting, diarrhea have not appeared)
- For an appropriate number of days
- And documented as ineffective using a flow sheet

mented a marked release of catecholamines, glucagon,[3] growth hormone,[5] cortisol, aldosterone, and other corticosteroids[19,25] as well as the suppression of insulin secretion.[5] These responses resulted in the breakdown of carbohydrate and fat stores, leading to severe and prolonged hyperglycemia and marked increases in blood lactate, pyruvate, total ketone bodies, and nonesterified fatty acids.[5,11] In combination these effects are not to be taken lightly and serve as further evidence of the fact that children's pain must be relieved for physiological and psychological reasons.

Maintaining Blood Levels of Analgesics

To achieve effective pain relief in severe pain, one must give analgesics around the clock to maintain blood levels of the drugs. Peaks and troughs of analgesia are eliminated by around-the-clock administration, and pain-associated anxiety is decreased or eliminated (see Chapter 7).

When attempting to discern whether a child might benefit from around-the-clock (ATC) administration, one should ask the question, "Is there a period of time when the child with these problems would not be in pain?" It is helpful to remember that pain is caused by chemicals, specifically the pros-

◆ COMMUNICATION ABOUT INEFFECTIVE ANALGESIA

Documentation should include:

- Patient's name
- Period of time drug has been tried
- Current drug(s) amount, frequency of administration, last change in dosage
- Rating scale being used
- 24-hour average pain rating, including highest and lowest rating
- (If narcotics) Respiratory rate, level of awareness, whether the child can sleep/rest
- Drug side effects child is currently experiencing on this dosage
- Nondrug measures currently being used for pain relief
- Request for suggestions from physician for more effective use of current drugs; if the physician has no suggestions, be prepared to *suggest* alternative

taglandins, histamine, and bradykinin (see Chapter 7). For example, the pain chemicals associated with a child 10 hours after surgery for a broken arm or with terminal cancer will still be causing pain. A child whose arm was broken, smashed by metal and trapped until freed by an ambulance crew would have pain from:

1. Cutaneous
2. Nerve
3. Vascular
4. Three separate sources from the broken bones
5. Swelling

Treatments such as surgery and/or wound care exacerbate the existing pain. It is highly unlikely that this child would be pain free unless appropriate interventions were undertaken. Some children may be able to use distraction, hypnosis, and other techniques to significantly alter the pain experience, but most children must have their pain reduced with analgesics so that they can concentrate to learn these valuable techniques. For some children who do not have these alternative methods at their disposal, analgesics may be their only alternative for pain relief.

Standard Doses

Standard doses are helpful general guidelines that need to be evaluated individually for each patient (see Table 12-2). In pediatrics, standard doses based on milligrams/kilograms have often resulted in unrelieved pain, and the American Pain Society has recommended pediatric doses that are easier to remember and result in improved pain control (see box). Pain must be reassessed after administration of analgesics to determine the resulting degree of pain relief. This may seem obvious, but the effects of analgesics are frequently not evaluated.

In pediatrics, standard doses of drugs are used when indicated, but if a standard dose will not achieve the desired therapeutic benefit the dose must be altered. If a "well" child develops a strep throat, ordinary doses of an antibiotic will be prescribed to eliminate the strep. A child with cancer and leukopenia will be placed on large doses of intravenous antibiotics at the first sign of the strep infection. A child with a simple arm fracture will most likely have pain relieved from ordinary doses of analgesics, but a child with an aggressive

◆ **Table 12-2**
Equianalgesic doses

Drug	IM dose (mg)	Oral dose required to equal IM dose (mg)
Dilaudid	2	4
Morphine	10	20–60
Methadone	10	5–20
Meperidine	75	Not recommended
Codeine	120	200
Nalbuphine (Nubain)	10	Unavailable
Butorphanol (Stadol)	2	Unavailable
Buprenorphine (Temgesic)	0.4	Sublingual not available in U.S. Not available orally

◆ **AMERICAN PAIN SOCIETY RECOMMENDATIONS FOR CHILDREN**

Children 13 years and older	Full adult dose
Children 7–12	One half adult dose
Children 2–7	One fourth adult dose
Children under 2	Use mg/kg guidelines

cancer may require aggressive increases in dosage because of the nature of the advancing disease process.

◆ PROCEDURAL PAIN

Preventing Procedural Pain

Too frequently the time between analgesic administration and the procedure is too short for the analgesic to take effect. If morphine sulfate has been ordered, the time required for peak analgesia is (1) 20 minutes via the IV route, (2) 30 to 60 minutes via the IM route, and (3) 50 to 90 minutes via the subcutaneous route.[14] The peak effect is directly related to the binding of the drug to plasma lipids. Although the times listed do not seem long, the clinical condition may not allow enough time to wait for the peak blood level or physicians may not leave enough time in their schedule to wait.

Sublimaze (Fentanyl) is a short-acting synthetic opioid 80 to 100 times more potent than morphine and has an immediate onset when given intravenously, with a duration of 30 to 60 minutes. When the drug is administered intramuscularly it has a 7 to 8 minute onset with a duration 1 to 2 hours. Sublimaze also is short acting and can be useful for frequent dressing changes, where a long duration of effect would not be desirable. Meperidine (Demerol) is also useful for procedures because it is highly soluble with a rapid onset; however, its duration is longer than that of sublimaze.

Many emergency rooms now have standing orders to place 3 ccs of TAC(tetracaine HCl, adrenaline, and cocaine)-soaked gauze into minor wounds before wound cleaning and suturing.[9,23,24] The TAC is absorbed through the walls and floor of the wound, making cleaning and suturing much more tolerable for all concerned. If more anesthetic is required it can be injected into the walls of a wound that is already anesthetized. TAC is prepared by the pharmacy in 5 ml portions of 5% tetracaine 25 mg/5 ml, adrenalin 1:2000, and cocaine 11.8%, 580 mg/5 ml. Cocaine is used in the solution as an anesthetic and for its vasoconstrictive properties. Concern has been raised over the use of it in this solution, and it can be left out without compromising the solution's efficacy. A death was reported with the use of TAC when a *three times normal dose* was accidentally used for suturing an infant's lip laceration.

◆ SPECIFIC PHARMACOLOGICAL AGENTS

Local Anesthetics

Some physicians are reluctant to use local anesthetics because children complain that their burning and stinging sensations are worse than the procedure itself. There is no question that local anesthetics burn and sting when injected, but the duration of the stinging is less when chloroprocaine HCl (Nesacaine) is used rather than lidocaine HCl (Xylocaine) or procaine (Novocaine). The onset of chloroprocaine HCl is almost instantaneous with stinging that lasts 1 to 2 seconds, and the duration of effect is 15 to 20 minutes. Lidocaine HCl and procaine sting for about 30 seconds and provide 2 to 3 hours of anesthesia. Most pediatric procedures can be completed in 15 to 20 minutes, and the failure to use chloroprocaine HCl is probably the result of the habit of using the other drugs and the failure to disseminate information about chloroprocaine HCl.

Antianxiety Agents

There is still great debate in pediatrics over whether to prescibe antianxiety agents for children who undergo repeated procedures. Children who have a chronic illness requiring many procedures may find the thought of additional procedures particularly distressing. A child who is not in control of his emotions and who has experienced multiple unpleasant experiences will be fearful and less cooperative, will be more anxious about the next procedure, and may have a series of nightmares about the procedure. Over time it is possible that the child may not require the medication. Some professionals feel that it is dangerous to sedate a child who will be traveling to the clinic, but when children are accompanied by adults this is not an issue. Others say that the use of antianxiety medications teaches children to use medications as a crutch or encourages them to escape reality. The child is escaping no reality. The children and their families are dealing with extraordinary circumstances that are not part of everyday life, and procedures have to be done. Administering an appropriate amount of an oral antianxiety agent, such as diazepam (Valium), hydroxyzine pamoate (Vistaril), or midazolam HCl (Versed), before the clinic visit is an appropriate intervention.

Specific Analgesics

What follows are some specific considerations for analgesics in children. The list is not intended to be all-inclusive, and readers are referred to other references for more complete information.

Aspirin

Availability. Oral chewable tablets, gum, and bicarbonate solution (which many children do not like).

Disadvantages. Not recommended for children under the age of 13 because of the association with Reye's syndrome.

Interferes with platelet aggregation and has significant gastrointestinal side effects.

Advantages. Has both analgesic and antiinflammatory properties.

Acetaminophen

Availability. Various forms including elixir, chewable tablets, tablets, and rectal suppository. Be alert to the facts that the different forms have different potencies and that overdose can result in serious hepatotoxicity.

Disadvantages. Acetaminophen has no antiinflammatory properties.

Advantages. Children usually find the taste acceptable; it can be combined with narcotic analgesics in young children for pain relief superior to either drug used individually. Little or no gastrointestinal upset.

Trisalicylate (Trilisate)

Availability. Oral tablets, cherry-flavored liquid.

Disadvantages. Currently not recommended for children under 12 years because it may be associated with Reye's syndrome although there have been no reported cases so far. Trilisate is a very large tablet that most children cannot swallow.

Advantages. Drug can be given twice a day instead of every four hours. Chemical action is similar to that of aspirin but it does not appear to cause problems with platelet aggregation, and the incidence of gastrointestinal side effects is quite low.

Other Nonsteroidal Antiinflammatory Drugs (NSAIDs)

A number of NSAIDs are currently undergoing the clinical trials necessary to make them available for use with children. Many of the NSAIDs have been shown to be superior to aspirin or acetaminophen in their ability to relieve pain and reduce inflammation. The reader should refer to the current literature and product updates as they become available for use in pediatrics.

Opioid Analgesics

Narcotic analgesics are appropriate for many types of pediatric pain. Currently several new routes of administration, including transdermal, oral sprays, lollipops, and sublingual, are under investigation that will make the task of administering narcotic analgesics even more acceptable to children, their parents, and nurses. Table 12-3 lists the various available forms of morphine sulfate and other drugs frequently used for severe pain as well as their disadvantages, taste, and advantages.

The advent of patient-controlled analgesia (PCA) devices, which administer a constant dose of intravenous narcotic analgesics, has been one of the most significant developments in pediatric pain control in recent times. The devices themselves are quite safe, are locked with narcotic keys, and are programmed to deliver a prescribed amount of drug each hour with bolus doses of drug for periods of increased pain. The PCA devices appear to be the means by which the practice world will finally implement intravenous analgesic administration in both pediatric and adult patients.

Heroin. Parents of children with terminal illness may ask if their children would receive improved pain relief if they were given herion. Heroin is biotransformed morphine and has been shown to have no superior pharmacokinetic or pharmacodynamic advantages over morphine.[13,15] Hydromorphone recently became available in concentrated solution (Dilaudid H-P, 10 mg/ml) and can be used with equal success,[7,20] and it is available in a concentrated form that makes it particularly appropriate for implanted infusion pumps.

◆ TEACHING FAMILIES AND CHILDREN WITH CANCER ABOUT MORPHINE

Terminally ill children and their families need to know certain information about taking morphine. This information was adapted from tables originally prepared by Twycross and Lack[26] (see boxes).

◆ SUMMARY

This chapter has provided some basic information about the pharmacological control of pediatric pain and has expanded on the more general topics of Chapter 7. It has iden-

◆ **Table 12-3**
Advantages and disadvantages of various forms of morphine

	Oral	Slow release	Quick release	Suppositories
Disadvantages	Frequent administration required	Expensive	Expensive	Children hate them
Taste	Awful taste	No taste	Taste okay	NA
Advantages	Cheapest form	Bid or Tid administration Dissolved over time — maintains even blood levels of the drug	Absorbed quickly Designed for break-through pain	Any amount can be put into them

◆ FOR THE CHILD WHO HAS NOT TAKEN MORPHINE BEFORE

1. The dose of morphine on which you have been started is a usual starting dose and may need adjusting.
2. If it doesn't work right away it just means the dose needs to be carefully increased.
3. If your head feels very "weird," you get dizzy, or your brain feels like there's a "cloud" in it, call the hospice nurse or doctor. The dose probably needs to be changed a little.
4. If you haven't been sleeping "all right," when the pain is better you'll sleep a lot until you catch up.
5. If you have been sleeping okay and with morphine all you want to do is sleep, call the hospice nurse or doctor and tell them.
7. If you stick with it for 2 to 3 days the "weird, dizzy, cloudy," feelings will go away. Hang in there.
8. Make sure you continue to go to the bathroom for a bowel movement as often as you have before you started taking morphine.
9. Morphine makes some people feel like they want to throw up. If this happens to you we can give you an "anti-throw up" drug.
10. Don't expect miracles right away as you start to take morphine; give yourself some time to get used to it.
11. Tell the people who come to see you, like friends, aunts, uncles, or grandparents, that you may be feeling a little weird or sleepy but it will go away.
12. Some adults really don't know what to say when they find out you're on morphine. Be patient with them; there are a lot of strange stories about morphine they may have heard that aren't true.
13. Some kids won't understand why you are taking morphine either. Try explaining it to them, but if they still don't understand, it's okay; some things are just hard to understand.

From Eland JM. (1989). Pharmacologic management of pain. In Martin B (ed), *Pediatric hospice care: what helps*. Children's Hospital of Los Angeles.

◆ PATIENT/FAMILY TEACHING ABOUT MORPHINE

1. You are taking morphine for the control of pain.
2. The fact that your child is taking morphine does not mean that he will die soon.
3. Take the morphine as often as it says on the bottle. Don't skip doses.
4. The effects on the body when morphine is used in this way are different from its effects on abusers. You won't get "high."
5. Remember to keep taking the other drugs your doctor has prescribed.
6. If you have trouble getting your prescription filled notify the hospice nurse.
7. If you are completely pain free call the hospice nurse and discuss the possibility of decreasing the dose. Don't stop taking the drug on your own.
8. Your body will *not* become accustomed to the medicine so that it will no longer work.
9. If you get to feeling better you will probably start moving around more and the dose may need to be adjusted.
10. If your pain gets worse the amount of medicine you take can be increased. Talk with your hospice nurse or physician about this.
11. If for some reason your pain goes away you will be able to gradually decrease the morphine without problems. You will *not* become an addict and be unable to stop the drug.

From Eland JM. (1989). Pharmacologic management of pain. In Martin B (ed), *Pediatric hospice care: what helps.* Children's Hospital of Los Angeles.

tified the clinical roadblocks to effective pain relief and has provided explanations and strategies to assist nurses to remove them. New developments in the area of analgesic management have also been identified and explained. Finally, pediatric considerations regarding specific analgesics have been identified. An attempt has been made to provide the latest information in this ever-changing area, but the reader is challenged to make every effort to keep current in nursing practice. Permanent change in nursing and medical practice occurs slowly, and the reader is reminded to persist in attempting to persuade others to more actively eliminate pediatric pain.

REFERENCES

1. American Pain Society. (1986). *Principles of analgesic use in the treatment of acute pain and chronic cancer pain—a concise guide to medical practice.* Washington, D.C.
2. Anand KJS and Hickey PR. (1987). Pain and its effects in the human neonate and fetus. *N Engl J Med, 21,* 1317-1321.
3. Anand KJS. (1986). Hormonal and metabolic functions of neonates and infants undergoing surgery. *Curr Opin Cardiol, 1,* 681.
4. Anand KJS, Brown MJ, Bloom SR, and Aynsley-Green A. (1985). Studies on the hormonal regulation of fuel metabolism in the human newborn undergoing anaesthesia and surgery. *Horm Res, 22,* 115.
5. Anand KJS, Brown MJ, Causon RC, et al. (1985). Can the human neonate mount an endocrine and metabolic response to surgery? *J Pediatr Surg, 20,* 41.
6. Beyer JE, Ashly LC, Russell GA, and DeGood DE. (1984). Pediatric pain after cardiac surgery: pharmacologic management. *Dimen Crit Care Nurs, 3,* 326.
7. Burchman SL. (1989). Hospice care of the cancer pain patient. In Abram SE (ed), *Cancer Pain* (p. 161). Boston: Kluwer Academic Publishers.
8. Eland JM. (1989). Pharmacologic management of pain. In Martin B (ed), *Pediatric hospice care: what helps.* Los Angeles: Children's Hospital of Los Angeles.
9. Eland JM and Herr KA. (1988). Does suturing have to hurt so much? *Child Nurse, 6,* (5) 1-3.
10. Eland JM and Anderson JE. (1977). The experience of pain in children. In Jacox AK (ed), *Pain: a sourcebook for nurses and other health professionals.* Boston: Little, Brown.
11. Elphick MC and Wilkinson AW. (1981). The effects of starvation and surgical injury on the plasma levels of glucose, free fatty acids, and neutral lipids in newborn babies suffering from various congenital anomalies. *Pediatr Res, 15,* 313.
12. Foley KM. (1985). Pharmacologic approaches to cancer pain management. In Fields HL (ed), *Advances in pain research and therapy, vol 9* (p. 641). New York: Raven.
13. Inturrisi CE, Max MB, Foley KM, et al. (1984). The pharmacokinetics of heroin in patients with chronic pain. *N Engl J Med, 210,* 1213-1217.
14. Jaffe JH and Martin WR. (1980). Opioid analgesics and antagonists. In Gilman AG, Goodman LS, and Gilman A (eds), *The pharmacological basis of therapeutics.* (pp. 506-509). New York: MacMillan Publishing.
15. Kaiko RF, Wallenstein SL, Rogers AG, et al. (1981). Analgesic and mood effects of heroin and morphine in cancer patients with postoperative pain. *N Engl J Med, 304,* 1501-1505.
16. Kaiko RF, et al. (1982). Central nervous system excitatory effects of meperidine in cancer patients. *Ann Neuro, 113,* 180-185.
17. Mandell GL and Sande MA. (1980). Antimicrobial agents. In Gilman AG, Goodman LS, and Gilman A (eds), *The pharmacological basis of therapeutics.* New York: MacMillian Publishing.
18. Miller RR and Jick H. (1978). Clinical effects of meperidine in hospitalized medical patients. *J Clin Pharmacol, 18*(4), 180.
19. Obara H, Sugiyama D, Maekawa N, et al. (1984). Plasma cortisol levels in paediatric anaesthesia. *Can Anaesth Soc J*, 31:24.

20. Payne R. (1989). Oral and parenteral drug therapy for cancer pain. In Abram SE (ed), *Cancer Pain.* (p. 29). Boston: Kluwer Academic Publishers.
21. Pinter A. (1973). The metabolic effects of anaesthesia and surgery in the newborn infant: changes in the blood levels of glucose, plasma free fatty acids, alpha amino-nitrogen, plasma amino-acid ration and lactate in the neonate. *Z Kinderchir, 12,* 149.
22. Porter J and Jick H. (1980). Addiction rate in patients treated with narcotics. *N Engl J Med, 302,* 123.
23. Pryor GJ, Kilpatric WR, and Opp DR. (1980). Local anesthesia in minor lacerations: topical TAC versus lidocaine infiltration. *Ann Emerg Med, 9*(11), 568-571.
24. Shannon M. (1988). Topical TAC anesthesia for lacerations: efficacy and potential toxicity. *Pediatr Alert, 13*(6), March 18, 1988, 1-2.
25. Srinivasan G, Jain R, Pildes RS, and Kannan CR. (1986). Glucose homeostasis during anesthesia and surgery in infants. *J Pediatr Surg, 21,* 718.
26. Twycross RG and Lack SA. (1983). *Symptom control in far advanced cancer: pain relief.* (pp. 309, 310). London: Pitman.

13

Pain in the Elderly

Betty R. Ferrell
Bruce Ferrell

◆ INTRODUCTION

A chief priority in geriatric care is the control of chronic disease symptoms, improvement of comfort, and preservation of dignity for the elderly person.[17] However, in the authors' review of 11 leading textbooks of geriatric medicine, only two have devoted chapters to assessment and management of pain. Similarly, in a review of eight geriatric nursing texts encompassing more than 5,000 pages of text, less than 18 pages were devoted to discussion of pain. It is ironic that so little emphasis is given to chronic pain in a population that is at high risk for chronic and painful illnesses. With the "geriatric imperative" for health care among the increasing elderly population, we can no longer ignore the problem of chronic pain in this population.

Until recently, the study of pain was largely limited to cancer pain in acute care settings. More recent studies have focused on the special needs of patients in alternative care settings such as home care[9] and hospice,[25] which are common sites for care of the elderly. Heavy reliance on family and nonprofessional staff for provision of care, limited access to diagnostic facilities, and limited pharmacy services influence pain management in these care settings. Similar problems exist in the nursing home setting.[17]

Research in the area of pain management in general has increased, as evidenced by the 1986 NIH Consensus Conference on the "Integrated Approach to the Management of Pain".[26] Advances have been evident in the areas of pain assessment,[35] pain technologies,[21] and organization of pain services or clinics.[18] Major emphasis has been focused on disease-specific areas such as cancer pain.[10] More recently, pediatrics has been identified as a special population for pain research.[15] Pain in the elderly, however, is largely an unexplored area for clinicians and researchers alike.

The purpose of this chapter is to explore the subject of pain in the elderly population and to promote advances in knowledge and treatment of pain in older persons. Included is an overview of the problem of pain in elderly persons, the nursing process applied to pain in the elderly, and implications for future work.

◆ BACKGROUND

Epidemiology

The prevalence of pain in the elderly population is not accurately known. Bonica estimated that the prevalence of all pain in the American population may be as high as 35%.[1] In a random survey of 500 households in Burlington, Ontario,[3] the morbidity associated with pain was two times greater in subjects over age 60, (250 per thousand), compared with 125 per thousand for subjects under age 60. Our own studies of pain among nursing home residents suggest that over 70% of this frail elderly population have significant pain problems.[6] There is abundant literature regarding the symptoms of pain associated with specific diseases, but this literature generally has not attempted to compare pain characteristics by age group. The NIH consensus conference recognized the need for "conduct of epidemiological studies of the incidence and prevalence of pain."[26] Similar to the work that led to major advances in understanding cancer pain, there is a need for basic epidemiological and descriptive research to explore pain in this specific group.

Pain Perception in the Elderly

It has been suggested that there is an age-associated decline in pain sensitivity and perception. Several induced-pain studies, using a variety of stimuli, for example, cutaneous heat,[34] achilles tendon pressure,[37] and electrical tooth shocks,[13] have demonstrated decreased sensitivity and tolerance to pain among elderly subjects. There is not a clear consensus among investigators on these observations.[14] No longitudinal pain perception studies have been reported to date, and most of the cross-sectional studies have failed to exclude subjects with confounding problems, such as subjects taking analgesic medications, subjects with diabetes, or subjects who have chronic pain. In the final analysis, whether any physiological decline in pain perception is related to normal aging, as opposed to coexisting disease or occult disease, remains to be clearly shown. Studies that have been confined to the laboratory setting may have limited application to clinical pain.

Clinical investigators have reported a variety of observations regarding pain perception among elderly patients. Results of the National Hospice study of terminal cancer patients suggested that although 77% of elderly subjects experienced pain, the presence of pain and its severity were negatively correlated with age.[12] The Nuprin Pain Report, a Harris national telephone survey, also suggested an age-related reduction in pain reports at all sites with the exception of joint pain.[31] Case reports of unusual presentations of common problems in the aged frequently suggest alterations in pain perception. For example, elderly patients not uncommonly present with "silent" abdominal catastrophes,[29] myocardial infarctions,[22] and life-threatening infections.[38] However, Portenoy and Farkash[30] warn that most of the literature on the subject is based on observations and anecdotes rather than empirical data.

Our research,[4,8,7,9,9c] has documented the significant relationship between pain, functional status, and overall quality of life. An individual's ability to remain mobile and carry on daily activities can be influenced by the presence of pain. This is apparent in younger adults who have pain-induced interruptions in their work schedules, recreational activities, or family roles. Data from our investigation of pain in the nursing home[8] indicates that this is also true for elderly patients residing in long-term care facilities. Table 13-1 is a summary of the self-reported effects of pain by 65 residents of a long-term care facility who reported having chronic pain.[8]

In summary, the data regarding age-associated changes in pain perception is controversial. The assumption that aging per se results in decreased pain perception is dangerous and may result in inaccurate assessment and needless suffering. Pain is an individual experience, and assessment of pain is best based on a thorough assessment of that individual rather

◆ Table 13-1
Self-reported effects of pain among elderly nursing home residents (n = 65 subjects with pain)

Effect	Frequency
Impaired enjoyable activities (recreational activities and social events)	35 (54%)
Impaired ambulation (walking, transfers, etc.)	34 (52%)
Impaired posture	32 (49%)
Sleep disturbance	29 (45%)
Depression	21 (32%)
Anxiety	17 (26%)
Impaired bowel function (constipation)	10 (15%)
Impaired appetite	9 (14%)
Impaired memory	8 (12%)
Impaired bladder function (incontinence)	5 (8%)
Impaired dressing or grooming	5 (8%)
None of the above	15 (23%)

Numbers total more than 100% because some subjects indicated more than one effect of pain.
From: Ferrell BA, Ferrell BR, and Osterweil D. (1990). Pain in the nursing home. *J Am Geriatr Soc* 38(4), 9-14.

than on assumptions based on age. Summaries of the major misconceptions about pain in the elderly are listed in the box on p. 353. These misconceptions are more fully discussed in Chapter 3. This information is vital for health care providers as well as for the patient and family.

◆ NURSING CARE OF ELDERLY PATIENTS IN PAIN

Providing optimum care for patients in pain requires planned interventions and recognition of the many special needs of this group. This can be best illustrated through the use of the nursing process as a guide to professional nursing practice. The process of assessment, planning, intervention, and evaluation is presented for nursing care of the elderly patient in pain.

Assessment

Assessment of chronic pain in the elderly is important for several reasons.[6] First, pain is the most common symptom of

◆ MISCONCEPTIONS ABOUT PAIN IN THE ELDERLY

MYTH: Pain is expected with aging.

FACT: Pain is not normal with aging. The presence of pain in the elderly necessitates aggressive assessment, diagnosis, and management similar to that of younger patients.

MYTH: Pain sensitivity and perception decrease with aging.

FACT: This assumption is dangerous! Data are conflicting regarding age-associated changes in pain perception, sensitivity, and tolerance. Consequences of this assumption are needless suffering and undertreatment of both pain and the underlying cause.

MYTH: If a patient does not complain of pain, he must not have much pain.

FACT: This is erroneous in all ages but particularly in the elderly. Older patients may not report pain for a variety of reasons. They may fear the meaning of the pain, diagnostic workups, or pain treatments. They may think pain is normal.

MYTH: A person who has no functional impairment, appears occupied, or is otherwise distracted from pain, must not have significant pain.

FACT: Patients have a variety of reactions to pain. Many patients are stoic and refuse to "give in" to their pain. Over extended periods of time, the elderly may mask any outward signs of pain.

MYTH: Narcotic medications are inappropriate for patients with chronic nonmalignant pain.

FACT: Opioid analgesics are often indicated in nonmalignant pain.

MYTH: Potential side effects of narcotic medications make them too dangerous to use in the elderly.

FACT: Narcotics may be used safely in the elderly. Although elderly patients may be more sensitive to narcotics, this does not justify withholding narcotics and failing to relieve pain.

disease. Accurate assessment of pain is essential in making an accurate diagnosis. Since treatment of underlying conditions is the most important aspect of pain management, an accurate diagnosis cannot be overemphasized. Second, assessment is important for the evaluation of the effect of therapy. Frail elderly are vulnerable to both undertreatment and overtreatment of pain. The therapeutic window, the margin of safety, for all analgesic drugs is more narrow for elderly patients.[19] In other words, the difference between the therapeutic dose of a medication and the toxic dose is smaller in the elderly. Third, assessment is important to differentiate acute, endangering pain from longstanding chronic pain. Progression of disease and acute injuries may go unrecognized if new symptoms are attributed to preexisting disease. Only systematic assessment can avoid this problem. Finally, the successful management of pain must be approached as would management of any other symptom of disease, beginning with an accurate assessment and continuing with modifications in treatment based on periodic reassessment.

Because pain is such an individual experience, a multidimensional approach to assessment is usually required (see Chapter 4). Physical, functional, and psychological evaluation should be combined to ensure appropriate assessment. This section will review salient features of multidimensional pain assessment, including the use of specific pain assessment scales.

The Pain History

Since acute and chronic pain often coexist in the elderly, it is extremely important that pain assessment begin with an accurate history to establish the medical diagnosis and a baseline description of the pain experience. Most clinicians are familiar with the "what, when, where, and how" approach to the pain complaint. The character of the pain should be described using the patient's own words, which will serve as a description for future reference. Exacerbating or relieving influences should include a description of activities and physical limitations. For the frail elderly, any history of trauma should be thoroughly evaluated.[28] Sudden changes in the character of the pain may indicate deterioration or new injury and should be carefully evaluated.

It is important to remember that elderly patients may present special problems in the obtaining of an accurate pain history. Memory impairment, depression, and cognitive impairment may hinder history-taking.[6] More important, patients may associate pain with aging and their other chronic diseases and underreport their symptoms as a result. Cancer patients may not report pain because they fear the meaning of pain. They also may think pain cannot be relieved and therefore do not report pain. Many elderly patients may not report pain because they "just don't want to bother anyone."[8] The importance of family and caregivers as a source of information about elderly patients cannot be overemphasized. Family members can often provide useful information about the patient's function, pain trajectory, and use of medications for pain relief. However, the clinician must carefully interpret the family members' assessments. For example, an adult child may deny that an elderly parent has pain as a mechanism of the child's own coping with the reality of an aging parent or feelings of helplessness as the child observes the loved one in pain.[9a,b]

Because elderly patients suffer multiple illnesses, care must be taken to avoid attributing acute pain to preexisting chronic illness. Making this problem worse is the fact that chronic pain is usually not constant. Both character and intensity of chronic pain may fluctuate with time. Injuries caused by trauma are easily overlooked in this setting. Bones may fracture, and muscles and tendons may strain, under very minor trauma. Only astute questioning and compulsive evaluation will enable one to avoid overlooking these acute episodes of pain in elderly patients.

Physical Examination

A thorough assessment of pain includes a comprehensive physical examination. Physical examination should serve to confirm suspicions elicited by the history as well as help evaluate functional limitations.

Because of the frequency of painful traumatic and degenerative musculoskeletal problems in the elderly, the physical examination should probably be focused on musculoskeletal and nervous systems.[6,28] Most important during the physical examination is palpation for trigger points and inflammation. A trigger point is an area sensitive to pressure of palpation, resulting in the production of a characteristic pain sensation. Trigger points may result from tendonitis, muscle strain, or nerve irritation. Other specific maneuvers that reproduce the pain, such as straight leg raising and joint range of motion exercise, may be useful in diagnosis as well as functional assessment. Additionally, a thorough neurological examination should be conducted, including attention to signs of autonomic, sensory, and motor deficits suggestive of neuropathic conditions and nerve injuries.

Evaluation of Function

Functional impairment is a major problem for elderly patients. Evaluation of function is important so that mobility and independence are maximized for elderly patients. The contribution of chronic pain to functional impairment may be quite important for elderly patients. The Iowa Rural Health Survey[20] found pain among older people with low back pain was more likely to result in impaired ambulation and increased health services utilization.

Functional assessment may include information from the history and physical examination as well as several available functional assessment tools. These tools (see Chapter 4), which primarily assess activities of daily living, may not always be sensitive to the effect of pain on function.[8] However, they have been shown to be useful in a variety of geriatric settings not only to document progression of disability but also to identify the need for supervision and nursing care. Tools such as the Tinetti Gait Evaluation Tool and the Lawton or the Katz activities of daily living scales may be useful and are easy to administer.[17]

Psychological Evaluation

Evaluation of mood should be conducted because of the psychological conditions that are strongly associated with chronic pain.[11] Most patients with chronic pain will have significant depressive symptoms at some time and may benefit dramatically from psychological or psychiatric intervention. Likewise, anxiety may be a significant psychological factor in the management of chronic pain. Caution must be exercised in attributing pain exclusively to a psychological cause. Failure to recognize the organic source of pain may result in needless suffering.

Another major psychological issue to be recognized in pain assessment is the relationship between cognitive impairment and pain.[11] No significant data exists on this important geriatric topic. Elderly patients may represent special problems in assessment and management of pain because of cognitive impairment. Clinical evidence suggests that cognitive impairment may be exacerbated by pain and its treatment. A critical question is whether pain assessment in the cognitively impaired is possible using existing assessment technology, which depends on the active involvement of and self-reporting by the patient (see Table 13-1). Better understanding of the behaviors associated with pain in this population may provide some assistance in pain assessment (see Chapter 3).

Psychological assessment should include at least a thorough mental status examination and evaluation for depression. Tools such as the Folstein Mini Mental State for cognitive impairment and the Hamilton, Beck, or Yesavage inventories for depression are easily implemented for these purposes.[17] Formal psychological tests, including the MMPI, which has been validated for use in older populations, may also be useful in some patients by identifying personality traits that might benefit from specific psychological or psychiatric therapy. For example, awareness of an extreme anxiety disorder or severe depression in an individual may assist the clinician in diagnosing and treating pain.

Assessment of Other Constructs

Another pain assessment technique is the measurement of related outcomes. Researchers are using established tools in other areas to gain insight into the patient's pain. One example is the validation of a quality of life tool for use in evaluating patients in pain.[4] The use of quality of life (QOL) measurement provides valuable insight into the multidimensional nature of pain and the effect of pain on the entire individual. This QOL was later implemented in clinical research in a study of controlled-release analgesia.[5] The study results indicate that QOL is indeed a useful outcome measure for evaluating clinical trials. The QOL tool provided a multidimensional assessment of outcomes associated with long-acting analgesics rather than evaluating the drugs on a single dimension of pain intensity.

Other constructs of interest include instruments that measure outcomes such as chronic illness adaptation or sickness impact.[32] These assessments allow us to view pain not as an endpoint in and of itself but rather as a symptom of underlying illness with resultant effect on multiple dimensions of the person. We have found that often, although a patient may report pain intensity as being mild to moderate, the patient also reports major life disturbances because of the distress associated with pain. "Moderate" pain in an elderly nursing home patient may be significant enough to interfere with important daily activities such as being able to play bingo, enjoy social outings, or participate in group meals.

Specific Pain Assessment Scales

Pain assessment instruments (tools or scales) have been developed to help both clinicians and researchers more accurately measure, document, and communicate the patient's pain experiences. These tools can be divided into qualitative and quantitative approaches. Qualitative instruments attempt to describe the patient's pain using tools such as pain diaries, pain logs, or pain graphs, or by observation. These tools rely on the patient's own description of the pain and communicate the patient's individual pain experience.

Pain logs or diaries (Figure 13-1) are used by having the patient record the intensity of pain during his or her daily routine to assess possible relationships between pain, medication use, and daily activities. Figure 13-2 illustrates the use of a pain graph. Here the physician or nurse may help the patient graphically illustrate his or her daily pain experience. These tools can be particularly useful in determining possible interferences with adequate pain management, such as the patient who refuses to take any pain medication until the pain is severe. Documentation of pain is useful in any age patient but is particularly helpful in the elderly because they often have confounding illnesses and symptoms and because they often depend on others for management of pain. The tools can be effectively used by caregivers when the patient is unable to write or maintain the logs or diaries.

Date/time	Activity	Pain intensity	Action	Outcome

FIGURE 13-1. Example of a pain diary.

An important qualitative technique is simple observation of the patient in pain. Recent work has attempted to validate pain behaviors such as facial grimace and agitation as valid behavioral cues for pain. This will be an important area of continued study with respect to elderly patients who are unable to verbally communicate their pain because of cognitive impairment. Assessment of behavior should be used with caution, however, because it is widely known that patients in pain often have no outward signs of distress. For example, chronic pain is a frustrating and fatiguing experience. Patients with chronic pain may have no energy to show outward behaviors or signs of pain.

Some interesting work is going on in the field of pediatrics in adapting common pain instruments for use with children.[15,35] (See Chapter 10.) One example uses a "happy face" scale, with varying degrees of smiling faces corresponding to a rating scale. Similar work is needed in the elderly to adapt existing tools to the special needs of this population.

Assessment of any symptom depends on psychometrically established tools with documented reliability and validity for the population in question. Unfortunately the establishment of pain tools has not yet been well documented for the old-old population (>85 years) or the cognitively impaired. Table 13-2 summarizes the major components of a comprehensive clinical assessment of pain in the elderly.

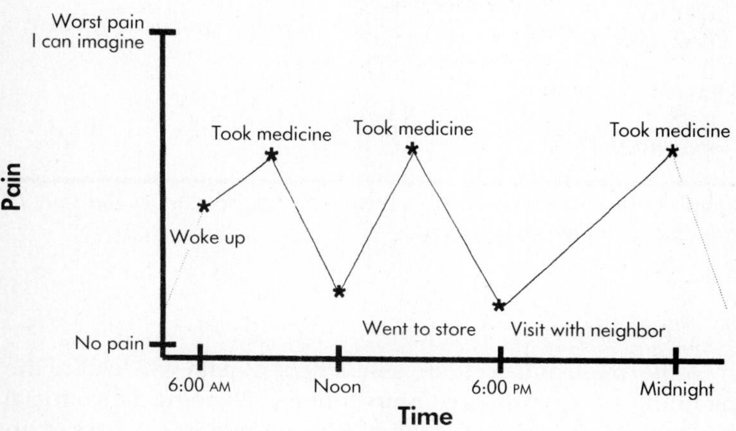

FIGURE 13-2. Pain graph.

◆ **Table 13-2**
The clinical assessment of pain

History	Physical exam	Pain assessment tools	Assessment of other constructs
MEDICAL HISTORY	**ROUTINE EXAM**	**VISUAL ANALOG SCALE**	**DEPRESSION SCALES**
	SIGNS OF TRAUMA		Hamilton Yesavage Beck
PAIN HISTORY Location Frequency Duration Severity Interventions Exacerbations Alleviations	**MUSCULOSKELETAL EXAMINATION** Trigger points Swellings Masses Tender spots Inflammation	**NUMBER OR WORD DESCRIPTOR SCALES**	**ACTIVITIES OF DAILY LIVING SCALES** Katz Lawton
HISTORY OF TRAUMA		**MCGILL-MELZACK PAIN SCALE**	**MOOD OR QUALITY OF LIFE SCALES**
MEDICATIONS Drug Dose Route Frequency Efficacy Reactions	**RANGE OF MOTION** Joints Muscles		
	FUNCTIONAL IMPAIRMENT		
PREVIOUS PAIN EXPERIENCES			

From Ferrell BR and Ferrell BA. (1990). Comfort. In Corr D and Corr C. *Nursing care in an aging society*.

Planning

A thorough and accurate assessment of pain will lead to the planning of appropriate interventions. Planning is a crucial prerequisite in caring for the elderly. Often, it is necessary to involve other family members or caregivers in planning pain management. Indeed, family members play a critical role as caregivers in pain assessment, in decisions about pharmacological management of pain, and in nonpharmacological interventions. This involvement may have a positive effect on these caregivers as it allows them to be actively involved in the patient's comfort and minimizes the feelings of helplessness that are common in caregivers.

Caregiver burden is a significant but understudied problem in relation to patients with pain. Caregivers often experience tremendous anxiety about the pain, sleep disturbance, financial strain, and daily disruption in their own lives as a result of caring for an elderly loved one in pain. Our recent research on pain from the perspective of the family demonstrates the impact of pain on family caregivers and interventions that support caregiver involvement.[9a-c]

Planning pain intervention for the elderly also requires progressing more slowly to introduce one change at a time or to avoid overwhelming the patient or family. The elderly consume multiple medications, and each change in medication must be evaluated with regard to the total medication profile. Drug-food interactions, timing of medications, and drug-drug interactions become important considerations.

Patients and families should be involved in establishing realistic goals for pain treatment. Goals for pain management may be related to desired mobility. For example, a patient goal in a nursing home setting may be to achieve a level of pain control to be able to ambulate to the dining hall for meals.

The process of planning implies patient involvement. This is certainly applicable to pain management, a personal experience that requires active patient involvement. For example, commonly suggested nondrug interventions, such as relaxation or imagery, may be inappropriate techniques for many elderly patients. Our experience[9] suggests that patients prefer such common nondrug interventions as hot baths, cold packs, praying, and simple distraction to relieve pain.

The most important consideration in planning pain interventions is individual consideration. Patients vary greatly in their medication requirements, choices of nondrug interventions, and trajectory of pain. Active involvement of patients and caregivers is essential during the planning phase of the nursing process.

Intervention

This section will explore specific principles of commonly used pharmacological and nonpharmacological pain management strategies as they apply to the elderly.

Few studies have actually evaluated specific pain management strategies for older people. Instead, the efficacy of various pain interventions has largely been extrapolated from studies of younger patients and patients with malignant pain. Although true for younger patients, use of multiple strategies seems particularly pertinent to the elderly. Using a combination of pharmacological and nonpharmacological techniques on an individual basis will result in more effective pain control, less reliance on medications, and fewer side effects in the elderly.

Pain Medications in the Elderly

The National Nursing Home Survey of 1977 (DHHS, 1981) reported that 36.6% of residents overall were receiving analgesic medications. The frequency increased to 48% for those residents with arthritis or rheumatism. In a comparative analysis, the National Hospice study suggested elderly patients required less analgesic medications for terminal cancer pain than did younger patients.[12] This does not mean that older patients experience less pain. Although pain perception is not significantly different in the elderly, these patients do require different approaches to drug management.

Clinical experience suggests that elderly patients are particularly sensitive to the effects of opiate analgesic drugs. Elderly people often respond with unpredictable sensitivity and frequent side effects to many classes of drugs, analgesics included. However, there is no data to suggest that analgesic drugs are any less efficacious in elderly patients. To the contrary, it has been shown that elderly patients experience greater pain relief from opiates than do younger patients.[16] This effect has been shown for postoperative pain as well as chronic cancer pain. It has also been shown that these effects may be related to altered pharmacokinetics and excretion of these drugs in elderly patients.[16] The effects vary widely among individuals, and therefore it is not possible to generalize or predict responses in all elderly patients.

Although opiates are frequently associated with side effects such as sedation or respiratory depression in the elderly, there are few studies that explore the avoidance or management of these undesirable effects. It should be emphasized that these drugs can be used safely in the elderly and that fear of side effects does not justify withholding analgesics and failing to treat pain.

The choice of opioid drugs to use in the elderly requires special consideration. Pentazocine (Talwin) and meperidine (Demerol) have been associated clinically with increased frequency of confusion and psychotic behavior in the elderly. Methadone should always be used cautiously because its extremely long half-life (12 to 48 hours) can lead to accumulation in all patients. It is of special concern in the elderly since they may have reduced metabolism and excretion. In the final analysis, most varieties of morphine and codeine in appropriate doses can be safely used in older patients.

Narcotic drugs do have some potential to become habit forming. Misconceptions continue to be prevalent that narcotics are habit-forming and that medical use of opioids is similar to street use of drugs. Because of cultural and social influences, the geriatric staff and elderly patients may be overly concerned about the possibility of drug addiction. The practitioners and patients should be assured that addiction is not a consideration in the appropriate use of medications for pain (see Chapters 3 and 7).

The common opioid side effect of constipation is a particular concern in elderly patients because many of these individuals have preexisting bowel problems. Careful assessment of bowel patterns and a history of current use of stool softeners and laxatives is important when beginning opioid therapy, as most patients will require some form of bowel management. The potential of opiates for urinary retention and incontinence should also be anticipated.

Nonsteroidal antiinflammatory drugs are known to be quite effective for mild to moderately severe pain in the elderly. These drugs are especially effective in arthritic pain and bone pain caused by malignant metastasis. Aspirin, acetaminophen (Tylenol), ibuprofen (Motrin, Advil, etc.), naproxen (Naprosyn), and fenoprofen (Feldene) are examples of drugs that block pain by inhibiting pain reception at the local (peripheral) level. Unfortunately, they have been associated with a variety of adverse effects in the elderly, including stomach ulcers, kidney insufficiency, and a propensity for bleeding. The analgesic use of these medications is also limited by a ceiling effect. In other words, raising the dose beyond a given point will not result in any additional analgesia. The most common complaint associated with nonsteroidal antiinflammatory drugs is indigestion. Taking the medication with antacid or food may reduce this symptom somewhat; however, severe ulceration may occur in the elderly in the absence of any symptoms, resulting in catastrophic bleeding or perforation of the stomach. Although previously considered the safest form of analgesia, recent studies are beginning to question their overall safety for the frail elderly.[2,23,30a] Acetaminophen has not been associated with renal or gastric problems but is known to result in severe hepatitis when taken in extreme doses.

Adjuvant analgesic drugs are medications without inherent analgesic properties themselves but that have been found to be helpful in treating certain types of chronic pain. These drugs include antidepressants, anticonvulsants, and some sedatives. For example, treatment of underlying depression or mood disorders may enhance other pain management strategies. Anticonvulsants, or drugs usually used to treat seizures, are often helpful in controlling painful neuropathies, such as herpes zoster (shingles), diabetic neuropathies, and phantom limb pain. Mild sedatives or tranquilizers are helpful in reducing anxiety, stress, and tension and allowing the patient to get a good night's sleep. Each of these drugs is fraught with side effects in elderly patients, including increased confusion, constipation, and the blood dyscrasias associated with use of anticonvulsants.

Nondrug pain management

Advances in pain management strategies have strongly supported the combination of drug and nondrug strategies for pain relief. These strategies include physical therapy, transcutaneous electrical nerve stimulation (TENS), biofeedback, hypnosis, and other nonpharmacological therapies. Indeed, clinical experience suggests many of these techniques are quite effective in individual cases.

Transcutaneous electrical nerve stimulation (TENS) has been used successfully in the elderly for a variety of chronic pain conditions. Painful diabetic neuropathies, shoulder pain or bursitis, and fractured ribs have been shown to respond to TENS therapy.[33] TENS therapy consists of a small electrical device with electrodes taped to the skin overlying a nerve. The TENS unit provides an adjustable electrical current to stimulate the underlying nerve. The result of this electrical stimulation is relief of pain. The procedure is virtually harmless, but the degree and duration of pain relief varies. The duration of effectiveness in the elderly remains controversial; however, some patients have obtained pain relief with TENS for years. Successful long-term use is more common with intermittent rather than continuous TENS use. An important issue in the success of TENS therapy is the appropriate placement of the electrodes and adjustment of the electrical current amplitude and pulse pattern. This involves meticulous searching for the settings that produce an individual's optimum comfort. It may take several weeks of continuous TENS before optimum pain control is reached or before one should abandon treatment.[33]

The importance of physical methods, including heat, cold, and massage, in the management of pain in the elderly cannot be overstated.[24] These measures relax tense muscles and are soothing for a variety of complaints. A heating pad or ice pack can be managed by the patient, thus giving the patient and family a sense of control over their symptoms and treatment. However, caution must be taken to avoid thermal burns with elderly patients during prolonged use of either heat or ice. Physical therapy directed at stretching and strengthening specific muscles and joints may also be useful in reducing muscle spasm and improving functional activity. Elderly patients, however, are at risk for injury from overzealous stretching and exercise. Referral to and instructions from a trained physical therapist should be obtained before stretching and exercise for painful conditions in older patients.

The feeling of being in control is an especially important issue for elderly patients in pain. Patients should be involved in pain management strategies and have some responsibility for the strategy's implementation. This applies to both drug and nondrug pain management. This involvement is essential from the assessment phase through the evaluation of strategies that the patient has helped choose. Elderly patients demonstrate a variety of cultural and personality characteristics that may affect the implementation of a pain management strategy. Some patients may exhibit stoic behavior, suggesting a high need for self-control and involvement in their care. On the other hand, many patients prefer high external control of their health care. Patients may resist efforts to increase their involvement and may prefer a dependent position in which responsibility to provide pain relief is delegated to others. These preferences are typically life-long patterns and represent overall health beliefs rather than only pain behaviors. For this reason, elderly patients may need particular attention and individualized care and instruction. The importance of trusting, professional relationships cannot be overemphasized.

A variety of psychological maneuvers may be quite effective in controlling pain (see Chapter 8). Biofeedback, relaxation, and hypnosis may be helpful for some patients. It is important to remember that these methods usually require higher levels of cognitive function and may not be appropriate for patients with significant cognitive impairment. In addition, a trained psychologist or therapist should be consulted for these techniques. Because of preconceived social or cultural attitudes, some elderly patients may be reluctant to try these treatments. However, age or culture alone should not be a barrier to offering the patient a variety of treatment options.

Finally, a variety of distractions may be effective in decreasing the perception of pain. Many patients find comfort in prayer, meditation, or music. Indeed, elderly patients may be more sensitive to comforts through religious pursuit, teachings, or fellowships. Involvement in activities, exercise, and recreation should also be encouraged as much as tolerated, emphasizing that care should be given to avoid overexertion. Inactivity and immobility may contribute greatly to depression and functional decline, and may exacerbate pain experiences.

Evaluation

Evaluation is the final but perhaps most critical step of the nursing process. Evaluation of the effects of an intervention should be based on comprehensive reassessment of pain. For elderly patients, frequent and systematic evaluation is even more critical because the clinician is repeatedly required to alter medications to accommodate the complex illnesses of the older patient, interactions, and variable side effects.

There are a few other concerns in pain management in older patients. Financial considerations are particularly worrisome in this population, and third-party reimbursement organizations, such as Medicare, have restricted payment schedules. Interventions should be carefully evaluated for cost and benefits to the patient.

As with all patients, a conservative approach to technology is advised. It is important to remember that the vast majority of patients can be effectively treated with oral analgesics. Oral medications are much preferred over any parenteral form of analgesia from the perspectives of cost, comfort, complications, and caregiver burden. Elderly persons can benefit greatly from attempts to maintain pain control with oral analgesia if possible.

◆ CONCLUSION

Pain is a distressing problem at any age. Principal goals of care for all elderly people are the provision of comfort and control of pain. The older patient offers many challenges to the clinician and researcher, yet successful management of pain can greatly improve overall quality of life and function.

REFERENCES

1. Bonica J. (1977). Basic principles in the management of chronic pain. *Arch Surg* 112:783-787.
2. Butt JH, Barthel JS, and Moore RA. (1988). Clinical spectrum of the upper gastrointestinal effects of nonsteroidal antiinflammatory drugs: natural history, symptomatology and significance. *Am J Med* 84 (2A) 5-14.
3. Cook J, Rideout E, and Browne G. (1984). The prevalence of pain complaints in a general population. *Pain* 2:49-53.
4. Ferrell BR, Wisdom C, and Wenzl C. (1989). Quality of life as an outcome variable in management of cancer pain. *Cancer* 63(11):2321-2327.
5. Ferrell BR, Wisdom C, Wenzl C, and Brown M. (1989). Effects of controlled release morphine on quality of life for patients with cancer pain. *Oncol Nurs Forum* 16(4):521-552.
6. Ferrell BA and Ferrell BR. (1989). Assessment of chronic pain in the elderly. *Geriatr Med Today* 8(5):123-134.
7. Ferrell BA and Ferrell BR. (1988). The experience of pain and quality of life in elderly cancer patients. (Abstract) *Gerontologist* 28:76.
8. Ferrell BA, Ferrell BR, and Osterweil D. (1990). Pain in the nursing home. *J Am Geriatr Soc* 38(4):9-14.
9. Ferrell BR and Schneider C. (1988). Experience and management of cancer at home. *Cancer Nurs* 11(2):84-90.

9a. Ferrell BR, Rhiner M, Cohen M, and Grant M. (1991). Pain as a metaphor for illness. Part I: Impact of cancer pain on family caregivers. *Oncol Nurs Forum* Vol 18:8.

9b. Ferrell BR, Cohen M, Rhiner M, and Rozak A. (1991). Pain as a metaphor for illness. Part II: Family caregivers' management of pain. *Oncol Nurs Forum* Vol 18:8.

9c. Ferrell BR, Ferrell BA, Rhiner M, and Grant M. (1991). Family factors influencing cancer pain. *Postgrad Med J* 67(2):S64-S69.

10. Foley KM. (1985). The treatment of cancer pain. *N Engl J Med* 113:84-95.
11. Fordyce WE. (1978). Evaluating and managing chronic pain. *Geriatrics* 33:59.
12. Goldberg RJ, Mor V, Wiemann M, Greer DS, and Hiris J. (1986). Analgesic use in terminal cancer patients: a report from the national hospice study. *J Chron Dis* 39(1):37-45.
13. Harkins SW and Chapman CR. (1977). The perception of induced dental pain in young and elderly women. *J Gerontol* 32:428-435.
14. Harkins SW, Kwentus J, and Price DD. (1984). Pain in the elderly. In: Benedetti C (ed), *Advances in pain research and therapy vol. 7.* New York: Raven Press.
15. Hester NO and Barcus C. (1986). Assessment and management of pain in children. *Pediatr Nurs Update* 1:2-7.
16. Kaiko RF, Wallenstein SL, Rogers AG, Gabinski PY, and Houde RW. (1982). Narcotics in the elderly. *Med Clin North Am* 66(5):1079-1989.
17. Kane RA, Ouslander JG, and Abrass IB. (1988). *Essentials of clinical geriatrics,* ed 2. New York: McGraw-Hill.
18. Kroening RJ. (1985). Pain clinics structure and function. *Semin Anesthesiol* 4:231-23.
19. Lamy PP. (1984). Pain management, drugs and the elderly. *Am Health Care J* 10:32-33.
20. Levasky-Shulan M et al. (1985). Prevalence and functional correlates of low back pain in the elderly. *J Am Geriatr Soc* 33(1):23-28.
21. Loesser JD, Black RG, and Christman A. (1975). Relief of pain by transcutaneous nerve stimulation. *J Neurosurg* 42:308-314.
22. MacDonald JB. (1984). Presentation of acute myocardial infarction in the elderly. *Age Ageing* 13:196-200.
23. Maniglia R, Schwartz AB, Moriber-Katz S. (1988). Non steroidal antiinflammatory nephrotoxicity. *Ann Clin Lab Sci* 18(3):240-252.
24. McCaffery M and Beebe A. (1989). *Pain: clinical manual for nursing practice.* St. Louis: CV Mosby.
25. Morris JN, Mor V, Goldberg RJ, et al. (1987). The effect of treatment setting and patient characteristics on terminal cancer patients: report from the national hospice study. *J Chron Dis* 39(1):27-37.
26. National Institutes of Health, Consensus Development Conference Statement: The integrated approach to the management of pain. US Government Printing Office: 1986-491-292:41148.
27. National Nursing Home Survey of 1977: Characteristics of nursing home residents' health status and care received, *National Health Survey Series* 13 #51, DHHS Publication #(PHS)81-1712, April, 1981.
28. Newton PA. (1984). Chronic pain. In: Cassel and Walsh J (eds), *Geriatric medicine,* 1984. New York: Springer-Verlag.
29. Oliver N. (1981). Abdominal pain in the elderly. *Aust Fam Phys* 13(6):402-404.
30. Portenoy RK and Farkash A. (1988). Practical management of non-malignant pain. *Geriatrics* 42(12):75-87.
30a. Roth SH. (1989). Merits and liabilities of NSAIDs therapy. *Rheum Dis Clin North Am* 15(3):479-498.
31. Sternbach RA. (1986). Survey of pain in the United States: the Nuprin pain report. *Clin Pain* 2:4.
32. Stromborg M. (1988). *Instruments for clinical nursing research.* Norwalk, Conn: Appleton and Lange.

33. Thorsteinsson G. (1987). Chronic pain: Use of TENS in the elderly. *Geriatrics* 43(5):29-47.
34. Tucker MA, Andrew MF, Ogle SJ, and Davison JG. (1989). Age-associated change in pain threshold measured by neuronal electrical stimulation. *Age Aging* 18:241-246.
35. Wong D and Baker C. (1988). Pain in children. *Pediatr Nurs* 14(1):9.
36. Wong D and Whaley L. (1986). *Clinical handbook of pediatric nursing,* ed 2. St. Louis: CV Mosby.
37. Woodrow KM, Friedman GD, Seigelaub AB, and Collen MF. (1972). Pain tolerance: differences according to age, sex, and race. *Psychosom Med* 34:548-556.
38. Yoshikawa TT and Norman DC. (1987). *Aging and clinical practice: infectious diseases in the elderly.* New York: Igaku-Shoin.

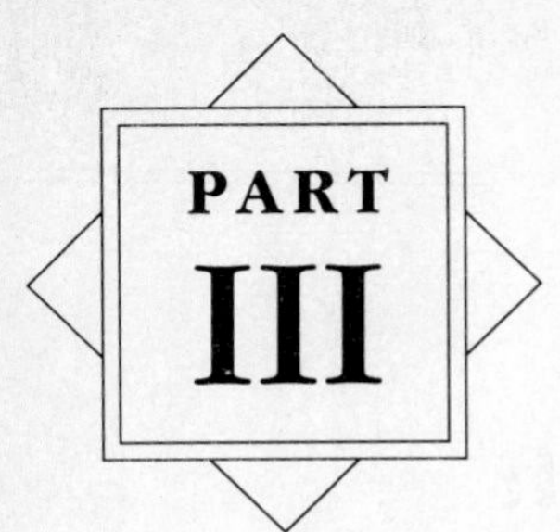

PART III

PAIN ISSUES FOR SELECTED PATIENTS

14

Patients with Cancer Pain

Judith A. Spross
Marybeth Singer

◆ INTRODUCTION

Patients with pain caused by cancer or its therapy are often underassessed and undertreated.[4,12a,27a] Unrelieved cancer pain is both a social and a clinical problem. Studies have shown that 25% of patients experience chronic pain as a result of antineoplastic therapy.[17,33] In advanced disease, there can be multiple sources of pain[40] with accompanying symptoms of nausea, constipation, and insomnia that can further compromise patient comfort. The purposes of this chapter are to describe the social and epidemiological aspects of cancer pain, to identify issues specific to the problem of cancer pain, and to describe selected cancer pain syndromes and therapeutic approaches.

◆ BACKGROUND

Misconceptions and Obstacles Hampering Pain Assessment and Management in Persons with Cancer

Barriers to cancer pain management have been conceptualized into three areas: those that arise from beliefs and attitudes held by persons with cancer and their families; those that arise from beliefs and attitudes of health professionals; and those that result from organizational, regulatory, and legislative processes.[11a] These barriers are listed in the accompanying box. A knowledge of these barriers is essential, and their

◆ BARRIERS TO EFFECTIVE MANAGEMENT OF CANCER PAIN

HEALTH PROFESSIONALS

- Lack of understanding of the pathophysiology of cancer pain
- Lack of knowledge of the clinical pharmacology of narcotic analgesics
- Lack of knowledge of new methods of pain relief, including the use of adjuvant drugs and neurosurgical procedures
- Insufficient professional education in cancer pain therapy
- Lack of knowledge of the difference between physical dependence and addiction
- Excessive concern about development of tolerance to narcotic analgesics
- Excessive concern about addicting patients to narcotic analgesics
- Excessive concern about the side effects of narcotic analgesics
- The belief that cancer pain should be moderate to severe before patients receive medication
- The belief that patients are not good judges of the severity of their pain
- Assignment of low priority to pain management
- Lack of thorough and frequent reevaluation of patients' pain status
- The difficult and frustrating nature of certain pain management problems

PATIENTS AND FAMILY MEMBERS

- Lack of awareness that cancer pain can be managed, with the result that patients may suffer in silence
- Fear that use of narcotic analgesics will lead to addiction
- Fear that use of narcotic analgesics will lead to mental confusion, disorientation, personality change
- Failure to report pain because of the desire to be a "good patient" and not distract the physician from the primary task of treating the disease
- Underreporting of pain because increasing pain suggests the disease is progressing

Reprinted with permission from: Dahl JL, Joranson DE, Engber D, and Dosch J. (1988). The cancer pain problem: Wisconsin's response. *J Pain Symp Manag 3*(1):S2-S8. (p. 53). (Elsevier Science Publishing Co., New York).

Continued.

◆ BARRIERS TO EFFECTIVE MANAGEMENT OF CANCER PAIN—cont'd

THE HEALTH CARE SYSTEM

- Lack of accountability for pain management because hospitals operate on an acute, disease-oriented model
- Lack of coordination of care as patients are moved from one setting to another, e.g., from hospital to nursing home
- Fragmentation of care because treatment of cancer has become highly specialized. It is not uncommon for a patient to consult with three to 15 different specialists. These consultations result in multiple sources of information and opinions for patients and families.
- Unwillingness of pharmacies in large cities to stock narcotics because of the risk of theft. In less urban areas, resources for relief of pain of neurosurgical and neurolytic procedures are not available.

effect on individual pain problems and pain problems in groups of cancer patients must be assessed. A thorough clinical assessment and well-designed care plan can be undermined by social or organizational barriers, such as a lack of collegial support in implementing the care plan or the unavailability of a drug in the community pharmacy.

In addition to barriers listed here and in Chapter 3, health professionals often express unfounded fears that opiate administration for cancer pain is synonymous with euthanasia.[18] Large doses of narcotics are rarely given to opioid-naive cancer patients. However, few cancer patients reporting pain are opioid-naive. Doses may be escalated rapidly in persons experiencing cancer-related pain. Clinical judgment of patients' responses relies primarily on effects of medications on pain. Prolonged sleep may occur. This is often a reflection of the body's attempt to catch up on sleep lost over a period of weeks or months while the person was in pain.

Staff members often worry that if death occurs after the administration of an opiate, and the death resulted from the drug, they will be held accountable. They should be reassured that, in persons with advanced disease who have been on opiates, the cancer process is the likely cause of death and that a death that occurs near the time of opiate administration is likely coincidental. Patients may need large doses of opiates to control pain. The authors have cared for many patients who have required about 1,500 mg of long-acting oral morphine sulfate (MS) daily or 1,000 to 2,000 mg of IV MS in 24 hours. Doses may be higher (one report cites 10,000 mg IV in 24 hours). The second author cared for a patient who received 7,000 mcg of Fentanyl/hour—the equivalent of 16,800 mg MSO_4 in 24 hours. These are not common doses, but they do illustrate the importance of titrating opiates to provide relief and the fact that when such titration is done, large doses can be administered safely. "Treatment of pain is never a form of euthanasia" (Foley,[19] p. 2258). The goal is always the management of symptoms. The issue is further discussed in this chapter under Clinical Judgment and in Chapter 6.

Standards of Care for Cancer Pain

It is important for nurses to be aware of available standards and guidelines for cancer pain management. Standards and guidelines can be useful in establishing goals for individual patients and groups of patients; in establishing organizational goals related to cancer pain; in developing policies and procedures on cancer pain assessment and management; and in developing clinical and quality improvement programs to improve the management of cancer pain. Table 14-1 presents organizations and a description of resources related to standards and appropriate references. Readers are encouraged to use these resources to establish cancer pain as a clinical and organizational priority. Establishing quality improvement programs, a mandated activity for most health agencies, is an appropriate way to evaluate and monitor the assessment and management of cancer pain. An example of standards related to pain and instruments to document the implementation of the standard is included in Appendix A.

In addition to these standards, alliances of consumers and professionals are improving cancer pain relief efforts by establishing statewide Cancer Pain Initiatives (CPIs). The first CPI was established in Wisconsin as a demonstration project of the World Health Organization.[11a] The purpose of such initiatives is to mobilize health professionals and the public to make treatment of cancer pain a priority by educating professionals and the public, eliminating legislative and regulatory barriers, and promoting provider-patient communication through effective use of advocates and media.

◆ **Table 14-1**
Existing standards/guidelines and other information

Organization	Information available	Reference
Oncology Nursing Society 501 Holiday Drive Pittsburgh, PA 15220 (412) 921-7373	1. Process and outcome standards that include comfort and coping	
	2. *Position paper on cancer pain* (a comprehensive treatise on problems of cancer pain and its assessment and management) (this is also available as a monograph for $6.00)	Spross J, McGuire D, and Schmitt R (1990). Oncology Nursing Society: position paper on cancer pain assessment and management. *Oncol Nurse Forum* Part I, Vol, 17, No. 4; Part II, Vol. 17, No. 5; Part III, Vol. 17, No. 6.
American Pain Society P.O. Box 186 Skokie, IL 60076-0816	1. Guidelines for use of analgesics and adjuvant medications in cancer pain 2. Standards for postoperative and cancer patients (draft)	American Pain Society: *Principles of analgesic use in the treatment of acute pain and chronic cancer pain* (ed 2). Skokie, Ill: APS, 1989.
Association of Community Cancer Centers 11600 Nebel St., Suite 201 Rockville, MD 20852	1. Standards for community cancer centers that identify the need for policies, procedures, and rehabilitation services regarding pain and articulate the nurse's role in pain management	Enck RE (1987). ACCC standards: past, present, and future. *J Cancer Prog Manag* 2(1):11-21.
National Health and Medical Research Council P.O. Box 100 Woden, ACT (Australia) 2606	1. Overview of approaches to acute and chronic pain problems; professional and public education information	National Health and Medical Council. *Management of Severe Pain*, Canberra, Australia: Australia Government Publishing Service, 1989.

Health and Welfare Canada Room 21-B/HPB Bldg Ottawa, Ontario, Canada, K1A, 0L2	1. A monograph on the management of cancer pain
National Hospice Organization Suite 307 1901 N. Fort Mayer Drive Arlington, VA 22209 (703) 243-5900	1. Standards on symptom control
Wisconsin Cancer Pain Initiative University of Wisconsin 3675 Medical Sciences Center 1300 University Avenue Madison, WI 53706 (608) 262-0978	1. *Cancer Pain Can Be Relieved* (booklets for adults, teens, and children) 2. Handbook on analgesic medications 3. Information on statewide CPI

Nurses, physicians, and others need to collaborate to initiate, develop, and adopt interdisciplinary standards and protocols to promote effective assessment and treatment of cancer pain. For example, establishing institutional protocols and standing orders for dose escalation of opiates and management of constipation that can be activated by nurses may assist in achieving the goal of effective pain management. Accountability for pain management can be established through job descriptions and in team conferences (for individual patients).

Epidemiology

It has been estimated that 50% of all patients with cancer and over 70% of patients with advanced disease experience pain. Using these statistics, Portenoy estimates that in 1983, 247,000 Americans terminally ill with cancer suffered from pain and over one million cancer survivors experienced pain.[33] It was estimated that in 1984, 19 million people worldwide experienced pain caused by cancer. Clinical studies provide documentation that cancer pain is often undertreated. Leaders in the field of cancer pain maintain that most patients experiencing pain caused by cancer should be able to obtain better relief.[45]

Prevalence of cancer pain can be correlated with disease stage, disease extent, and cancer type. Patients in earlier stages of cancer have less pain than those with advanced disease. Patients with larger, more extensive tumors have more pain than those whose cancers are smaller and more confined. Cancers of the breast, lung, prostate, and pancreas are more often associated with pain than leukemia or lymphoma. The most common cause of pain in cancer patients is bone pain. At least one study documented that patients with advanced disease have more than one pain.[39]

◆ CAUSES OF PAIN IN CANCER

Causes of pain in cancer can be classified according to syndrome and duration. An understanding of the many possible etiologies of pain in patients with cancer is essential to directing evaluation and treatment. Pain may be associated with direct involvement of tissue by tumor. Bones, nerves, viscera, blood vessels, and mucous membranes are susceptible to invasion and/or compression by tumor. Cancer therapy may cause acute or chronic pain. In addition to acute, postoperative pain, surgery may produce chronic pain syndromes resulting from injury to nerves or other tissues. Patients may experience pains that are indirectly related or unrelated to cancer. These pains include preexisting pain problems (e.g., low back pain) and pain or discomfort that arises from symptom management, such as opiate-induced constipation. Table 14-2 identifies common examples of acute and chronic cancer pain.

Selected Cancer Pain Problems

Mucositis, bone pain, and deafferentation pain will be examined in detail as illustrations of types of cancer pain.

◆ **Table 14-2**
Causes of pain in cancer

	Examples	
Duration	**Acute**	**Chronic**
Syndrome associated with direct tumor involvement progression	Pathological fracture Bowel obstruction Superior vena cava syndrome	Bone pain caused by metastases or primary tumor Pancreatic cancer Nerve plexopathies
Syndrome associated with cancer diagnosis	Bone marrow biopsy	
Syndrome associated with cancer therapy	Stomatitis/mucositis Postoperative pain	Postmastectomy syndrome Postamputation syndrome Phantom sensations Postradiation neuropathies
Pain indirectly related or unrelated to cancer	Herpes zoster Headache	Postherpetic neuralgia Constipation Migraine Osteoarthritis Diabetic neuropathy

Acute Cancer-Related Pain: Mucositis

Radiation therapy and chemotherapy can cause cutaneous and mucosal irritation and ulceration. Chemotherapy-induced mucositis will be described as a model for acute cancer-related pain.

Populations at risk. Oral mucositis occurs in more than 40% of all patients receiving chemotherapy.[7] Chemotherapeutic agents that commonly cause mucositis include: doxorubicin, daunorubicin, cyclophosphamide (Cytoxan), Ifosphamide, cytarabine, methotrexate, 5-fluorouracil, procarbazine, lomustine, hydroxyurea, 6-thioguanine, 6-mercaptopurine, dacarbazine, and mitomycin-C. Many of these drugs are used together in certain drug regimens, compounding the risk of mucositis. Mucositis can occur along the entire gastrointestinal tract, resulting in ulceration and tissue sloughing following cellular destruction. Populations at risk include:

1. Patients receiving chemotherapeutic agents known to cause mucositis
2. Patients receiving radiotherapy directed at a field that includes part of the gastrointestinal tract
3. All bone marrow transplant patients.

Pain mechanism. The mechanism for injury from chemotherapy or radiotherapy results from the direct effect of the therapy on rapidly dividing cells in the gastrointestinal tract. As these cells break down, they release chemical mediators of pain—histamine, bradykinin, and potassium. Secondary infection or hemorrhage caused by myelosuppression can delay healing and increase discomfort.

Damage to the mucosa results in noxious stimulation of sensory receptors. These sensory receptors are most prevalent in skin, mucosa, muscle, connective tissue, and thoracic and abdominal viscera.[32] From the site of this peripheral damage, myelinated and unmyelinated fibers carry pain messages to the spinal cord. Myelinated receptors respond to noxious mechanical stimuli, causing sharp, stinging pain. Unmyelinated, polymodal nociceptors respond to mechanical, thermal, and chemical noxious stimuli and are associated with dull, burning, aching pain.[32] These receptors can also be sensitized by chemical mediators released as a result of tissue injury (e.g., bradykinins, prostaglandin, potassium). Noxious impulses caused by tissue injury are conducted to the central nervous system via the spinal cord, where they enter via the dorsal root and synapse into the dorsal horn, thereby activating the ascending nociceptive system.[32] Pain caused by mucositis is probably mediated by a variety of nociceptive inputs (chemical input resulting from mucosal injury; mechanical input such as chewing; and thermal input such as food temperature).

The descending analgesic pathway may be activated by many physiological, psychological, and pathological stimuli. In the case of pain associated with chemotherapy or radiation-induced mucositis, patients may view the pain as part of the price paid for a chance at cure. This may account for an individual's ability to endure significant pain caused by oral mucositis.

Characteristics. Characteristics of mucositis pain vary with site(s) of pain and with the degree of mucosal injury. Oral mucositis is common, although mucositis can occur anywhere along the gastrointestinal tract. Early baseline assessment and continuing assessment of changes are necessary to identify appropriate interventions. Characteristics of mucositis pain include:

- Sensitivity to hot and cold
- Pain on swallowing
- Stinging pain at sites of ulceration, fissures
- Pulling, burning
- Localization of pain to affected area (e.g., mouth, rectum)
- Inability to swallow saliva because of generalized, severe oropharyngeal pain
- Pain on talking
- Severity of mucositis pain often associated with degree of myelosuppression
- Resolution/healing occurring with bone marrow recovery[11]
- Loss of gag reflex possibly occurring in cases of severe mucositis

Therapeutic approaches. Medical and nursing approaches focus on supporting the patient through mucositis by effective use of systemic and local analgesics and prevention and management of secondary complications. Symptomatic treatment includes the appropriate use of narcotic, nonnarcotic, and topical anesthetics and analgesics. In cases where swallowing is moderately to severely painful, parenteral narcotics are the treatment of choice. For patients on patient-controlled analgesia (PCA) or intravenous continuous infusions (IVCI) opiates, if pain occurs before meals, a bolus dose

15 minutes before meals is recommended. One should be sure to assess effectiveness. For patients who are unable to swallow, continuous intravenous morphine infusions have been used with good effect. This can be accomplished via a PCA delivery system or rate-calibrated delivery system. In many bone marrow transplant units, PCA is used. As symptoms improve, analgesics can be converted to oral doses and gradually reduced. Oral analgesics may be used if the patient can swallow. Topical application of dyclone, viscous xylocaine, or mixtures of 1:1:1 Kaopectate, Benadryl, and viscous xylocaine may be helpful. The accompanying box lists available topical agents.

Nursing interventions include vigilant assessment of the

◆ TOPICAL ANALGESICS FOR ORAL MUCOSITIS

VISCOUS XYLOCAINE (2%)

Can be applied directly to ulcerations with cotton tip applicator

Can be swished and swallowed diluted or undiluted (can diminish gag reflex)

Can be used in equal parts with benadryl elixir and Kaopectate or Maalox

Author uses Benadryl:Kaopectate:xylocaine

Any of these applications can be used 10-15 min before meals

CETACAINE SPRAY (0.1%)

Spray buccal mucosa or pharynx to relieve pain. Diminished gag reflex can result.

May be contraindicated in presence of clots (pressure of spray can dislodge clots and cause bleeding).

DYCLONE (0.5%)

Can be swabbed on lesions or gargled for pharyngeal pain. Swallowing, gargling may diminish gag reflex.

Note: Many of the topical agents are difficult for BMT patients to use because a lack of saliva and degree of ulceration causes more discomfort. Artificial saliva, frequent saline rinses, and systemic (parenteral) analgesics are most beneficial.

McDermott B (1982). Standards of clinical nursing practice: the side effects of chemotherapy in the treatment of leukemia, *Cancer Nurs 5*, (4):317-323.

oral mucosa and of pain. The nurse should collaborate with other providers and coordinate plans to manage pain associated with mucositis. Early detection of infection and bleeding can be accomplished through continuous assessment. Nurses play a pivotal role in evaluating the effectiveness of analgesic regimes and recommending changes. Patient teaching is an integral part of managing mucositis pain, with special emphasis on hygiene measures, narcotic and topical analgesics, and anticipated side effects. Focusing on the time-limited course of injury and healing can assist the patient in coping. Management of nausea and vomiting, particularly with bone marrow transplant (BMT) patients, can further increase comfort by decreasing mechanical and chemical irritation to damaged mucosa. If the patient is able to swallow, medicating with analgesics before meals can improve oral intake. Topical anesthetics should be used 15 minutes before meals; oral systemic analgesics should be taken 1 hour before meals.

Chronic Cancer-Related Pain: Bone Pain

The causes of chronic pain syndromes in cancer are most commonly related to direct tumor invasion of bone and neural structures.[33] Bone pain, secondary to metastatic lesions or primary disease, is the most common cause of pain in cancer patients.[20]

Populations at risk. Foley[20] found that 65% of patients with primary bone tumors, 52% of patients with breast cancer, and 45% of patients with lung cancer had significant pain. These findings were determined by evaluating analgesic use, and certainly imply the need for further epidemiological study. The populations at risk for developing pain secondary to bony metastasis include patients with:

1. Primary bone tumors (e.g., osteogenic sarcoma)
2. Breast carcinomas
3. Lung carcinomas
4. Prostate carcinomas
5. Renal cell carcinomas
6. Multiple myeloma

Pain mechanism. The mechanisms of injury that occur with bone pain result from the destruction of bone and new bone formation. As the tumor grows, it stretches the periosteum, causing pain. The periosteum is rich in both myelinated and unmyelinated afferent fibers. Prostaglandins are necessary for both osteoclastic and osteolytic bone changes and are known to sensitize nociceptors to noxious stimuli. This provides a physiological explanation of the efficacy of prostaglandin inhibitors in relieving bony pain.[32] Osteoclast activating factor chemically stimulates nociceptors.[32]

Once nociception has occurred, the pathway to the central nervous system is the same as that described with transmission of pain impulses related to mucositis. Both types of pain represent nociceptive or somatic pain.

Characteristics. The characteristics of bone pain are related to the specific physiology and site of metastasis. Bone pain is often described as a dull ache that increases in intensity over the course of the day. The pain may be fleeting or constant.[6] The pain is well localized; however, if multiple sites are involved, the pain may be described as aching all over. The quality of bone pain is described as constant and aching or gnawing in nature.[32] Because of the risk of pathological fracture, particularly in weight-bearing bones, care must be taken in avoiding torsion or excessive pressure. Pathological fractures have occurred in patients with bone lesions who have held stair railings tightly, landed on a toilet seat or commode "too hard," brushed their hair, or been transferred from bed to stretcher. New onset of severe, sharp pain can indicate fracture.

When back pain is present from vertebral body metastasis, nurses must be alert to signs and symptoms of epidural spinal cord compression. Back pain is the presenting symptom for 90% of patients with epidural spinal cord compression.[35] This is a cancer emergency. Back pain from spinal cord compression is often exacerbated by lying down and may be at least partially relieved by standing or sitting. Sensory changes, such as burning or tingling in dermatomal distribution, may also be early warning signs. Motor signs, such as leg weakness, loss of bowel and bladder control, and paralysis, are late findings and are often irreversible. Early recognition of impending spinal cord compression and emergent treatment may avert devastating neurological sequelae such as irreversible paralysis.[35]

Therapeutic approaches. Effective management of bone pain requires collaboration among several disciplines: radiation therapy, medical oncology, nursing, and physical therapy. Collaborative interventions address three purposes:

1. Antitumor therapy to address the cause of pain

2. Symptomatic control of pain
3. Prevention and early detection of complications

Antitumor therapy to control the course of bone pain includes hormonal therapy, chemotherapy, and radiotherapy. Hormonally responsive tumors, such as those caused by primary breast and prostate carcinomas, can be successfully palliated by ablative hormonal therapy. Ablation can be accomplished with medications, surgery, or radiation therapy. In breast cancer, tamoxifen is the most extensively used agent.[37] Patients with bone pain who begin tamoxifen therapy should be assessed for flare in bone pain. Anticipating this potential side effect can assure that patients have analgesics on hand at home. The author knows of one case in which the severity of tamoxifen flare required hospitalization for pain control. Aminoglutethamide is a drug used to suppress adrenal function.

In prostatic carcinomas, primary androgen ablation to palliate bone pain is accomplished chemically by flutamide and leuprolide. In treating prostatic carcinoma, hormonal therapy or surgical castration is standard therapy for bony metastasis. Leuprolide and flutamide offer advantages over diethylstilbestrol (DES) because of their less serious side effects. Prednisone[38] and etidronate[30] have been reported to provide some pain relief for patients refractory to hormonal therapy. Depending on the tumor, surgical ablation of hormone production can be achieved by oophorectomy, orchiectomy, or hypophysectomy.

Surgical intervention for stabilization of weight-bearing bones plays an important role in the management of bone metastasis. Surgical stabilization is usually followed by radiation therapy, again reducing pain and improving functional mobility.[37] Such stabilization is often done prophylactically.

Localized radiation therapy to painful bony lesions has produced partial or complete responses in 73% to 96% of patients.[24] It is important to mention that some patients experience a worsening of bone pain during initial treatment, because of inflammation. This will get better, and improved relief may be expected within 3 to 10 days of initiation of therapy. Pain relief from osseous metastasis after radiation therapy can last anywhere from 3 months to 12 months or more, depending on tumor type and extent of disease.[31,37] Increased mobility and decreased need for analgesic medication often occurs after successful treatment.[31]

Physical therapists can provide strategies for safe mobility and pain reduction to patients with bone metastasis. Ambulation assistance devices, such as walkers, canes, and braces, are often useful. In some institutions the physical therapist is responsible for application of transcutaneous electrical nerve stimulators (TENs) for pain management (see Chapter 8).

Pharmacological strategies for managing bone pain related to cancer are used concomitantly with antitumor therapies. Kantor[23] estimates that up to 50% of all cancer pain could be controlled using nonsteroidal antiinflammatory drugs (NSAIDs) alone. Ventafridda[42] and Kantor[23] have found tumor growth and calcium levels to decrease with the use of NSAIDs. A recent study evaluated the effect of two different doses of naproxen sodium on bone pain resulting from metastasis from breast cancer. They concluded that both 550 mg tid and 275 mg tid provided relief in approximately 80% of subjects. However, the amount of relief was significantly higher with the higher dose. There were no differences between groups in the number of gastrointestinal complaints.[25] For additional information regarding the WHO analgesic ladder and nonopiate and opiate analgesics, the reader is referred to Chapters 7 and 12.

The combination of a nonnarcotic or nonsteroidal antiinflammatory drug with an opiate significantly improves analgesia. Effective therapy for patients with bone metastases involves finding an individual approach that combines effective antitumor therapy and appropriate analgesics. For instance, patients with leukemias often present with bone pain and arthralgias as a result of leukemic infiltration. This pain resolves rapidly with chemotherapy. However, when the pain results from endstage disease, treatment with analgesics is generally required for the remainder of the patient's life and incorporates the principles outlined in the WHO analgesic ladder (Chapter 7). In both situations, pain is continually assessed and pain relief measures evaluated to ensure optimal analgesia and quality of life.

Deafferentation Pain: Postmastectomy Pain Syndrome

Populations at risk. Postmastectomy pain syndrome (PMPS) has been reported to occur as a result of surgical interruption of the intercostal brachial nerve, in some cases resulting in neuroma formation.[22] Postmastectomy pain syndrome can occur in patients with breast cancer who have had a range of surgical interventions from lumpectomy with lymph node dissection to radical mastectomy. Axillary lymph node dissection has been identified as a probable cause, and it was recently suggested that the syndrome be changed to post–axillary dissection pain.[41] The incidence of the syndrome in breast cancer patients has been reported to range from 4%[22] to 14%.[44] Patients at highest risk for developing PMPS syndrome are those with postoperative complications, such as infection, which can cause fibrosis of nerves. It is important to note that breast reconstruction does not alter the postmastectomy pain syndrome.[22] Other cancer populations at risk for deafferentation pain include those with limb amputations (phantom limb pain); colon resections (phantom anal pain); other surgeries in which nerves are resected or damaged; and postherpetic neuralgia.

Pain mechanism. The pain associated with PMPS results from direct injury to the intercostal brachial nerve during surgical treatment for breast cancer. Pain caused by deafferentation often is severe and described as a constant dull ache, with or without superimposed paroxysms of burning or shock-like pain.[32] Disruption of nerves can cause abnormal spontaneous firing, resulting in epileptiform activity, accounting for the paroxysmal nature of this type of pain. Myelinated and unmyelinated nociceptors play a role in deafferentation pain. Chemical mediators of pain (kinins, prostaglandins) may sensitize nociceptors after injury and may provide an explanation for the development of chronic neuropathic pain. Reflex sympathetic dystrophy (RSD) can develop as a result of PMPS and the decreased mobility of the affected arm and shoulder.

Characteristics. PMPS pain is characterized by constricting, tight, burning pain in the axilla and posterior arm on the operative side. The pain can radiate across the anterior chest. Hyperpathia is often present and can lead to development of frozen shoulder.[22,37] PMPS pain can occur during the immediate postoperative phase or as late as 6 months postoperatively. Patients describe not being able to tolerate being touched on the affected area and report that getting dressed takes longer, both because of pain of movement and the increasing pain experienced when clothing touches the affected area.

Therapeutic approaches. Since local and regional nodal metastasis may account for pain in patients at risk for PMPS, it is advisable to rule out local tumor recurrence in this disease.

Clinical data suggest that it may be possible to prevent postoperative pain by providing preoperative analgesia.[43] In addition, intraoperative and postoperative prevention of sensitization of the neurons through regional and local anesthetics intraoperatively, and good postoperative pain control are thought to be important in preventing PMPS. Effective use of analgesics preoperatively and postoperatively, and postoperative physical therapy can play a role in preventing the syndrome. Treatment of PMPS involves the use of adjuvant analgesics. Deafferentation pain syndromes are generally unresponsive to opiates. However, in the clinical experience of the authors, a low dose of an opiate may contribute to overall pain management, but dose escalations do not increase the amount of relief. Amitriptyline, a tricyclic antidepressant, may be used for the burning component of pain. For patients who are having concomitant sleep disturbances, it will improve sleep.[19,37] Baclofen may provide additional analgesic effect in refractory pain.[37] Anticonvulsant drugs are indicated for paroxysmal pain, although controlled studies on this population have not been done. A recent report on the topical application of capsaicin in postmastectomy patients showed significant promise, and this treatment needs to be further evaluated with a larger population.[44] Since deafferentation pain can be very difficult to treat with available therapies, the positive effects of capsaicin are a helpful advance in efforts to improve pain relief for this population. Sympathetic blockade or oral sympatholytic therapy (phenoxybenzamine) may provide relief, particularly when used early in the pain experience[37] (see also Chapter 7). If RSD occurs, sympathetic blocks and physical therapy may relieve pain and improve function.[5,37]

Physical therapy to maximize mobility and prevent frozen shoulder should be instituted early. Appropriate analgesia enhances the patient's ability to comply with plans to increase the mobility of the affected shoulder and arm. One patient found the use of a support sleeve helpful in reducing PMPS pain.

Nursing approaches involve identifying patients at risk and coordinating early intervention. In the early postoperative phase, around-the-clock analgesia improves comfort and compliance with exercises and may be essential to the prevention of chronic pain. Teaching about pain and its management as well as adjuvant pain control strategies improves the patient's sense of control. Believing the complaints of pain and treating the associated symptoms are crucial. Watson[44] reports that many of the patients referred for capsaicin therapy had been diagnosed as having "emotionally derived pain" after mastectomy although there was a direct physical cause of pain.

Overview of Pharmacological Considerations Specific to Patients with Cancer

The previous chapter on pharmacology includes the WHO analgesic ladder, which provides a basic approach to analgesic therapies in cancer pain management (see Chapter 7). Nonopioid analgesics, especially aspirin, NSAID analgesics, and acetaminophen, are important first-line analgesics for managing mild to moderate pain in persons with cancer. If a sufficient trial of these drugs in adequate doses and at regular intervals is ineffective, one selects analgesics from the next "rung" of the ladder. It is important to note that for severe pain it is necessary to select strong opiates immediately, rather than progress through each rung of the ladder in sequence. Cancer pain can be effectively managed for the majority of patients if the right drug(s) are taken in the right doses at the right times. Patients with chronic cancer pain should have an around-the-clock pain regimen with rescue or breakthrough doses available as needed between regularly scheduled doses. If the gut works, the oral route should be used. If the oral route is unavailable then sublingual, rectal, and parenteral routes may be used. The choice of route should be based on individual patient concerns, i.e., ease of use, indications, clinical condition, cost, and supportive home care (support services).

Nonopiates and NSAIDs

In cancer patients, adding an NSAID or acetaminophen to an opiate regimen can increase analgesia without increasing sedation. Adequate hepatorenal function is necessary. The concern for fever suppression and bleeding for patients undergoing active myelosuppressive therapy will affect drug choices. Knowledgeable nurses can offer counsel in decision-making.

Opiates

Opiates are the mainstay of treatment of cancer pain. The nurse caring for the oncology patient experiencing pain needs to know about several clinical issues in opiate use in this population. Concerns for addiction should not play a role in cancer pain management. The incidence of addiction is extremely small in patients.[29] Many health care providers withhold medication or give less than prescribed doses because of fear of respiratory depression.[25a] Respiratory depression is rare, and tolerance to this effect develops rapidly. It is often progression of disease rather than drug tolerance that creates a need for more analgesia, but tolerance should not be ruled out. Patients with rapidly advancing disease may have intractable pain requiring rapid titration of narcotics.

Switching opiate analgesics or analgesic routes because of inadequate pain relief or untoward side effects can offer advantages. At various points in their illness, patients may need alternate routes of analgesic delivery (oral, rectal, subcutaneous, intravenous, intrathecal).[10] Guidelines for administration of opiates via various routes are available.[2,34]

Nurses have a responsibility to monitor for side effects in patients receiving opiates. The most critical need is the prevention of constipation. Educating the patient and family about medication and side effect management is an essential part of nursing care (see Appendices B and C and Chapter 5).

Coanalgesics (Adjuvant)

Tricyclic antidepressants have been reported to be effective in managing burning dysesthesia associated with neuropathic (deafferentation) pain or in normalizing sleep patterns in chronic cancer pain.[17] The dose usually is less than that recommended for depression, with starting doses of 10 mg to 25 mg of amitriptyline at bedtime. In the clinical experience of the authors, giving the dose 3 hours before bedtime helps to reduce early morning sedation. Anticholinergic side effects exacerbate constipation and urinary retention when used with opiates (see also Chapter 7).

Anticonvulsants have been reported to decrease pain in patients experiencing lancinating or paroxysmal shock-like pain. Dosing is similar to that for seizure disorders. Bone marrow depression can be a limiting side effect, and evaluation of risks and benefits is necessary. Carbamazepine has been used most frequently.[17]

Steroids

Corticosteroids have been used to manage the pain associated with bone metastasis as well as nerve compression, e.g., epidural spinal cord compression. In advanced disease, the added benefits of increased appetite, improved sense of well-being, and euphoria can improve the quality of life for patients. Limited data are available, however an excellent review of the literature is presented by Ettinger and Portenoy[14] (see also Chapter 7).

Stimulants

Stimulants can be helpful for patients experiencing intolerable sedation from opiates despite attempts at dose reduction. Age and cardiac status need to be considered. Dextroamphetamine and methylphenidate (Ritalin) are available for use; starting dose of dextroamphetamine is usually 2.5 mg po bid, and the second dose should not be administered later than 3 PM. In postoperative studies dextroamphetamine increased the analgesic effect of morphine.[21] A recent study evaluated the use of methylphenidate as an adjuvant to narcotic analgesics and found it to be very effective in selected patients.[3] Four out of 50 patients in this study had acute psychiatric toxicities requiring discontinuation of the drugs, but the majority of patients tolerated methylphenidate quite well.[3] Toxicities with the use of methylphenidate occurred early.

Phenothiazines

Phenothiazines are used for managing nausea, a common side effect of narcotic analgesics. Methotrimeprazine is the only phenothiazine with known analgesic properties.[19,26] It is not recommended for ambulatory patients. Phenothiazines, commonly thought to potentiate analgesic effects of narcotics, have now been shown to have little or no analgesic effects and to exacerbate side effects, such as depression, sedation, hypotension, and respiratory depression.

Issues

High Tech vs. Low Tech

There are a variety of drugs and routes of administration to treat cancer-related pain. In general, the simplest, least invasive approach that is *effective* should be used. For example, if the gut works, the oral route should be used. Other factors that enter the decision include: patient preference, length of time the patient has been in pain, cost, insurance coverage, patient's and family's cognitive and psychomotor skills, availability of support for high-tech procedures, and the pain diagnoses. More research is needed to determine when certain pain interventions are most appropriate and most effective.

Clinical Judgment

Many of the issues related to cancer pain are related to effective use of pharmacological agents. Selected problems identified in the discussion of barriers are addressed in this section. Parameters for clinical judgment are outlined (see box).

◆ THE ROLE OF THE NURSE IN CANCER PAIN MANAGEMENT

The National Institutes of Health (1986) issued a consensus development conference statement that emphasized the key role nurses play in caring for people with acute and chronic pain. Since nurses may be the first provider to encounter persons experiencing pain or to identify that a problem of uncontrolled pain exists, their skill in pain assessment and management are critical.[28] Nurses caring for persons with cancer pain should incorporate a systematic pain assessment as a regular part of nursing assessment (e.g., every 4 hours around the clock or every shift). Patients may not volunteer information about their pain, so directed questions are often needed. Nurses must identify and address the barriers to cancer pain assessment and management (see accompanying box and Chapters 1 and 3) that contribute to ineffective pain management in their settings.

With regard to intervention, nurses should understand the WHO analgesic ladder and how to use it. Effective use of the ladder includes being able to evaluate side effects and to exercise appropriate clinical judgment as outlined previously (see box).

Nurses have considerable power to influence treatment plans. Patient and family education is one important intervention and should include content about self-administration of medications or other therapy, anticipatory guidance regarding patients' fears, expected therapeutic and side effects and self-

◆ PARAMETERS FOR CLINICAL JUDGMENT

NURSE'S CONCERN: RESPIRATORY DEPRESSION

PARAMETERS FOR CLINICAL JUDGMENT

- Risk of respiratory depression is low in cancer patients who have been on opioids; risk is higher (although still relatively low) with first dose of opiate in opiate-naive patients, in patients with elevated intracranial pressure, in patients with respiratory compromise, with administration of intraspinal narcotics, and (probably) in patients with significant hepatic and renal dysfunction. Patients who have received an effective nonopiate intervention, such as radiation therapy or nerve block, may need their opiate requirements reevaluated to avert respiratory depression.
- There is no constant definition of respiratory depression; therefore systematic initial baseline (what is normal for a particular patient) assessment of respirations and ongoing, *systematic* evaluation of an individual's respiratory pattern is probably ***most important*** in making the clinical determination that respiratory depression exists. Using a pain flow sheet or the existing graphic sheet for capturing this information can promote accuracy in clinical evaluation of respiratory depression.
- Collaborate with attending physician to establish the lowest acceptable respiratory rate (RR) based on baseline rate. (Lowest absolute rate is 6/min)
- If patient's RR falls below lower limit, rouse patient; encourage patient to breathe. When patient's RR reaches baseline and time for next scheduled dose occurs or pain returns, administer medication. (If pattern of med administration and subsequent RR depression persists, consider reduction in dose or increase in interval between doses, if this does not compromise analgesia.) If analgesia will be compromised, a nalaxone drip has been used along with the analgesic to strike a balance that maintains pain control but maintains an acceptable RR (see Narcan guidelines below). Collaborate with medical and nursing staff to develop a *rational* plan for using naloxone *before* such intervention is needed (see guidelines for Narcan use).

Continued.

◆ PARAMETERS FOR CLINICAL JUDGMENT—cont'd

- Do not precipitate opiate withdrawal by continuing to withhold opiates after RR rises to lower limit or administering naloxone too precipitously or at too high a dosage. Remember to assess *pain*, not just respiratory depression (decreasing dose slightly or increasing interval may be sufficient).
- "The only safe and effective way to administer a narcotic is to *watch the individual's response,* especially to the first dose" (McCaffery and Beebe[27], p. 72).
- Severe pain appears to counteract the respiratory depressant effects of opiates in patients with severe pain.
- Tolerance to narcotic analgesia usually is associated with tolerance to respiratory depression (the risk of respiratory depression, although small, is greater with intraspinal analgesics than with peripheral analgesics).
- Whenever you are evaluating patients for opiate-induced respiratory depression consider other factors that may contribute to the change in patient's condition (e.g., metabolic dysfunction such as hypercalcemia, administration of other sedating medications such as lorazepam, brain metastases). For patients who have been on well-established opiate regimens or whose opiate escalations have been slow, it is more likely that other factors explain the phenomenon.
- Although sedation and respiratory depression can influence each other, they are not the same clinical phenomena and should be evaluated differently.

NALAXONE GUIDELINES

- Significant respiratory depression is best treated by slow infusion of dilute naloxone (Narcan). To avoid acute narcotic withdrawal, dilute one 0.4 mg ampule of naloxone into 10 cc of saline and slowly infuse IV until respirations increase. A constant IV infusion of low-dose naloxone may be temporarily necessary to maintain analgesia but prevent recurrent respiratory depression (add 5 ampules of naloxone to 500 cc of D_5W to achieve a final concentration of 4 μg/cc; start the infusion at a rate of 2.5 to 3.0 μg/kg/hr; titrate as needed to maintain adequate respirations with retention of analgesia). Patients who are comatose should be intubated to prevent aspiration from naloxone-induced salivation and bronchial spasm. Naloxone may also precipitate seizures, especially in patients receiving meperidine.

NURSE'S CONCERN: FEAR OF CAUSING ADDICTION

PARAMETERS FOR CLINICAL JUDGMENT

Patients Without History of Substance Abuse

- Extremely unlikely in this population (less than 1/1,000). Is not a reason for undermedicating or withholding medication.

Recovered Substance Abusers

- The patient is responsible for his or her recovery from substance abuse. The health team consults with the patient about the *use of narcotics for pain relief.*
- Collaborate with the patient in developing a care plan for opiate use and use of adjuvant, noninvasive measures during pain trajectory. If pain is likely to decrease/disappear, develop a plan for tapering narcotics based on patient's wishes *and* report of pain decrement. These patients can be *gradually* withdrawn from opiates as effectively as the opiate-naive patient. If patient is likely to experience increased pain with advancing or terminal disease, patient may need significant coaching to accept pain relief and long-term and/or escalating doses of narcotics.
- Do not "punish" patient by withholding needed analgesics. Base care plan on accurate assessment, patient wishes, and standard approaches to measuring pain in cancer populations.
- Patients on maintenance doses of methadone will need this therapy continued *as well as* additional analgesics for the pain problem.

Active Opiate Substance Abuser*

- Determine accuracy of label "addict"; use of opiates for *pain relief* is not addiction.
- If goal of hospitalization and/or treatment is not substance abuse rehabilitation, focus should be on pain relief and prevention of withdrawal.
- These patients will need larger doses of opiates for pain relief. One physician should be responsible for prescribing these medications. (Obtain consultation from an expert in addictions medicine).
- Care plan will need to be explicit regarding rules and expectations (e.g., contracts). Consideration needs to be given to the expected duration and trajectory of the pain problem in outlining plan.
- Opiates should not be withheld as a punitive or rehabilitative measure in the person who has pain.

*An excellent and detailed approach to the concern about addiction with additional references can be found in McCaffery M and Beebe A. *Pain: a clinical manual for nursing practice,* St. Louis: CV Mosby, 1989.

Continued.

◆ PARAMETERS FOR CLINICAL JUDGMENT—cont'd

NURSE'S CONCERN: OVERSEDATION

PARAMETERS FOR CLINICAL JUDGMENT

- Know baseline mental status.
- Know prior sleep pattern—if patient has had poor sleep over weeks or months, patient is likely to sleep a lot during initial opiate therapy. Sedation usually subsides after 2 or 3 days of therapy.
- If patient is able to be roused, usually what seems like excessive sleepiness is a normal response to finally experiencing pain relief.
- This pattern may recur with dose escalation.
- If respirations are within acceptable limits and if sedation is acceptable to the patient, continue with opiate regimen and allay family's fears. If not, decrease the opiate dose and give more frequently.
- If excessive sleepiness occurs suddenly after patient has been on stable opiate doses investigate other causes (e.g., metabolic causes; metastases; elevated liver function tests; or abnormal renal function tests).
- If tolerance to sedation does not develop and no other cause of excessive sedation is identified yet decreasing the analgesic dose increases pain, consider addition of a stimulant.

NURSE'S CONCERN: CONFUSION, DELIRIUM, DYSPHORIA

PARAMETERS FOR CLINICAL JUDGMENT

- If it occurs immediately after opiate administration, opiate may be cause.
- Appearance of these symptoms after patient has been on stable doses of oral or intravenous opiate (with or without dose escalation) with relief of pain, the cause is unlikely to be the opiate. Metabolic causes such as hypercalcemia, sepsis, bleeding, uremia, or pathological causes, such as brain metastases or carcinomeningitis, should be investigated.

Guidelines to Narcan Use, source: Handbook of cancer pain management. Published by the Wisconsin Cancer Pain Initiative in Madison, Wisc., 1988.

care, and resources to call for questions and complications. Such education can determine the success or failure of a pain treatment plan (see Appendices B and C).

Nurses also can initiate many noninvasive measures that can alleviate pain (see Chapter 8). In addition to therapeutic communication, which can reduce anxiety and improve coping, nurses can coach patients in relaxation, guided imagery, focused breathing, self-talk or affirmation, meditation, and cutaneous techniques. Research has shown that cognitive strategies can make a difference in an individual's experience of pain.[12,15] Development of standards of care that incorporate the use of these independent nursing interventions in the treatment of pain can encourage nurses to use these measures more consistently and enhance pain relief.

Finally, nurses make a very significant contribution to the interdisciplinary care of persons with cancer experiencing pain. They communicate the patient's reports of pain and related concerns to colleagues, contribute to the diagnostic workup, and suggest therapies that might be useful based on assessment. They are often the sole providers available to evaluate the efficacy of pain therapy and satisfaction with pain relief.

Implications for Further Research

Nurses play an important role in pursuing areas of clinical investigation. Clinical issues requiring further research include:

- Identifying trajectories associated with various types of cancer pain (somatic, visceral, and deafferentation) and developing nursing interventions specific to these.
- Evaluating collaborative, interdisciplinary approaches to pain management and identifying criteria for support and success.
- Assessing and evaluating patterns of therapeutic communication: What is it about the nurse-patient relationship that instills hope, courage, empowerment?
- Developing prevention and early detection strategies for identifying and managing cancer pain and the ensuing clinical implications. Can severe pain be prevented by early detection and treatment of known cancer pain syndromes?
- Evaluating effectiveness of patient education in improv-

ing pain relief and in reducing side effects and complications of pain therapy.

◆ SUMMARY

This chapter has reviewed problems and issues associated with cancer pain and the epidemiology and causes of cancer pain. In addition, selected common cancer pain problems have been used as models for understanding risk factors, pain mechanisms, and therapeutic approaches. An overview of pharmacotherapy of cancer pain was provided as well as clinical approaches to common concerns that nurses have about analgesic therapy. The pivotal role nurses play in effective assessment and management of cancer pain was described. Finally, several areas warranting further nursing research were described.

BIBLIOGRAPHY

1. Barkas G and Duafala ME. (1988). Advances in cancer pain management: a review of patient controlled analgesia. *J Pain Sympt Manag 3,* 150-160.
2. Bruera E, Brenneis C, Michaud M, et al. (1987). Continuous subcutaneous infusion of narcotics using a disposable portable device. *Cancer Treat Rep 71*:635-637.
3. Bruera E, Brenneis C, Paterson AH, and MacDonald RN. (1989). Use of methylphenidate as an adjuvant to narcotic analgesics in patients with advanced cancer. *J Pain Sympt Manag 4,* 3-6.
4. Camp L D. (1988). A comparison of nurses' recorded assessments of pain with perceptions of pain as described by cancer patients. *Cancer Nurs 11,* 237-243.
5. Campbell JN. (1989). Pain in peripheral nerve injury. In Foley KM and Payne R (eds), *Current therapy of pain.* Toronto: BC Decker, 158-169.
6. Carr D and Carr J. (1983). Role of opiates in pain relief. In Stoll BA and Parbhoo S (eds), *Bone metastases: monitoring and treatment.* New York: Raven Press, 375-394.
7. Chapman CR, Korneu J, and Syrjal KL. (1987). Painful complications of cancer diagnosis and therapy. In McGuire DB and Yarbro CH (eds), *Cancer pain management.* Orlando, Fla: Grune and Stratton, Harcourt Brace Jovanovich Publishers, 47-67.
8. Clark J, Landis L, and McGee R. (1987). Nursing management of outcomes of disease, psychological response, treatment, and complications. In Ziegfield CR (ed), *Core curriculum for oncology nursing.* Philadelphia: WB Saunders, 304.
9. Coyle N. (1985). A model of continuity of care. In Foley KM. *Management of cancer pain—syllabus of the post graduate course.* New York City: Memorial Sloan-Kettering Cancer Center.
10. Coyle N. (1989). Continuity of care for the cancer patient in pain. *Cancer 63,* 2289-2293.

11. Daeffler RJ. (1985). Protective mechanisms: mucous membranes. In Johnson BL and Gross J. (eds), *Handbook of oncology nursing.* New York: John Wiley & Sons, 253-274.
11a. Dahl JL, Joranson DE, Engber D and Dosch J. (1988). The cancer pain problem: Wisconsin's response. *J Pain Sympt Manag 3*(1), S2-S8.
12. Dalton J. (1987). Education for pain management. *Pat Ed Counsel 9,* 155-165.
12a. Daut RL and Cleeland CS. (1982). The prevalence and severity of pain in cancer. *Cancer 50,* 1913-1918.
13. Donovan MI. (1985). Nursing assessment of cancer pain, *Semin Oncol Nurs 1,* No. 2., May, 109-115.
14. Ettinger AB and Portenoy RK. (1988). The use of corticosteroids in the treatment of symptoms associated with cancer. *J Pain Sympt Manage 3,* 99-103.
15. Fernandez E and Turk DC. (1989). The utility of cognitive coping strategies for altering pain perceptions. *Pain 38,* 123-136.
16. Ferrell BR, Wisdom C, Wenzl C. (1989). Quality of life as an outcome variable in management of cancer pain. *Cancer 63,* 2321-2327.
17. Foley KM. (1985). Adjuvant analgesic drugs in cancer pain management. In Aronoff G (ed), *Evaluation and treatment of chronic pain.* Baltimore: Urban and Schwarzenberg.
18. Foley KM and Payne RM. (1989). *Current therapy of pain.* Toronto: BC Decker.
19. Foley KM. (1985). The treatment of cancer pain. *N Engl J Med 313,* 84-95.
20. Foley KM. (1979). Pain syndromes in patients with cancer. In Bonica JJ and Ventafridda V (eds), *Advances in pain research and therapy,* vol 2. New York: Raven Press, 59-75.
21. Forrest WH, Brown BW, Brown CR, et al. (1977). Dextroamphetamine with morphine for treatment of postoperative pain. *N Engl J Med 296,* 712-715.
22. Kanner R. (1985). Post surgical pain syndromes. In Foley KM, *Management of cancer pain—syllabus of the post graduate course.* New York City: Memorial Sloan Kettering Cancer Center, 65-72.
23. Kantor TG. (1982). Control of pain by nonsteroidal anti-inflammatory drugs. *Med Clin North Am 66,* 1053-1059.
24. Kersh CR and Harzra TA. (1985). Radiation therapy in the management of oncologic pain. *Clin Cancer Briefs,* March 3-11.
25. Levick S, Jacobs C, Loukas DF, et al. (1988). Naproxen sodium in treatment of bone pain due to metastatic cancer. *Pain 35,* 253-258.
25a. Marks R and Sachar E. (1973). Undertreatment of medical inpatients with narcotic analgesics. *Ann Intern Med 78,* 173-181.
26. McCaffery M. (1979). *Nursing management of the patient with pain.* Philadelphia: JB Lippincott, 11.
27. McCaffery M and Beebe A. (1989). *Pain: clinical manual for nursing practice.* St. Louis: CV Mosby.
27a. McGuire DB and Yarbro CH (eds). (1987). *Cancer pain management.* Orlando, Fla: Grune and Stratton.
28. McMillan SC, Williams FA, Chatfield R, and Camp LD. (1988). A validity and reliability study of two tools for assessing and managing cancer pain. *Oncol Nurs Forum 15,* 735-744.
29. Miller RR and Jick H. (1979). Clinical effects of meperidine in hospitalized patients. *J Clin Pharm 18,* 180-189.

30. Nocks BN. (1989). Pain in the male genitourinary system. In Foley KM and Payne R (eds), *Current therapy of pain.* BC Decker: Toronto.
31. Nussbaum H. (1983). Quality of life in patients with bone metastases. In Stoll BA and Parbhoo S (eds), *Bone metastases and treatment.* New York: Raven Press, 311-320.
32. Payne R. (1989). Anatomy, physiology, and pharmacology of cancer pain. *Cancer 63,* 2266-2274.
33. Portenoy RK. (1989). Cancer pain: epidemiology and syndromes. *Cancer 63,* 2298-3307.
34. Portenoy RK. (1989). Intravenous infusion of opioids for cancer pain. In Foley KM and Payne R (eds), *Current therapy of pain.* BC Decker: Toronto.
35. Posner JB. (1985). Back pain and epidural spinal cord compression. In Foley KM (ed), *Management of cancer pain—syllabus of the post graduate course.* New York City: Memorial Sloan Kettering Cancer Center, 1985.
36. Spross JA and Hope A. (1985). Alterations in comfort: pain related to cancer. *Orthop Nurs 4,* 48-52.
37. Stillman MJ. (1989). Pain in breast cancer. In Foley KM and Payne R (eds), *Current therapy in pain.* Toronto: BC Decker, 361-384.
38. Tannock I, Gospodarowicz M, Meakin W, et al. (1989). Treatment of metastatic prostatic cancer with low dose prednisone: evaluation of pain and quality of life as pragmatic indices of response. *J Clin Oncol 7,* 590-597.
39. Twycross RG and Fairfield S. (1982). Pain in far advanced cancer. *Pain 14,* 303-310.
40. Twycross RG and Lack SA. (1983). Symptom control in far advanced cancer: pain relief. London: Pitman Books.
41. Vecht CJ, Van de Brand HJ, and Wajer OJM. (1989). Post axillary dissection pain in breast cancer due to a lesion of the intercostobrachial nerve. *Pain 35,* 171-176.
42. Ventafridda V, Fochi C, Delonno D, et al. (1980). Use of nonsteroidal anti-inflammatory drugs in the treatment of pain in cancer. *Br J Clin Pharmacol 10,* 3435-3465.
43. Wall PD. (1986). The prevention of postoperative pain (editorial). *Pain 33,* 289-290.
44. Watson CPN, Evans RJ, and Watt VR. (1989). The post-mastectomy pain syndrome and the effect of topical capsaicin. *Pain 38,* 177-186.
45. World Health Organization. (1986). Cancer Pain Relief. Geneva: WHO.

Acknowledgment

The authors wish to acknowledge Valerie Grande, who patiently prepared the manuscript for this chapter.

15

Surgical Pain Management

Tracy J. Wasylak

◆ INTRODUCTION

Surgery is the second-most-common reason for admission to the hospital. In the United States and Canada, more than 3 million people have surgery performed every year. Pain is the number one complaint patients have after surgery. It is second to death and disability as a feared phenomenon preoperatively.

The pain experience usually begins when surgery is performed. Therefore it is considered iatrogenic and is directly related to the degree of tissue and nerve ending trauma. Surgery results in the liberation of pain-producing substances that migrate into the surrounding tissue and circulation. These substances alter the normal environment of the nociceptor and trigger a sensation that is interpreted as pain.[16] Similar responses also occur when surgical patients are subjected to procedures such as a dressing change, central line insertion, catheter placement or removal, or debridement of the wound. Consequently pain stimuli for surgical patients may be generated from a variety of sources, ranging in severity and duration and requiring numerous strategies to alleviate and/or prevent them.

The purpose of this chapter is to discuss the mechanisms of surgical pain and review the current issues in the treatment of postoperative pain and their implications for clinical practice. As well, current therapy and practices useful in treating postoperative pain will be addressed.

Definitions

Surgical pain can be defined as iatrogenic and acute, of relatively short duration, usually well localized, and directly related to incision type and length, as well as the degree of surgical trauma. Surgical pain or postoperative pain is most often described according to the surgical procedure being performed (e.g., appendectomy, hemicolectomy, thoracotomy) and/or the anatomical location of the incision (e.g., thoracic, upper or lower abdominal). Unfortunately, this provides limited information for practitioners about the type of pain patients are experiencing. In assessing and treating surgical pain, practitioners must gather additional data that includes:

1. Pain intensity and duration
2. Pain location
3. Factors influencing the pain (e.g., time of day, previous experience with pain)
4. Pain's influence on activities of daily living (e.g., eating, sleeping, and ambulation)
5. The patient's knowledge about his or her surgery and its implications

Pain is far more complex than many practitioners realize. Treatment therefore requires a broader understanding of etiology, transmission, and characteristics, such as prevalence, intensity, duration, and time course of postoperative pain.

Pain Etiology

Postoperative pain is initiated by excitation of peripheral pain receptors, known as nociceptors, located in the skin, muscles, ligaments, and organs. Of these cutaneous nociceptors, 50% are sensory nerves and travel alongside efferent fibers of the sympathetic nervous system.[22,37,93] These peripheral nociceptors transmit pain along fibers called A-delta or C-fibers, (a more comprehensive discussion of these mechanisms can be found in Chapter 2). Generally speaking, A-delta fibers are responsible for the transmission of sharp, well-localized pain sensation. C-fibers are responsible for transmission of dull, burning, or diffuse pain sensation. C-fibers include a group of fibers called efferent sympathetic fibers, which are responsible for increasing peripheral nociceptors' sensitivity to pain stimuli and may play a role in chronic pain.[93] It is also postulated that increases in sympathetic drive (e.g., from surgery, stress, trauma) may contribute to increasing levels of pain by repeated stimulation of nociceptors. This may partially explain why many nonpharmacological measures assist in alleviating postoperative pain.

Surgical manipulation of the body results in numerous changes to the body's equilibrium, which include:

1. Changes in the body's chemical environment (e.g., fluid and electrolyte shifts, changes in acid-base balance)
2. Release of endogenous algesic substances into the microcirculation (i.e., serotonin, bradykinins, prostaglandins)
3. Alterations in the microcirculation and changes in capillary permeability
4. Increases in efferent sympathetic activity (general adaptation syndrome, alterations in hormonal balance).

These changes play a role in lowering nociceptive threshold to pain both directly and indirectly. For example, algesic substances have a direct effect on nociceptors by increasing their excitability (lowering their threshold), making them more likely to fire. Indirectly, these same substances have vasoactive properties potentially altering the nociceptive environment (i.e., the cellular microcirculation), increasing cellular excitability and the triggering of pain.[22,93]

Somatic and Visceral Pain

Pain transmission after surgery involves both somatic and visceral sensations, depending on the location of the pain and the organ(s) affected.

Somatic pain is defined as localized, sharp, or precise pain and is usually described as sharp or stinging. The transmission of this type of pain occurs mainly along the A-delta fibers. Somatic pain sensations can be triggered when an area of trauma, such as an incision line, is stimulated. Removal of the stimulus will result in cessation of the painful sensation.[93]

Visceral pain is more complex than somatic pain. It is poorly localized, vague, and more intricate. Visceral pain is usually described as colicky, cramping, dull, or aching pain and may be referred to other areas, making it more difficult to treat (e.g., uterine pain is often referred to the back). The viscera is insensitive to burning and cutting but is very sensitive to inflammation, tearing, stretching, intense contraction, necrosis, or compression of ligaments or vessels.[22] For example, a preoperative patient with bowel obstruction may present with very severe diffuse pain throughout the abdomen and back. Postoperatively, the pain becomes more localized and somatic as the visceral component has been alleviated.

Visceral and somatic pain reception are closely associated and triggered via similar mechanisms. Therefore, when patients have surgery, more than one mechanism of pain transmission may be functioning. This is especially true if patients experience complications postoperatively. The occurrence of infection, inflammation, or compression may incite visceral mechanisms.

Pain after surgery is serious and if not treated properly may hinder recovery. Recent studies have demonstrated that effective pain control after surgery can decrease morbidity and shorten hospital stay.[16,22,88,92]

Physiological Effects of Pain

The stress response to surgical trauma is characterized by a number of neuroendocrine activities that affect most systems in the body. Pain increases activity in the sympathetic nervous system, causing increased levels of antidiuretic hormone, epinephrine, aldosterone, and cortisol. Other substrates, such as bradykinins, serotonin, and prostglandins, are liberated in the postoperative period and result in altered metabolic activity and increased modulation of nociceptive transmission. Pain in the postoperative period also leads to increased suffering and anxiety. Sleeplessness, feelings of loss of control, and restlessness accompany moderate to severe pain.

Increases in sympathetic drive occurring as a result of the stress of surgery and pain result in adverse effects for the cardiovascular and respiratory systems. Patients in pain experience increases in heart rate, stroke volume, myocardial oxygen consumpton, and peripheral vascular resistance. In healthy patients this added stress is usually tolerated. However, more and more surgical patients have underlying medical conditions that put them at risk with surgery. Moderate to severe pain postoperatively can be seen as a risk factor for these patients and may result in grave sequelae such as myocardial infarction and/or respiratory failure.[22]

Pain associated with thoracic and abdominal surgery leads to splinting with resultant decreases in tidal volume, vital capacity, and functional residual capacity, leading to alveolar hypoventilation. This pattern of breathing results in microatelectasis, placing the patient at risk for atelectasis and pulmonary infection.[23]

Pain causes an increase in gastrointestinal secretion, and at the same time decreases intestinal tone, slowing gastric emptying. The risk for the patient includes a higher chance of nausea and vomiting with or without aspiration as well as gastric irritation and ulceration.

Pain affects sphincter tone in the bladder, consequently increasing atony and urinary retention. Pain induces muscle spasm in the areas of trauma, potentiating immobility and splinting. Major determinants of urine production are cardiac output and peripheral vascular resistance. Although not scientifically linked, pain's direct effect on the cardiovascular system may also reduce blood flow to the kidneys, resulting in diminished renal activity.[22,92]

Despite the increasing evidence of the deleterious effects of pain in the postoperative period, the literature suggests that the undertreatment of surgical pain continues to be a major problem in almost all acute care settings. In fact, it has been suggested that undertreatment of pain has reached epidemic proportions.[39]

Undertreatment of Postoperative Pain

The problems of postoperative pain have to be drawn from the findings of several small clinical studies because no comprehensive epidemiological studies on the prevalence, intensity, and duration of postoperative pain across the entire surgical population have been reported.

Marks and Sachar[46] interviewed 37 medical patients to ascertain the level of pain and the adequacy of the medication regime. A questionnaire was sent to physicians to elicit their attitudes and knowledge about narcotic analgesics. The results showed that 73% of the patients experienced moderate to severe pain despite the analgesic regime utilized. The data clearly demonstrated a general pattern of undertreatment of pain with narcotic analgesics. Physicians were found to underprescribe narcotic dosages, providing ineffective treatment, and nurses further reduced the amount of analgesics given. Marks and Sachar[46] suggest that these behaviors were due to an exaggerated fear of respiratory depression and narcotic addiction.

Cohen[18] studied the incidence of pain in postoperative

patients by chart review and questionnaires sent to the nursing staff. The purpose was to ascertain the nurses' attitudes and knowledge about narcotic analgesics. Her results showed that by the third postoperative day, 75% of the patients continued to report moderate to severe pain. Her findings showed a discrepancy between the amount of analgesic prescribed and the amount of analgesic the patient received. The nurses' responses to the questionnaire revealed their inadequate knowledge of narcotic analgesics, their choice of inappropriate dosages, and an exaggerated fear of narcotic addiction.

Donovan, Dillon, and McGuire[26] queried whether the problems identified by Marks and Sachar[46] still existed, and examined the current prevalence of pain in hospitalized patients. They interviewed a random sample of 353 hospitalized patients about their levels of pain and a number of other factors perceived to influence pain. The patients' charts were also audited to ascertain the amount of medication prescribed, the analgesic consumed, and the pain documented as a problem by health care staff. Their results concurred with the previous literature's findings, as more than 75% of the patients reported experiencing pain within 72 hours of the interview. A total of 90% of the patients had moderate to severe pain that was periodic to continuous. Further, 203 patients reported experiencing horrible or excruciating pain some time during their hospitalization.[26] The authors concluded that pain management has not improved significantly in the past decade and that patients continue to receive inadequate analgesics to control their pain. The persistence of this problem is further documented in numerous reports and editorials circulated through the literature.* Chapman and Bonica[16] concur with these statements and add that with the plethora of pharmacological agents and the advances in technology today, no patient should experience the degree of pain that many are presently experiencing.

Pain Prevalence

Although postoperative pain prevalence has not been systematically measured, Chapman and Bonica[16] compiled data from numerous studies to estimate pain resulting from sur-

* References 1, 14, 48, 50, 72, 87.

gery. They calculated prevalence, intensity, and time course of postoperative pain by examining patients' demands for analgesia. They suggest that regardless of surgical procedure, it seems that 30% of all patients experience mild pain, 30% experience moderate pain, and 40% experience severe or very severe pain. Extensive reporting of clinical practice indicates that postoperative pain occurs more often and is more severe after intrathoracic, intraabdominal, and renal surgery; and extensive surgery of the spine, major joints, and large bones in the hand and foot.[5,16]

Duration of Pain

Time profiles for the onset and duration of postoperative pain demonstrate wide variations within the surgical population. Although in general major surgery causes greater initial pain than minor surgery, many minor surgical procedures produce pain intensities equal to those seen after major surgery.[10] However, the rate of decline in pain after minor surgery is usually much greater than the rate of disappearance of pain caused by extensive surgery.[5,10]

The duration of moderate to severe pain after intrathoracic and upper abdominal surgery ranges anywhere from 2 to 7 days (mean = 4.5 days). On the other hand, the duration of moderate to severe pain after lower abdominal surgery is anywhere from 1 to 4 days (mean = 2.5 days).[5] Melzack and others[51] found that 31% of the requests for analgesic medication on a surgical ward were made by patients who had their surgery more than 4 days previously. These authors found that patients with delayed pain resolution were generally older and received lower medication doses despite high pain levels. Paul[60] observed a similar trend in a group of hysterectomy patients. She reported that 60% of the hysterectomy patients complained of mild or discomforting pain 10 days postoperatively. The time course of postoperative pain is affected by the type and nature of pain treatment utilized as well as by the site and extent of surgery. Current practice dictates that after 48 to 72 hours of receiving parenteral analgesics, most patients are switched to less potent analgesics, usually by the oral route. The oral route may be appropriate but the doses of prescribed analgesic are of concern, especially if the studies reported above are generally applicable, and many patients continue to experience high levels of pain beyond the average time course. These findings substantiate the need for greater individualization of postoperative care.

Aggressive treatment of pain in the early stages postoperatively can reduce subsequent pain and improve recovery. Wood, Lloyd and others[91] used paravertebral blockage with bupivacaine in a group of patients undergoing inguinal herniorrhaphy and found significantly lower use of analgesic in the first 24 hours compared with a control group. The experimental group subsequently required less analgesics over the next 3 days than did the control group. In the author's own work, hysterectomy patients were aggressively treated early in the postoperative period with a loading dose of morphine followed by use of patient-controlled analgesia (PCA).[81] This was compared to a control group who received standard intravenous morphine in the recovery room and intermittent intramuscular injection of morphine on the ward. The group receiving PCA had lower pain intensity and reduced variability of pain, as well as better recovery with less morbidity than the control group.

Factors Influencing Pain

The incidence and severity of postoperative pain is influenced by the physical, psychological, emotional, motivational, and personality characteristics of the patient.[5,76] Physical factors that are reported to influence the occurrence, intensity, and duration of postoperative pain include[5]:

1. The site, nature, and duration of the operation, the type of incision, and the degree of intraoperative trauma
2. The anesthetic management before, during, and after surgery
3. The quality of the postoperative care

Generally speaking, the degree of preoperative and postoperative anxiety and fear is considered an important predictor of postoperative pain. However, results of studies on anxiety as a predictor of pain show equivocal results. Chapman et al[16] found that anxiety increased over the postoperative period, especially in patients who were ill-prepared. Volicer[85] showed that admission to the hospital produced anxiety and stress that were highly correlated with the incidence and intensity of postoperative pain. Patients who scored high in "hospital stress" preoperatively had more pain and lower physical status (greater morbidity) postoperatively and less improvement after discharge than patients having a low stress score. Taenzer, Melzack, and Jeans[76] found that patients who reported greater pain in the postoperative period had higher levels of trait anxiety and neuroticism. Situational anxiety and fear of surgery assessed the evening before surgery were not significantly correlated with most pain measures and did not contribute to the prediction of pain levels.

Pain Assessment

Pain assessment is discussed in depth in Chapter 4. The following questions have been effective in eliciting basic and individualized information from surgical patients (see box).

Patients should be included in the assessment of their pain. Nurses should explain to patients the importance of their role in pain management, particularly in reporting their pain and evaluating the effectiveness of treatments. Many patients assume that the nurse will automatically detect the pain and successfully treat it. Preoperative explanations by the nurse of anticipated pain sensations, typical postoperative expectations (e.g., deep breathing and coughing exercises, ambulation, etc.), and the goals of pain therapy will facilitate the assessment and treatment of postoperative pain.

◆ QUESTIONS TO ASK WHEN ASSESSING POSTOPERATIVE PAIN

1. Are you having pain? Variations include: Are you having discomfort, cramps, aching sensations, etc.?
2. Where is the pain, discomfort, cramp? Check to see if the patient's sensation is occurring in more than one area.
3. Is the pain constant or intermittent?
4. Is this the worst your pain has been?
5. How would you rate your pain on a scale from 0 to 10?
6. Is/are there any word(s) that best describe your pain?
7. Have you been up at all today? What activities have you been able to engage in (ambulating, self-care activities)?
8. Does anything relieve your pain, discomfort?
9. Does pain interfere with your eating, sleeping, walking?
10. How do you feel about having surgery? Do you have any questions/concerns?

◆ STRATEGIES FOR TREATING POSTOPERATIVE PAIN

The goal of therapy in treating postoperative pain is maximal relief of pain with minimal or no side effects from the therapy. As previously mentioned, narcotic analgesics remain the first line of treatment for most types of postoperative pain[11] (see Chapters 7 and 12).

Parenteral Opioid Analgesics

Parenteral administration of narcotics is the most frequently utilized method of pain relief during the first 24 to 48 hours postoperatively. Intermittent intramuscular (IM) injection is the most frequently ordered route of administration. Unfortunately, intermittent IM injection has many inadequacies that result in poor pain control.

The pharmacokinetic and pharmacodynamic variability of intramuscular injections is high.[50,54] The resulting variation in absorption rates of narcotic analgesic produces fluctuating drug serum levels at the receptor site. Within an hour of the time of an IM injection, there is an initial relative overdosage. As pain builds and the analgesic is detoxified/excreted, a relative underdosage exists until the next injection is given. This regime leads to peaks and troughs of analgesia and pain. It also increases the risk of unwanted side effects such as somnolence and nausea. Planning and timing of nursing care interventions, such as ambulation, become a challenge for patients because of these side effects. In fact, many patients refuse analgesia for this reason alone. Clinically, injections are time-consuming for the nursing staff as they require on average 10 to 15 minutes of preparation time per injection.[62] This includes locating narcotic keys, drawing up of medication, bookkeeping of narcotic administration, and documentation of the event. On a busy surgical ward with an average nursing assignment of six to eight patients, this requires that a minimum of 2 hours be allocated for analgesic administration. This estimate does not include the assessment of pain and the evaluation of the effects of those pain injections. When compared with other forms of postoperative pain therapy (e.g. patient-controlled analgesia), IM injections were found to be less effective in controlling pain and more time-consuming for nursing personnel.[62]

Although meperidine is commonly prescribed in the postoperative period, recent studies have shown that normeperidine, an active metabolite of meperidine, may be responsible for potential central nervous system excitant activity.[22,36a] Normeperidine has an active half-life of 14 to 21 hours in patients with normal renal function. The active metabolite accumulates in the body after prolonged administration, producing untoward effects (including seizures); therefore normeperidine is losing the favor of many physicians, anesthesiologists, and pharmacologists.[22]

Recent studies comparing fixed-interval IM injections with other forms of analgesia have shown some positive results. McGrath and others[49] compared IM fixed-interval injections with PCA administration of meperidine. Their results showed no significant differences between groups on pain scores 4 and 24 hours after surgery. Patients receiving IM injections were scheduled to receive medication every 3 hours. The authors concluded that proficient pain assessment by nursing staff followed by regular analgesic administration could be an effective means of postoperative pain control. However, patients on PCA were given high demand boluses with accompanying long lockout intervals. These restrictions may have prevented the PCA group from adequately medicating themselves. Nonetheless, IM injections can be effective if based on a good assessment and followed by an evaluation of the patient's pain. For instance, the first dose of narcotic given should be monitored and assessed hourly for its effectiveness in relieving pain. Just observing a patient does not provide adequate information about the presence and intensity of the pain, as pain behaviors vary from one patient to the next. If pain relief is not achieved, the medication dosage should be increased and/or the interval between injections decreased. Second, patients should be assessed or medicated on a fixed interval (e.g., every 3 hours) rather than only when they ask for pain medication. Many patients deny pain or refuse medication until the pain becomes unbearable. This is problematic because severe or very severe pain requires more analgesic and is much more difficult to control than moderate pain. Patients need to know their role in postoperative pain management. Therefore the nursing staff should incorporate this type of information into their preoperative teaching plans. Patients should be told the type and intensity of pain they are likely to experience, the therapy to be utilized to decrease their pain, and their role in treating the pain (i.e., informing nursing staff when pain begins to increase). In the author's institution, nurses schedule IM injections every 3 hours. This ensures that the patient is assessed on a fixed interval and allows for better control of pain.

Intravenous (IV) administration of narcotics is another route used for intermittent scheduling of analgesics. The primary difference between IM and IV administration is the speed at which medication can reach the receptor sites in the central nervous system. IM injections require absorption of medication across the muscle and capillary wall before reaching the receptor site. Medications given IV are introduced directly into the systemic circulation, expediting transport to the receptor site. Although IV medications generally are faster acting, their duration of action is shorter than IM injections.

IV bolus administration of narcotics is commonly used in acute care settings, especially intensive care or special care units. Problems with IV bolus medications include hypotension, drowsiness, and nausea and vomiting. Although IV bolus medication provides rapid temporary pain relief, most bolus injections are given too infrequently to provide consistent pain control. The short duration of action of IV boluses makes their use on a general surgical ward unrealistic in view of the staffing patterns on most surgical wards. The use of bolus medications is best as an adjunct when the patient experiences breakthrough pain while receiving patient-controlled analgesia, continuous infusions, or epidural analgesia. IV bolus may also be used to prevent severe pain resulting from procedures or nursing care such as dressing changes, removal of chest tubes, etc. Like IM injections, IV bolus of narcotics results in a relative overdosage of medication followed by a period of relative underdosage until the next IV bolus is given.

Continuous infusion of analgesics is often utilized in specialty areas for patients with high levels of pain that is anticipated to last for long periods of time (e.g., burn and trauma victims, patients undergoing extensive surgery). Therapy involves a loading dose of analgesic followed by a maintenance infusion (e.g., a patient receiving a morphine infusion would receive 5 to 10 mg as a bolus followed by a 1 to 6 mg hourly infusion rate). The dose needs to be titrated to the individual patient; some patients with severe to very severe pain can tolerate very high doses of narcotic. Continuous infusions are more convenient for nursing staff because they take less time to prepare and administer. However, initially they may require more nursing time for titration and observation of the patient for therapeutic effect and possible side effects.

Drug Tolerance, Physical Dependence, and Addiction

Drug tolerance, physical dependence, and addiction are often mistakenly thought of as synonymous (see Chapter 7). Drug tolerance occurs when the usual analgesic dose becomes ineffective in relieving pain. Physical dependence is the alteration of the patient's physiological state such that withdrawal symptoms occur when the drug is no longer given.[47] Addiction, on the other hand, is a form of drug abuse and involves compulsive use of a substance. The incidence of addiction in patients receiving narcotics over the acute phase of their illness is less than .1%.[47] Portenoy and Foley[63] studied 38 patients receiving long-term opioid analgesic for nonmalignant pain. They concluded that opioid maintenance therapy was safe and effective in relieving pain without producing signs of addiction. Clinically, when patients are requiring high doses of opioid analgesics, tolerance and dependence may occur. As McCaffery and Hart[47] point out, physiological dependence and drug tolerance do not always occur after repeated doses of analgesics; however, when they do occur, they often coincide. Further, tolerance and dependence are less likely to occur with a continuous infusion than with IM or IV administration, because the peaking and troughing of analgesic levels accelerates this process. If patients develop tolerance (decreasing duration of action), the possibility of increasing the medication dosage must be evaluated. Weaning patients from high doses of opioid analgesics should be done slowly to prevent signs and symptoms of physiological dependence.

Patient-Controlled Analgesia

Patient-controlled analgesia (PCA) or demand analgesia, although not new, has recently received considerable attention.* PCA is a regime that allows the patient to self-

* References 6, 7, 11, 12, 25, 28, 30, 33, 35, 42, 44, 57-59, 62, 65, 66, 70, 79, 80, 88-90.

administer small prescribed doses of analgesia sufficient to maintain relatively constant plasma concentrations and analgesia.[77] Most machines operate in a manner that allows the patients to trigger their own analgesic by pressing a small push-button control (similar to a nursing call button). After the infusion of a small dose of analgesia called the demand bolus, a preset lockout delay is activated, ensuring that another dose of analgesic is not delivered until the preset lockout interval has elapsed. This is to ensure that the therapeutic effect of the narcotic has occurred, preventing overdosing. As most opioid analgesics exert their effect within 5 minutes, the lockout interval on most machines cannot be set below this interval.

Given the many factors affecting the intensity of an individual's pain, it seems logical to utilize a system that allows an individualized approach to pain relief. Summarized in the accompanying box are the advantages and disadvantages of the PCA system.

PCA is not the universal answer for postoperative pain management. The literature frequently reminds the reader that PCA is not effective 100% of the time. There is no individual therapy that is effective for all postoperative patients. Currently however, PCA is the most effective and individualized therapy available.

Some professionals have expressed fear about the inadvertent use of PCA with individuals with addictive personalities. It has been documented that these patients tend to use PCA inappropriately. Usually they tend to self-administer maximal doses of medication—providing not only pain relief, but extra central nervous system effects as well.[62] These patients can be detected very early in the treatment period and may either be discontinued from the machine or have their pump settings adjusted to prevent abuse.

Effective use of PCA requires the cooperation of the entire health care team, including the patient. Proper instruction and understanding of how the machine operates is essential. Patients should be instructed on how to use the machine, when to use the machine, and what to do if they do not get pain relief or experience side effects. Another tip for smooth operation of the PCA pump is to encourage patients to use the machine before painful procedures such as ambulation and physiotherapy. Nurses also require instruction on the PCA machine and how to assess and work with patients using PCA.

◆ **ADVANTAGES AND DISADVANTAGES OF PCA**

ADVANTAGES	DISADVANTAGES
IV administration of narcotics; no need for IM injections	Patent IV line necessary
Very effective pain control	Individual must be competent and able to understand how to operate unit
Self-administration of analgesics	Cost of equipment
Less analgesic intake over the postoperative period	Patient may not prefer this type of therapy
Individualized approach to pain control	
More comfortable and improved recovery	
Less interference with physical activity (e.g., ambulation)	
Shorter hospital stay	
Ability to utilize with most operative patients	
Incidence of respiratory depression not higher than with other forms of analgesics	
Incidence of addiction less than .1% (not greater than other forms of analgesic administration)	

Spinal Analgesia

Since the discovery of opioid receptors in the spinal cord, spinal analgesia has become a more popular method of treating postoperative pain.[22,32,53] Therapy consists of the placement of a small amount of analgesic or anesthetic into the intrathecal (i.e., subarachnoid) or epidural space (see Chapter 7). This results in selective binding of analgesics to the spinal opiate receptors, leading to blockage of the nociceptive pathways.[53] A major advantage of spinal analgesia is the ability to eradicate sensory pathways without affecting motor function. Epidural analgesics are capable of treating both visceral and somatic pain associated with surgery.

Efficacy of Epidural Analgesia

Numerous studies with small samples have compared epidural analgesia with other regimes commonly used to treat postoperative pain (IM, IV, PCA). Epidural analgesia is reported to produce better and longer pain relief with fewer complications and faster recovery.[27,66a,b,92]

Patients report less nausea and vomiting, demonstrate improved pulmonary function, consume fewer analgesics over the course of their hospitalization, and have a lower incidence of paralytic ileus, improved bowel function, and shorter duration of stay in hospital.*

Complications of Epidural Analgesia

The insertion and maintenance of epidural catheters for the infusion of analgesia are invasive techniques that are the responsibility of the anesthetist. Complications may arise as a result of the catheter placement or the medication being administered. Nursing staff members are responsible for monitoring the patient's level of consciousness, pain intensity, respiratory rate, and infusion rate/volume on the pump. The dressing site is examined for signs of infection or leakage of medication around the catheter.

Potential catheter-related problems include neurological damage to the nerve roots or spinal cord, infection, hematoma, and migration of the catheter. No nerve damage has been reported in the literature.[32] The incidence of infection is less than 1% and is related to insertion technique and the length of time that the catheter remains in situ. The risk of infection is known to be higher in patients receiving long-term therapy (e.g., chronic pain therapy, cancer therapy). Bleeding may occur during the insertion of the catheter, resulting in a hematoma. The presence of hematoma may exert pressure on delicate spinal structures and lead to more serious neurological sequelae. Finally, migration of the epidural catheter can occur after placement. Gregg[29] reports two cases of subdural migration resulting in loss of analgesia.

Side effects of epidural analgesia may result from the type and amount of medication infused. These include nausea and vomiting, pruritis, and urinary retention. Nausea and vomiting occur with drugs such as morphine, fentanyl, and pethidine,

* References 9, 20, 29, 32, 53, 66a, 92.

although their incidence is less than with IM or IV administration. Pruritus can be very distressing to the patient; some patients find this to be more distressing than the pain itself.[53] Presently, histamine release is thought to be responsible for the pruritis. Preservative-free narcotics are also recommended for epidural administration.

Gregg[32] suggests the use of very low-dose naloxone as an adjunct to alleviate side effects without altering the analgesic effects. However, naloxone therapy is also not without complications and has resulted in acute pulmonary edema and sudden death.[32]

Respiratory depression is a major concern with spinal opiates, and its appearance is very unpredictable.[53] Respiratory depression emerges 6 to 11 hours after intrathecal opioid administration and may continue for as long as 23 hours. Respiratory depression after epidural opioid administration may arise anywhere from an hour to 6 hours after injection. Cousins and Mather[21] reviewed most of the reported cases of respiratory depression and listed those factors predisposing to its development. These include[21]:

1. Advanced age
2. Use of lipophilic opiates such as morphine
3. Higher doses of opioid
4. Preexisting respiratory disease
5. Concomitant drug therapy (e.g., benzodiazepines)
6. Low patient tolerance to opiates
7. Raised intrathoracic pressure, which apparently aids the cephalad spread of drugs

Postoperative Protocol

Epidural infusions are becoming more frequently used for a variety of patients undergoing surgery. Catheter placement is often done before surgery, so that analgesia may be provided throughout the operation. After insertion, patients receive a test dose of analgesia and are observed for signs of reaction. After the operation, patients are monitored in the recovery room and then transferred to the ward. The nurses are responsible for monitoring vital signs, including respiratory rate, level of consciousness, blood pressure, heart rate, and side effects (e.g., nausea, vomiting, and pruritus). Respiratory rate is monitored hourly for the first 24 hours and with any changes in infusion or medication concentration. Nurses should observe the patient's respiratory rate first because arousing the patient to obtain blood pressure readings may provide enough stimulation to increase the respiratory rate momentarily. A pulse oximeter is useful for these patients. Unfortunately, they are not always available for patients outside of a specialty area. The accompanying box outlines the advantages and disadvantages of epidural analgesia.

Nonpharmacological Approaches to Postoperative Pain

Transcutaneous Electrical Nerve Stimulation (TENS)

Transcutaneous electrical nerve stimulation has been used in recent years to alleviate postoperative incisional pain. The procedure (see Chapter 8) involves placement of electrodes near the incision immediately after wound closure. After the

◆ **ADVANTAGES AND DISADVANTAGES OF EPIDURAL ANALGESIA**

ADVANTAGES	DISADVANTAGES
Very effective pain control	Requires specially trained personnel to insert catheter
Efficient/time-saving for nursing staff	Certification of nursing staff is required
Less analgesic consumption over the postoperative period	Risk of serious sequelae may be higher than with conventional analgesic administration
Fewer side effects than with conventional analgesics	Respiratory depression is unpredictable, related to analgesic being infused
Lower incidence of complications	May be contraindicated in some patients (e.g., trauma and burn victims)
Shorter hospital stay	
Better postoperative recovery	
Less risk of respiratory depression — ability to vary duration by use of various drugs, from short duration of fentanyl to long duration of morphine	

operation, the electrodes are attached to a TENS stimulator, and high-frequency, low-intensity stimulation is initiated. Smith and others[71] report that TENS significantly reduces the cutaneous component of postoperative pain associated with movement and is less effective in reducing deep pain or visceral pain.

Some studies report benefits associated with TENS other than reductions in pain intensity and analgesic intake. Ali et al[3] reported improved respiratory function in a TENS-treated group (increased vital capacity, increased functional residual capacity, and normal arterial oxygen levels) when compared with a control group. On the other hand, Cooperman et al[19] found no appreciable differences in respiratory function when comparing patients receiving TENS with those receiving meperidine. Stratton and Smith[75] used TENS in patients undergoing cholecystectomy and found no differences in peak flow rates between groups.

Overall TENS is considered an effective adjunctive therapy in the treatment of postoperative pain. Its ability to reduce narcotic intake and lower pain intensity with no apparent side effects make it a feasible and practical option in conjunction with narcotic analgesics. Potential drawbacks to utilizing TENS include the need for training of staff and purchasing of expensive, specialized equipment.

◆ SUMMARY

Postoperative pain is an important issue in today's health care settings. Despite the advanced technology and plethora of pharmacological agents available, postoperative pain management continues to be very inadequate for many patients. Although many efforts are being made to study and improve our knowledge of pain, this improved knowledge base is not reflected in current practice.

Nurses play an essential role in the delivery of health care and are responsible for assessing and treating postoperative pain. Unfortunately, many nurses lack the knowledge base to do this effectively. Current practice is dictated by poor analgesic regimes and exaggerated fears of addiction and respiratory depression. Nurses have to replace these deficits in their knowledge base with an attitude that acute pain can be treated effectively with the use of a variety of techniques. This requires effective skills in assessment and evaluation of postoperative pain. Nurses should be creative in their approach to treating surgical patients, and utilize all the strategies that may alleviate the patient's suffering. The use of narcotics through a variety of routes will continue to be the mainstay of therapy; however, adjuncts to therapy, such as TENS, distraction techniques (e.g., music, imagery, etc.), ice, massage, and heat should be investigated for their effectiveness postoperatively. Multiple-technique approaches may be the most effective. Nurses need to be actively involved in research to determine effective pain strategies. Most important, nurses need to utilize research findings to optimize current practice.

REFERENCES

1. Angell M. (1982). The quality of mercy. *N Engl J Med 306* 98-99.
2. Ali J, Weisel R, Layug A, Kripke B, and Hectman H. (1974). Consequences of postoperative alterations in respiratory mechanics. *Am J Surg 128,* 376-382.
3. Ali J, Yaffe C, and Senette C. (1981). The effect of transcutaneous electric nerve stimulation on postoperative pain and pulmonary function. *Surgery 89,* 507-512.
4. Ashburn M and Fine P. (1989). Persistent pain following trauma. *Mil Med 154,* 86-89.
5. Benedetti C, Bonica J, and Bellucci G. (1984). Pathophysiology and therapy of postoperative pain: a review. In Benedetti C et al (eds), *Advances in pain research and therapy: volume 7* (pp. 373-407). New York: Raven Press.
6. Bennett RL, Batenhorst RL, Bivins BA, et al. (1982). Patient-controlled analgesia. A new concept of postoperative pain relief. *Ann Surg 195*(6), 700-704.
7. Bennett R, Batenhorst RL, Graves D, et al. (1982). Morphine titration in postoperative laparotomy patients using patient-controlled analgesia. *Curr Ther Res 32*(1), 45-51.
8. Bennett R, Batenhorst RL, Griffen WO, and Wright BD. (1982). Postoperative pulmonary function with patient-controlled analgesia. *Anesth Analg 61*(2 Abstract), 171.
9. Bronge HA, Johansson K, Ygge H, and Lindhagen J. (1988). Effect of continuous epidural analgesia on intestinal motility. *Br J Surg 75,* 1176-1178.
10. Bullingham RES. (1984). Postoperative pain. *Postgrad Med J 60*(710), 847-857.
11. Bullingham RES, Jacobs OLR, McQuay HJ, and Moore R. (1986). The Oxford system of patient-controlled analgesia. In Foley KM and Inturrisi CE (eds), *Advances in pain research and therapy: volume 8* (pp. 319-324). New York: Raven Press.
12. Burns JW, Hodsman NBA, McLintock TC, et al. (1989). The influence of patient characteristics on the requirements for postoperative analgesia. A reassessment using patient-controlled analgesia. *Anaesthesia 44,* 2-6.
13. Camporesi EM, Nielsen CH, Bromage PR, and Durrant PAC. (1983). Ven-

tilatory carbon dioxide sensitivity after intravenous and epidural morphine in volunteers. *Anesth Analg 62,* 633-640.

14. Cartwright PD. (1985). Pain control after surgery: a survey of current practice. *Ann Royal Coll Surg Engl 67,* 13-16.
15. Chadwick HS and Ready LB. (1988). Intrathecal and epidural morphine sulphate for postcesarean analgesia—a clinical comparison. *Anesthesiology 68,* 925-929.
16. Chapman CR and Bonica JJ. (1983). *Current concepts in acute pain.* Michigan: Upjohn Co.
17. Chrubasik J, Wust H, Schulte-Monting J, Thon KT, and Zindler M. (1988). Relative analgesic potency of epidural fentanyl, alfentanyl, and morphine in treatment of postoperative pain. *Anesthesiology 68,* 929-933.
18. Cohen FL. (1980). Postsurgical pain relief: patients' status and nurses' medication choices. *Pain 9,* 265-274.
19. Cooperman A, Hall B, Mikalacki K, Hardy R, and Sadar E. (1977). Use of transcutaneous electrical nerve stimulation in the control of postoperative pain. *Am J Surg 96,* 649-659.
20. Cousins MJ and Bridenbaugh PO. (1986). Spinal opioids and pain relief in acute pain. In Cousins MJ and Phillips GD (eds), *Acute pain management* (pp. 151-185). New York: Churchill Livingstone.
21. Cousins MJ and Mather LE. (1984). Intrathecal and epidural administration of opioids. *Anesthesiology 61,* 261-275.
22. Cousins MJ and Phillips GD. (1986). *Acute pain management.* New York: Churchill Livingstone.
23. Craig DB. (1981). Postoperative recovery of pulmonary function. *Anesth Analg 60*(1), 46-52.
24. Cuschiere RJ, Morran CG, Howie JC, and McArdle CS. (1985). Postoperative pain and pulmonary complications: comparison of three analgesic regimens. *Br J Surg 72,* 495-498.
25. Dahlstrom B, Tamsen A, Paalzow L, and Hartvig P. (1982). Patient-controlled analgesic therapy, part iv: pharmacokinetics and analgesic plasma concentrations of morphine. *Clin Pharmacokinet 7,* 266-279.
26. Donovan M, Dillon P, and McGuire L. (1987). Incidence and characteristics of pain in a sample of medical-surgical inpatients. *Pain 30,* 69-78.
27. El-Baz N and Goldin M. (1987). Continuous epidural infusion of morphine for pain relief after cardiac operations. *J Thorac Cardiovasc Surg 93,* 878-883.
28. English MJM. (1987). Patient-controlled analgesia—new treatment modality for the relief of postoperative pain. *Tod Ther Trends* September, 15-29.
29. Fischer RL, Lubenow TR, Liceaga A, McCarthy RJ, and Ivankovitch AD. (1988). Comparison of continuous epidural infusion of fentanyl-bupivacaine and morphine-bupivacaine in management of postoperative pain. *Anesth Analg 67,* 559-563.
30. FitzGerald JJ. (1987). Let your patient control his analgesia. *Nursing 7,* 48-51.
31. Graves DA, Foster TS, Batenhorst RL, Bennett RL, and Baumann TJ. (1983). Patient-controlled analgesia. *Ann Intern Med 99,* 360-366.
32. Gregg R. (1989). Spinal analgesia. In Oden RV (ed), *Anaesthesiology clinics of North America, management of postoperative pain* (pp 79-100). Toronto: WB Saunders.
33. Hadaway LC. (1989). Evaluation of advanced IV therapy. Part 2: patient controlled analgesia. *JIN 12*(3), 184-191.

34. Harmer M, Slattery PJ, Rosen M, and Vickers MD. (1983). Intramuscular on demand analgesia: double blind controlled trial of pethidine, buprenorphine, morphine and meptazinol. *Br Med J 286,* 680-682.
35. Hodsman NBA, Kenny GNC and McArdle CS. (1988). Patient controlled analgesia and urinary retention. *Br J Surg 75,* 212.
36. Hjortso NC, Christensen T, and Kehlet H. (1985). Effects of extradural administration of local anaesthetic agents and morphine on the urinary excretion of cortisol, catecholamines and nitrogen following abdominal surgery. *Br J Anaesth 57,* 400-406.

36a. Inturrisi CE and Umans JG. (1983). Pethidine and its active metabolite, norpethidine. In Bullingham RES (ed), *Opiate analgesics, clinics in anaesthesiology* (p. 123). London: Saunders.

37. Janig W and Kollman W. (1984). The involvement of the sympathetic nervous system in pain. Possible neuronal mechanisms. *Arzneim-Forsch/Drug Research 34*(11), 1066-1072.
38. Jeans ME, Stratford JG, Melzack R, and Monks RC. (1979). Assessment of pain. *Can Fam Phys 25,* 159-162.
39. Jeans ME. (1986). The scope of pain and its variation. In: *Integrated approach to the management of pain.* Report of the National Institute of Health Consensus Development Conference. *6*(3), 24-27.
40. Jorgensen BC, Schmidt JF, Risbo A, Pedersen J, and Kolby P. (1985). Regular interval preventive pain relief compared with on-demand treatment after hysterectomy. *Pain 21,* 137-142.
41. Kay B. (1981). Postoperative pain relief. Use of an on-demand analgesia computer (ODAC) and a comparison of the rate of use of fentanyl and alfentanyl. *Anaesthesia 36,* 949-951.
42. Keeri-Szanto M and Heaman S. (1972). Postoperative demand analgesia. *Surg Gynaecol Obstet 134,* 647-651.
43. Lange PM, Dahn MS, and Jacobs LA. (1988). Patient-controlled analgesia versus intermittent analgesia. *Heart Lung 17*(5), 495-498.
44. Loper KA and Ready BL. (1989). Epidural morphine after anterior cruciate ligament repair: a comparison with patient-controlled intravenous morphine. *Anesth Analg 68,* 350-352.
45. Mann HJ, Fuhs DW, and Cerra FB. (1987). Pharmacokinetics and pharmacodynamics in critically ill patients. *W J Surg 11,* 210-217.
46. Marks RM and Sachar EJ. (1973). Undertreatment of medical inpatients with narcotic analgesics. *Ann Intern Med 78*(2), 173-181.
47. McCaffery M and Hart L. (1976). Undertreatment of acute pain with narcotics. *Am J Nurs 76*(10), 1586-1591.
48. McCaffery M. (1984). Pain in the critical care patient. *Dimen Crit Care 3*(6), 323-325.
49. McGrath D, Thurston N, Wright D, Preshaw R, and Fermin P. (1989). Comparison of one technique of patient-controlled postoperative analgesia with intramuscular meperidine. *Pain 37,* 265-270.
50. Melzack R. (1990). The tragedy of needless pain. *Sci Am* 262(2), 27-32.
51. Melzack R, Abbott FV, Zachon W, Mulder DS, and Davis MWL. (1987). Pain on a surgical ward: a survey of the duration and intensity of pain and the effectivness of medication. *Pain 29,* 73-83.
52. Meyers JR, Lembeck L, O'Kane H, and Baue AE. (1975). Changes in functional residual capacity of the lung after operation. *Arch Surg 110,* 576-583.

53. Morgan M. (1987). Epidural and intrathecal opioids. *Anaesth Inten Care 15*(1), 61-67.
54. Nimmo WS and Duthie DJR. (1987). Pain relief after surgery. *Anaesth Intens Care 15*(1), 68-71.
55. Oden RV. (1989). Management of postoperative pain. *Anaesth Clin North Am 7*(1), Toronto: WB Saunders.
56. Owen H, Glavin RJ, Reekie RM, and Trew S. (1986). Patient-controlled analgesia. Experience of two new machines. *Anaesthesia 41*(12), 1230-1235.
57. Owen H, Plummer L, Armstrong I, Mather LE, and Cousins MJ. (1989). Variables of patient-controlled analgesia. 1. Bolus size. *Anaesthesia 44,* 7-10.
58. Owen H, Szekely M, Plummer L, Cushnie M, and Mather LE. (1989). Variables of patient-controlled analgesia. 2. Concurrent infusion. *Anaesthesia 44,* 11-13.
59. Panfilla R, Brunckhorst L, and Dundon R. (1988). Nursing implications of patient-controlled analgesia. *J Intraven Nurs 11*(2), 75-77.
60. Paul P. (1980). *A study of postoperative pain and anxiety.* Unpublished master's thesis (applied), McGill University, Montreal, Quebec.
61. Phillips GD and Cousins MJ. (1986). Neurological mechanisms of pain and the relationship of pain, anxiety, and sleep. In Cousins MJ and Phillips GD (eds), *Acute pain management.* New York: Churchill Livingston.
62. Pierce JE. (1988). Viewpoint: from all perspectives, patient-controlled analgesia seen as beneficial and profitable. *Pharm Pract News,* February, 1988.
63. Portenoy RK and Foley KM. (1986). Chronic use of opioid analgesics in non-malignant pain: report of 38 cases. *Pain 25,* 171-186.
64. Raj PP, Knarr D, Runyon J, and Hopson CN. (1987). Patient-controlled analgesia for postoperative pain in orthopaedic patients. *Orthopaed Rev 16*(12), 69-75.
65. Raj PP, Knarr D, Vigdorth E, et al. (1985). Comparative study of continuous epidural infusions versus systematic analgesics for postoperative pain relief. *Anaesthesiology 63,* 698.
66. Rapp RP, Bivins BA, Littrell RA, and Foster TS. (1989). Patient-controlled analgesia: a review of effectiveness of therapy and an evaluation of currently available devices. *DICP, Ann Pharmacol 23* 899-904.
66a. Rawal N, Sjostrand UH, and Dahlstrom B. (1981). Postoperative pain relief by epidural morphine. *Anesth Analg 60:* 72b.
66b. Reiz S, Anlim J, Ahrenfeld B, et al. (1981). Epidural morphine for postoperative pain relief. *Acta Anaesthesiol Scand 25:* 11.
67. Rosenburg PH, Heino A, and Scheinin B. (1984). Comparison of intramuscular analgesia, intercostal block, epidural morphine and on-demand-i.v.-fentanyl in the control of pain after upper abdominal surgery. *Acta Anaesthesiol Scand 28,* 603-607.
68. Rutter PC, Murphy F, and Dudley HAF. (1980). Morphine: controlled trial of different methods of administration for postoperative pain relief. *Br Med J 5,* 12-13.
69. Sechzer PH. (1971). Studies in pain with the analgesia-demand system. *Anaesth Analg 50,* 1-10.
70. Sinatra RS, Lodge K, Sibert K, et al. (1989). A comparison of morphine,

meperidine, and oxymorphine as utilized in patient-controlled analgesia following cesarean delivery. *Anaesthesiology, 70,* 585-590.

71. Smith CM, Guralnick MS, Gelfand MM, and Jeans, ME. (1986). The effects of transcutaneous electrical nerve stimulation on post-cesarean pain. *Pain 27,* 181-193.
72. Sriwantankul K, Weis OF, Alloza JL, et al. (1983). Analysis of narcotic analgesic usage in the treatment of postoperative pain. *JAMA 250*(7), 926-929.
73. Stanski DR. (1987). The role of pharmacokinetics in anaesthesia: application to intravenous infusions. *Anaesth Intens Care 15*(1), 13-18.
74. Stanski DR. (1987). Narcotic pharmacokinetics and dynamics: the basis of infusion application. *Anaesth Intens Care 15*(1), 19-22.
75. Stratton SA and Smith MM. (1980). Postoperative thoracotomy. Effect of transcutaneous electrical nerve stimulation on forced vital capacity. *Phys Ther 60*(1), 45-47.
76. Taenzer P, Melzack R, and Jeans ME. (1986). Influence of psychological factors on postoperative pain, mood and analgesic requirements. *Pain 24,* 331-342.
77. Tammisto T and Tigerstedt L. (1982). Narcotic analgesics in postoperative pain relief in adults. *Acta Anaesth Scand 74* (supp 1), 161-164.
78. Tamsen A, Hartvig P, Dahlstrom B, Lindstrom B, and Holmdah MH. (1979). Patient controlled analgesic therapy in the early postoperative period. *Acta Anaesth Scand 5,* 464-470.
79. Tamsen A, Hartvig P, Fagerlund C, Dahlstrom B, and Bondesson U. (1982). Patient-controlled analgesic therapy: clinical experience. *Acta Anaesth Scand 74* (supp 1), 157-160.
80. Tamsen A, Sjoestroem S, and Hartvig P. (1986). The Uppsala experience of patient-controlled analgesia. In Foley KM and Inturrisi CE (eds), *Advances in pain research and therapy: volume 8* (pp 325-331). New York: Raven Press.
81. Teske K, Daut RL, and Cleeland CS. (1983). Relationships between nurses' observations and patients' self-report of pain. *Pain 16,* 289-292.
82. Thomas DW and Owen H. (1988). Patient-controlled analgesia—the need for caution. *Anaesthesia 43,* 770-772.
83. Traynor C and Hall GM. (1981). Endocrine and metabolic changes during surgery: Anaesthesia implications. *Br J Anaesth 53,* 153-160.
84. Vanstrum GS, Bjornson KM, and Ilko R. (1988). Postoperative effects of intrathecal morphine in coronary artery bypass surgery. *Anaesth Analg 67,* 261-267.
85. Volicer BJ. (1978). Hospital stress and patient reports of pain and physical status. *J Hum Stress 4*(6), 28-37.
86. Wattwil M, Thoren T, Hennerdal S, and Garvill J-E. (1989). Epidural analgesia with bupivacaine reduces postoperative paralytic ileus after hysterectomy. *Anaesth Analg 68,* 353-358.
87. Weis OF, Sriwantankul K, Alloza JL, Weintraub M, and Lasagna L. (1983). Analysis of narcotic analgesic usage in the treatment of postoperative pain. *Anesth Analg 62,* 70-74.
88. Wasylak T. (1988). *The impact of pain on postoperative physical functioning.* Unpublished master's thesis, McGill University, Montreal, Quebec.
89. White PF. (1985). Patient-controlled analgesia: a new approach to the management of postoperative pain. *Semin Anesth 4*(3), 255-266.

90. White PF. (1988). Use of patient-controlled analgesia for management of acute pain. *JAMA 259*(2), 243-247.
91. Wood GJ, Lloyd JW, Bullingham RE, Britton BJ, and Finch DR. (1981). Postoperative analgesia for day-case herniorrhaphy patients. A comparison of cryoanalgesia, paravertebral blockade and oral analgesia. *Anaesthesia 36*(6) 603-610.
92. Yaeger MP, Glass DD, and Neff RK. (1987). Epidural anesthesia and analgesia in high-risk surgical patients. *Anaesthesiology 66,* 729-732.
93. Zimmermann RM. (1984). Basic concepts of pain and pain therapy. *Arzneim-Forsch/Drug Research 34*(11), 1053-1059.

16

Chronic Pain and the Management of Conflict

Robin E. Weir
Joan M. Crook

◆ INTRODUCTION

Pain and its consequences pose some of the most common yet difficult and important problems faced by nurses in their day-to-day practice. Indeed, the symptom of pain is of great clinical importance in that it is often the reason that people seek health care, and more often than not it becomes the focus of treatment and ultimately the landmark for success or failure. For the average person, the probability of suffering from a pain problem is very high. VonKorff[34] estimates that 85% of people surviving to age 70 years will have experienced a problem with back pain. In addition, the lifetime occurrence of headache, abdominal pain, and chest pain conditions are predicted to exceed 40%. We are, in fact, confronted by pain problems on all fronts, be it in suffering from some painful condition ourselves or in being a caregiver to a pain sufferer.

Within the clinical situation, the nurse usually spends more time with the patient than any other member of the health care team and hence is more regularly confronted with the needs and requests for pain relief and the challenge of pain management. For example, it is reported that 35% to 75% of surgical patients have significant pain and inadequate pain relief during the first 48 postoperative hours.[13] How the nurse responds to this clinical situation is variable but very well may be central to the effectiveness of treatment. Consider the options that are possible: she may attend to the patient's need or request by administering the prescribed dose and schedule of analgesia or by helping him use other coping measures; or she may fail to anticipate or even be aware of the patient's condition of pain; or she may ignore the patient's need or request by delaying or withholding analgesia, information, support, or encouragement; or, finally, she may actively mismanage the patient's treatment by making inadequate treatment choices (giving too little too late) because of inaccurate or erroneous assumptions ("the patient cannot be having *that* much pain!") or insufficient information (not knowing the length of time between previous doses and/or the effectiveness of treatment).[8]

The factors that influence the nurse's choice of options are not predictably known. Studies concerned with postoperative pain management, for example, have shown that the administration of narcotic analgesia postoperatively is influenced by factors other than physician orders and the type of surgical treatment.[36] Indeed there is some suggestion that there are important variables in the relationship between patient and nurse that may influence treatment decisions. From this perspective, the patient and nurse are said to be engaged in some reciprocal relationship in which the behavior, beliefs, and circumstance of the patient influence the behavior and decision-making of the nurse.[17,29] On occasion this relationship may result in a struggle for control, particularly when the patient feels dependent on the "goodness" of his caregivers. The patient is in a vulnerable position as a "petitioner for aid" from those who have the power to provide relief. Treatment conceivably could be withheld, or other sanctions could be evoked against him, such as being "reported to some higher authority" or being labeled uncooperative or troublesome, or even being discharged.[29] The nurse's monopoly of resources and information in a particular area give her power over patients by giving her control over what is needed and wanted by them.[14] In this scenario, the patient is in a struggle for control of his pain and himself (his territory and area of expertise), and the nurse is in a struggle for control over the treatment (her territory and area of expertise). In the ensuing battle, the roles of the person in pain (as petitioner) on the one hand, and the nurse (as authority) on the other hand, reinforce each other and serve to maintain and perpetuate each other's inappropriate behavior. How this cycle of problematic behaviors, attitudes, and feelings can be broken is fundamental to the therapeutic process and the relief of suffering.

The purpose of this chapter is to offer a practical view of some of the factors that contribute to the conflict between the patient and nurse over pain management and to suggest some strategies for managing and resolving the conflict. The view taken here is not that conflict can always be avoided but rather, given a conflictive situation, can the nurse resolve the conflict? What are the alternatives to the feelings of martyrdom (the long-suffering nurse giving in to patient demands) or the need for omniscience (the expectation that the nurse must know what is best for him)? What kind of "cognitive shift" must the nurse make to alter her treatment approach when treatment goals are not being achieved? There is a need for more explicit description of this "shift" in thinking to guide practitioners through many of the essential steps of the therapeutic process.

◆ SOURCES OF CONFLICT: I. CLASSIFICATION OF TYPES OF PAIN

The treatment approaches most often chosen by clinicians working with patients suffering pain depend on the frame of reference they use in selecting the clinical data considered relevant to the problem and to the treatment.[21] An elaboration of this point may be useful to understand where some of the gaps in our knowledge and understanding exist.

In general, clinicians have found it useful to classify pain into three major categories based on etiology or time. The pain that accompanies acute injury, disease, or surgery is called acute pain; pain associated with cancer or other progressive disorders is called malignant or chronic malignant pain; and pain that cannot be explained by an active organic lesion is chronic nonmalignant or chronic benign pain.[24,23,19] Acute pain, particularly in the form of postoperative pain, should be the least complex to manage since its source is usually distinct and its course is self-limiting.[20] Indeed, there is ample evidence that effective postoperative pain control is possible.[6] Increased knowledge about the factors contributing to pain perception and pain relief and the development and availability of new technologies in pain management could be expected to reduce the incidence of suffering postoperatively.

Instead, the evidence continues to indicate that a significant proportion of surgical patients receive inadequate pain relief.[7,35,13] It has been shown that physicians prescribe less than the amount of analgesia needed, nurses administer less than the prescribed doses,[1,7,4] and certain patients (children, elderly, and females) are at risk for undertreatment.[4,16,30]

Another pain category is attributed to pain that persists after tissue damage has apparently healed or in the absence of evident tissue damage, and is classified as chronic or persistent pain.[23] In the community at large, this type of pain has a reported prevalence of 11%,[9] and clinicians working with chronic pain patients are beginning to recognize the multiple biological, psychological, and social dimensions to this pain phenomenon.[18] While the etiology of such pain is poorly understood, there is growing acknowledgement of its global effect on the sufferer in the form of compromised job performance, relationships, activities of daily living, and social and emotional functioning. For example, many patients with chronic pain who attend specialized pain clinics share some well-recognized characteristics: The onset of their pain is most often linked to a work-related injury; they have significant difficulties in performing regular activities of daily living; they report loss of appetite, loss of energy, and decreased libido; and other indications of depression include feelings of hopelessness and thoughts of death. The long-term consequences of their problem include job loss, lawsuits, drug and alcohol abuse, and frequent use of health services.[10]

Traditional medical interventions have often failed to alleviate persistent pain problems and the experience of suffering. In response to this difficult situation, some patients experience feelings of helplessness and hopelessness, and are demoralized about their problems.[33] Stuck in patterns of unproductive and frequently conflictive behavior, their continuing search for a cure frequently places them in frustrating and nontherapeutic relationships with their health care providers. Nurses and physicians may regard these pain sufferers with growing suspicion, which, not infrequently, leads to adversarial relationships. These efforts made by patients to deal with their pain have been called coping strategies. Both acute and chronic pain sufferers develop cognitive and behavioral coping strategies, and the type that is used may greatly affect their ability to adjust to their pain condition.[26] Indeed, there is some evidence that depressive withdrawal and an adversarial posture in patients make a crucial difference in their ability to adjust to their chronic condition. The success of behavioral approaches in enabling patients to adjust to chronic pain conditions may be explained by the way these approaches focus patients' attention on changing these self-defeating attitudes and behavior.[11]

The tendency to apply disease-model principles, which assume that symptoms are "caused" by some "underlying pathology" or prior event, forces the categorization of pain patients into either organic or psychogenic categories.[25] This system of thinking splits the psychological and social from what is objectively physical. Compounding the effect of such a point of view is the additional belief that physical problems are more "respectable" than the others.[32] Practitioners also have expectations about the amount of pain patients should have for a given problem, for how long, and with what acceptable behaviors.[15] Patients are subtly encouraged and sometimes blatantly required to conform to the practitioner's expectations. Such assumptions and expectations create a simplistic and unprofitable perspective, as represented in Figure 16-1. From this point of view there is only one appropriate, acceptable, and respectable category in which the patient can be placed.

The remaining options lead to the labeling of "nonconforming" patients as malingerers, troublesome, neurotic, psychogenic, or hysterical. In such instances, patients feel that they have to prove that their pain is real and at the same time, not be labeled as a complainer. Health professionals, sensing the patient's anxiety and defensiveness, feel frustrated and

Cause	**Symptom Expectation**	
	Appropriate	Inappropriate
Respectable (physical, organic)	*Accept*	Reject ? Neurotic
Not respectable (psychogenic, psychosocial)	Reject ? Psychogenic	Reject ? Hysterical

FIGURE 16-1. Categories of problem definition.

powerless to do what their roles demand, that is, relieve the pain. The ensuing battles may be manifest in a process of fruitless diagnostic and therapeutic maneuvers. Patients continue to be labeled pejoratively and may demonstrate excessive drug use or drug dependence, mood and personality changes, and exaggerated pain behavior.[25]

It is apparent from this brief review that pain, regardless of its source and manifestations, is a complex, challenging, and frustrating problem for the patient and clinician alike. It is also apparent that fundamental to the understanding and treatment of pain, whether it be acute or chronic, are the attitudes and expectations of the patient and the nurse, and the resulting quality of the nurse-patient relationship. Because of the importance of the nurse's role in implementing any treatment program with the patient, it may be useful to examine the nurse-patient relationship for some of the factors and events that occur within a conflict episode.

Although conflict can have constructive or destructive effects, depending on its management, the purpose of this analysis is to identify where strategic intervention could influence the constructiveness of the exchanges between patient and nurse, the essence of problem solving, to lead to treatment progress and adherence. The underlying assumption is that some theoretical orientation may reveal the various dimensions of the interaction and hence increase the range of alternatives available for intervention. When the rationale for an intervention is known, the outcomes are better understood and evaluated, and alternate intervention approaches can be identified.

◆ SOURCES OF CONFLICT: II. PROPERTIES OF THE PAIN EXPERIENCE

There are certain properties of the pain experience that are potential sources of conflict between helper and pain sufferer. Some of the more common properties are subjectivity, meaning and threat, expression, multidimensionality, and uncertainty.

Subjectivity

Pain is a personal, subjective experience that invades the sufferer's awareness effortlessly and with certainty. It is whatever the person says it is and exists whenever he says it does.[28] For the person in pain, the certainty of pain is uncontested, whereas, for the observer, the elusiveness of pain makes it unconfirmable. For persons around the pain sufferer it is relatively easy to remain unaware of the person's pain, even to doubt its very existence, or finally to deny its existence. Even with the best effort to try to relate to the pain, the observer can conceive of the adversities of the experienced pain only in the most removed way. "Whatever pain achieves, it achieves, in part, through its unsharability, and it ensures this unsharability through its resistance to language." Indeed, pain can actively destroy language, reducing sufferers in the most extreme instances to "an inarticulate state of cries and moans."[27]

It is revealing that no other interior state of consciousness—emotional, perceptual, or somatic—resists naming and description like pain. One explanation is that pain, unlike any other state of consciousness, has no object in the external world to which to refer.[27] Pain is not "of or for anything." All of our other interior states are accompanied by objects in the external world. For example, we have a feeling for something or somebody—love of, fear of, hunger for—which can be made knowable to another through description. In this way we enable others "to *see*" what we are thinking or feeling. Precisely because pain has no objective reference in the external world, it does not lend itself to verbal description. There is no alteration in the blood count, no change on the EKG, no pattern on the CAT scan. Alternatively, consider, for example, the experience of hunger. People are rarely challenged about the veracity of their report of hunger. Measures of intensity, duration, and frequency are not required before one provides the "sufferer" with a meal. Although it is generally accepted that hunger is a personal experience, it is also describable and sharable. "Hungry as a bear" or "I could eat a horse" convey a meaning and experience that is knowable. Food intake is quantifiable as are measures of utilization (blood sugars, metabolic tests, weight, etc.). Further, the failure to complain of hunger under certain circumstances (anorexia, starvation), is considered to be a dangerous signal. In contrast, the failure to report pain under circumstances when it is expected is usually greeted with relief, if not acknowledgement and reinforcement for bravery and stoicism! The major dilemma in this whole issue of pain is the challenge of expecting care givers to assess the quality and quantity of a patient's pain, that is, judge whether or not the patient has pain and how much, when pain can be known only by the person experiencing it. The potential for making an error in judgment is very high under these circumstances.

Meaning and Threat

Another source of conflict between patient and nurse concerns the meaning of the pain and the threat it poses to the individual who has it. Because the meaning and the threat are different for each person, it is inappropriate and most often inadequate to make inferences about pain behavior based on simplistic or stereotypic information. Although some differences in pain perception and responsiveness have been associated with culture, age, gender, and social class, these one-dimensional assessments are inappropriate to problems requiring more complex assessments. When pain is experienced as a punishment, threat, or warning and generates the fear of a future of constant suffering, debility, or even death, then it should come as no surprise that our usual treatments and remedies have little or no lasting effect. We eventually run out of prescriptions except the final one: "You'll have to learn to live with it!"

Expression

Pain complaints are a form of communication whereby patients may express their symptoms of pain to convey distress or gain desired benefits. Indeed, a chronic pain problem may set up familial and social patterns of attention and reward that reinforce the pain behavior even though the patient is unaware of the association between the two events. To the extent that the behavior is seen as sick rather than bad, certain advantages result. Treatment rather than punishment is the appropriate response. Mechanic[22] points out that illness behavior accompanying pain is a common method of coping with the pain because it is more socially acceptable than more direct expression, such as moaning. The language the pain sufferer uses to express his feelings and how he behaves in response to his pain (limping, grimacing, rubbing the site, etc.) are not typically noticed or consciously manipulated by him. Indeed, the illness behavior and the decision to seek help frequently are, from the patient's point of view, a rational attempt to make sense of his problem and cope with it within the limits of his intelligence and his social and cultural understandings.[22] Yet the illness behavior and its implicit appeal for attention or sympathy sometimes engender doubt in others, and the sufferer becomes engaged in a struggle to prove the legitimacy of the symptom. The limp, moan, or grimace that is perceived by others as "exaggerated" sets up another climate of suspicion, which may raise questions such as, "What is he trying to avoid or prove?" These suspicions lead to useless discrediting approaches, such as treating him as if he were lazy or weak, which have negative moral overtones.[3]

Multidimensionality

Additionally, pain is multidimensional in its effects. For the toothache sufferer, the report of pain is of the total experience: the pain, the inability to sleep, the resulting fatigue, the fear and worry about what the dentist will do, the total absorption of trying to live through the pain now, the pacing, the headaches, the difficulty in concentrating on anything else and do a job well, and the irritability with family, friends, and co-workers. When the pain becomes all encompassing, the person's entire life is given over to the experience of pain. Interventions that fail to acknowledge and address these social and personal definitions typically fail. Health care providers, in exasperation, tell these patients that their pain is "all in their head." The idea that it could be otherwise challenges all of our understanding of the structure and function of the human body! Pain *is* a central phenomenon, meaning that it is processed or experienced consciously—in the brain in the head. It is this very property of pain that contributes to the multidimensional aspects of the experience (the unique subjective experience with cognitive, affective, and sensory components in the context of the individual's background and ongoing life experience) and to the self-absorption of the person experiencing it.

Uncertainty

Finally, for the person with chronic pain, new and persistent symptoms take on a different meaning. New symptoms (aching, stiffness) or the reappearance of symptoms (irritability, fatigue), may signal the failure of treatment efforts and/or the progress of the pain problem. Perceived in this way, the symptoms may generate a wave of fear and panic and actually exacerbate the original symptoms. In addition, persistent symptoms, such as the pain itself, fatigue, muscle spasm, insomnia, etc., may take on a life of their own. In fact, pain and its accompaniments can begin to define one's very existence. All activities are experienced in relation to these symptoms, and even in the absence of continuous pain, activities are colored by its threat, sometimes by avoiding the activities or anticipating them with anxiety and despair.

Sharron

Sharron suffered a whiplash neck injury in a car accident 4 years ago. She was gradually recovering when 2 years later she was in another rear-end collision. Her neck and shoulders ache constantly, and the pain is aggravated by any physical activity. She has severe headaches, trouble concentrating, and memory lapses. Sharron's two major goals are to get to work and to "last" for the day. Her weekends are devoted to getting caught up on her housework and to preparing meals for the rest of the week. She has stopped having family and friends over to visit because she is too exhausted to think about planning an evening with them, let alone to prepare refreshments or a dinner!

During the course of Sundays she gradually becomes aware of a feeling of dread in anticipation of Mondays. She usually has a restless and disturbed night and begins yet another week feeling fatigued, painful, and fearful of whether she will be able to tolerate what the week has in store for her. Each day of the week she returns home from work more fatigued, in pain, and depressed than when she left. Each evening she makes supper for the family, cleans up and goes to bed—to try to get pain relief as well as to try to obtain some rest.

Sharron's life has become a constricted program of survival in which she is "stuck" in unproductive cycles of pain, anxiety, depression, and fatigue. Her choices, as she sees them, are to try to contain the symptoms, but with each passing day she feels less and less hopeful about being able to do even that and feels more and more out of control.

The uncertainty of the "cause" of the pain for many chronic pain sufferers, plus the uncertainty of when the pain will recur or escalate, influence the total pain experience. Patients worry about how long the episode will last, whether it will be reversible this time, and whether they can endure it. The person's sense of time in turn shapes the pain experience and the perception of the accompanying symptoms.[3] Sharron's "now" of pain seems to be endless: each moment in pain seems like an eternity. Her major concern is enduring the pain. "Time seems to have stopped for her and she feels flooded" with her pain, fatigue, and depression, and further distanced from hope for a recovered future.

◆ SOURCES OF CONFLICT: III. MODELS OF MANAGEMENT

Clinicians who work with complicated clinical problems, particularly those who work with chronic pain problems, need to be flexible because of the multiple dimensions of the problem. The therapeutic process by necessity, therefore, is made up of a variety of interventions that must be integrated under some "umbrella of meaning." These "umbrellas" or frameworks influence how one thinks about the problem of interest (chronic pain) and can expand or constrict the definition of the problem by determining what is treated and what is not. Because the nurse implicitly uses one or a combination of models in assessing and managing clinical situations, it is important to know what guides his or her decision-making and what can expand the choices. It is equally important to know the model from which the patient is making his interpretations and creating his expectations. Like the patient with whom she is working, the nurse also can become "stuck" in unproductive vicious circles that undermine her control, confidence, and hope, and create the ingredients for unproductive conflict.

These points are illustrated by applying three different models of management to the same middle-aged executive suffering from migraine headaches.

Biomedical Model

The biomedical model views pain as a signal that something is wrong. Practitioners using this model concern themselves with etiology, pathogenesis, signs and symptoms, differential diagnosis, treatment, and prognosis. Knowledge of the "cause" determines the treatment (Figure 16-2).

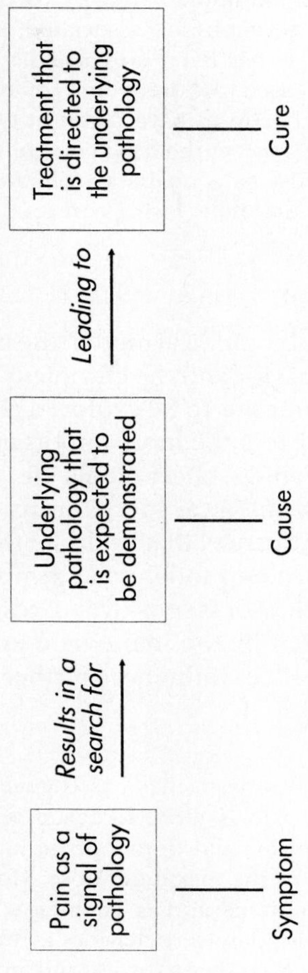

FIGURE 16-2. Andrew viewed from a biomedical perspective.

Andrew

Andrew has been studied at length in all the major migraine headache clinics in North America and by the leading experts. He has had multiple diagnostic tests, and brain tumors and vascular lesions have been ruled out. He presents as a fairly typical migraine sufferer, and the "cause" of his pain is theoretically explainable. Treatment consists of searching for additional triggers to his headaches and eliminating factors that he thinks are associated, such as food additives and air pollution. He has been prescribed a variety of medications, which have decreased the frequency of his headaches. Recently, however, he has begun to have different types of headaches. On occasion, he has had to go to the local emergency department for stronger analgesics because he is unable to tolerate the pain of these headaches, and he feels that he is losing control.

Behavioral Model

In contrast with the biomedical model, the behavioral model views the patient's behavior and the chronicity or time frame of the problem as the symptoms to be explored (Figure 16-3). The longer the pain has existed, the more important are psychological factors such as meaning, effect on his life, and uncertainty, in influencing the physiological mechanisms, such as muscle tension and sleep disturbance, that underlie the pain behavior. Behavior is to the learning model what symptoms are to the disease model. Pain behavior is sensitive to, responds to, and/or is particularly controlled by the immediate environment. The quality of the consequences influences further activity.[18]

Andrew (cont'd)

The quality of Andrew's headaches has changed over the past 3 months. He reports his pain is more localized at the onset of the migraine, with more intensity and duration. He has been warned to limit his Cafergot intake to the maximum dose. He has paid increasing attention to his symptoms and is keeping a diary. Treatment consists of reinforcing his adaptive behaviors in handling himself in spite of the headache, e.g., going to work and not focusing on his pain. Attention received from his family inadvertently reinforces his help-seeking behavior, e.g., going to hospital.

Cognitive-Behavioral Model

The cognitively oriented models explain behavior in terms of the meaning that individuals give to their experience. These

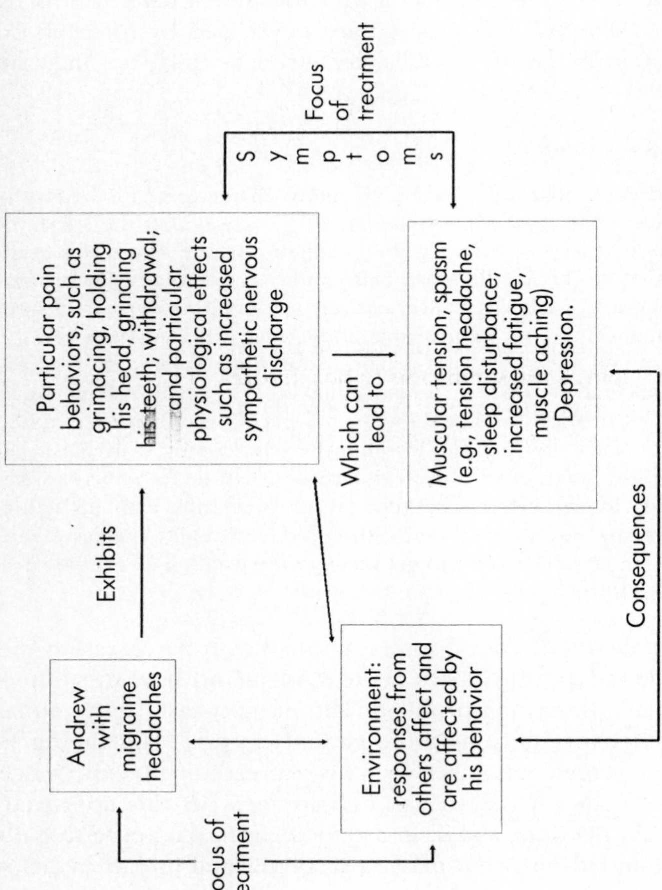

FIGURE 16-3. Andrew viewed from a behavioral perspective.

models postulate an association between thought content and behavior.[2] The focus of the assessment, therefore, is the thoughts and feelings that may be sources of apprehension, fear, beliefs, needs, and so on. The focus of treatment is to change the patient's internal dialogue and interpretation of his problems (cognitions) so that they are understood as being solvable and at least partly under the individual's control. A sense of control and mastery are developed by focusing on successes (behaviors), which are given as evidence that the problem is controllable (Figure 16-4).

Andrew (cont'd)

Andrew is worried that the changing character of his headache indicates "real" pathology (beliefs). He proposes that the spasm of the blood vessels is reducing the circulation to the side of his brain and right eye (hence the sharp pain) and that eventually this process could interrupt the circulation entirely (rationale to support his belief). In addition, he is concerned about what will happen when the Cafergot no longer controls his pain within the allowable dose schedule (anticipatory anxiety, catastrophizing). He organizes his treatment, i.e., medication, hot showers, hot packs, to enhance his ability to get to work and make it through the day (coping strategies). He has not lost much time from work (attitude) but he feels increasingly stressed, knows that he has become more irritable with his fellow workers, and he arrives home exhausted each night (negative self-appraisal). He tries to rest to get through the evening in a reasonable mood with the family (coping strategies).

Cognitive behavioral interventions begin by assessing the experiential world of patients to understand how they interpret their presenting problem. The primary task of the nurse in this instance is to help the patient express his meaning as well as to create a link between his expressed pain experience and the logic of the treatment approach. In this approach, there is a need for a shift in the focus from pain cure to pain management. This shift may be accomplished in part by helping Andrew examine his responses to his pain; for example, when his headache has escalated, he feels more tense as he tries to "cope" with it; it takes all of his energy to focus on getting his work done, so he is exhausted and even unable to be socially responsive. The potential for change, that is, breaking this cycle of tension-fatigue-irritability, raises the idea that change is possible (pain does not need to control his life) and generates hope that life could be different and more satisfy-

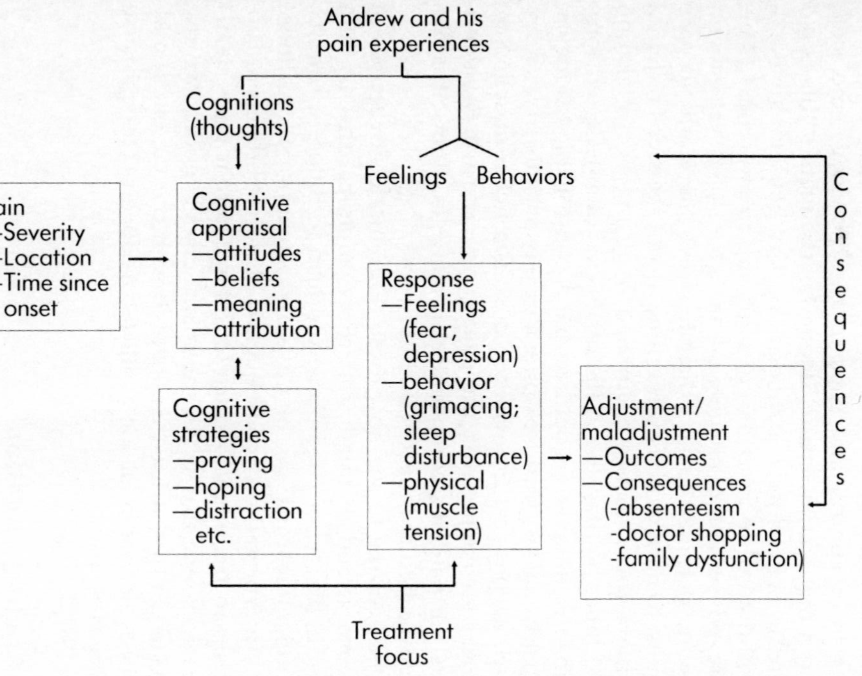

FIGURE 16-4. Andrew viewed from a cognitive-behavioral perspective.

ing. The logic of a treatment program that would assist skill development (e.g., relaxation techniques for muscle tension) and alternatives for managing pain (e.g., altering self-defeating thoughts) reinforces hope and confirms the necessary role the patient must play in gaining and establishing control. The redefinition of the patient's "problem" as his response to his pain rather than the pain itself, assists in the exploration of strategies of control and gaps in his knowledge and skill. Linkages then can be made among his thoughts ("this could kill me"), feelings (fear, helplessness) and behavior (irritability, withdrawal) to assist him in acquiring an awareness of his own responses and to create a rationale for skill development. Goals are identified (e.g., to handle stress differently, to pace activities, to have more family outings), and the steps required to achieve these goals are outlined (e.g., practice relaxation skills 3 times per day, use at the first signal of muscle tension). Gaining the ability to recognize what is controllable (thoughts, feelings, behavior) by developing a variety of skills (relaxation, distraction, physical fitness, etc.) creates a belief in self. New strategies for coping with the pain experience will be identified as the patient's competence in managing himself is further developed and his confidence grows.[33]

It is revealing to see how these three models or frames of reference attend to totally different symptoms, that is, pain report, behavior, or cognitions, and lead to different summaries and interpretations of the same situation. In addition, these interpretations consequently lead to different approaches to treatment because of their different goals. It becomes apparent that when the management models we use are congruent or at least compatible with the patient's models, then the potential for conflict is reduced. The converse must be true also.

A Conflict Situation

One might conclude from this exploration of some of the properties of pain and the management models that we use that conflict is inevitable because of the complexity of the pain problem, which by definition appears to prevent health care providers from being able to know what to do and how to do it. The social scientists, however, offer an additional perspective that could enable the health care provider as well as the patient to relate from another point of view. They distinguish between pain illness and pain disease.[5] Whereas pain disease refers to an objective biomedical account (pain as a symptom of underlying pathology) that guides some treatment decisions (surgical removal, anatomical injection, targeted drug), pain illness comprises the patient's subjective account—with all its dimensions—of the person's experience. Illness is acknowledged as a social process woven with meanings that may change over time as a result of circumstances and interactions with others. Patients shape their experience within the context of other people and events, and attempt to control the situation in keeping with biographically meaningful events. The context, therefore, becomes a dimension that limits the choices available to the patient. On the other hand, knowledge of the context for the caregiver may in fact expand the treatment options.

Linda

Linda was finally diagnosed as having atypical facial pain. She had had a tooth extraction, a root canal, a 3-year history of investigation, and a variety of treatment approaches, including nerve root injection, acupuncture, and medication (pain disease orientation). Her pain was disabling in that she feared losing control of herself and so became housebound to avoid "going crazy publicly." She no longer shopped for food or other necessities. She stopped driving her car, isolating herself further and relinquishing her role in helping her children meet their commitments; she felt she could not be certain of her ability to sustain herself to cook a meal or spend an evening with people and so isolated herself from friends and family; she became fearful of leaving her house and was so tired she had little energy to even want to leave. She felt guilty that she was no longer a contributing member of the family and at the same time felt inadequate and incompetent because she could not fulfill her usual role functions as wife, mother, homemaker, and seamstress. She became caught in vicious circles of pain-anxiety-fatigue leading to depression-further fatigue-increased pain-anxiety-insomnia and so on, until she feared that she would not be able to stand it any further and might go crazy (pain illness orientation).

Linda's experience had begun as a "normal" dental problem that had escalated into a nightmare of uncertainty and suffering. Hope for curative treatment in the beginning had involved a number of unsuccessful approaches by her own dentist, a variety of consultations with other health care professionals, and a gradual message that she would just have to learn to live with it because no one knew what to do for her.

All treatment approaches had failed, and she began to feel at fault for being unresponsive to treatment. Not only had she failed to respond to the treatments offered, she also began to feel inadequate in her roles as wife and mother as she found it increasingly difficult to perform her usual tasks and keep pace with the family activities. Her choices became more and more limited as her world became more and more constricted.

If the nurse and Linda's definition of the pain experience is pain-disease (biomedical model), then there is an assumption of a "knowable" underlying cause of the problem that can be altered or influenced with some predictable effect. In this model, it remains for the caregiver (nurse) to provide the treatment (cure) and for the patient to provide the appropriate response (proof) of the effectiveness of the treatment. If Linda's proof (her response or behavior) does not meet the nurse's expectations—such as Linda reporting more pain than the nurse expects the condition to warrant or behaving in a way that a nurse views as inappropriate or manipulative, or if the nurse's treatment does not "cure," then the exchanges between them will be conflictive. Linda's behavior around her pain complaint, that is, suffering in silence, isolating herself, and staying in bed, invites "solution attempting" behavior on the part of the nurse (professional activity) such as encouraging her to socialize, to get out of her house, and to get on with her life. Because this "treatment" is not congruent with the pain disease model, it in turn invites stronger efforts on the part of Linda to be believed and for the nurse to rescue Linda from her suffering. The resulting vicious circle can be interrupted only if the input of either or both of the participants is altered. This whole process is represented in a simpler form in Figure 16-5.

Process of Conflict

This process model of conflict[31] depicts five main events that occur within a conflictive episode from the point of view of one of the participants. These events occur consecutively and are the feelings of frustration that set off the situation, the explanation that the participants have for the situation, the ensuing behavior of one of the participants, the reaction of the other to the behavior, and, finally, the resulting outcome. For purposes of illustration, an adaptation of this model will be

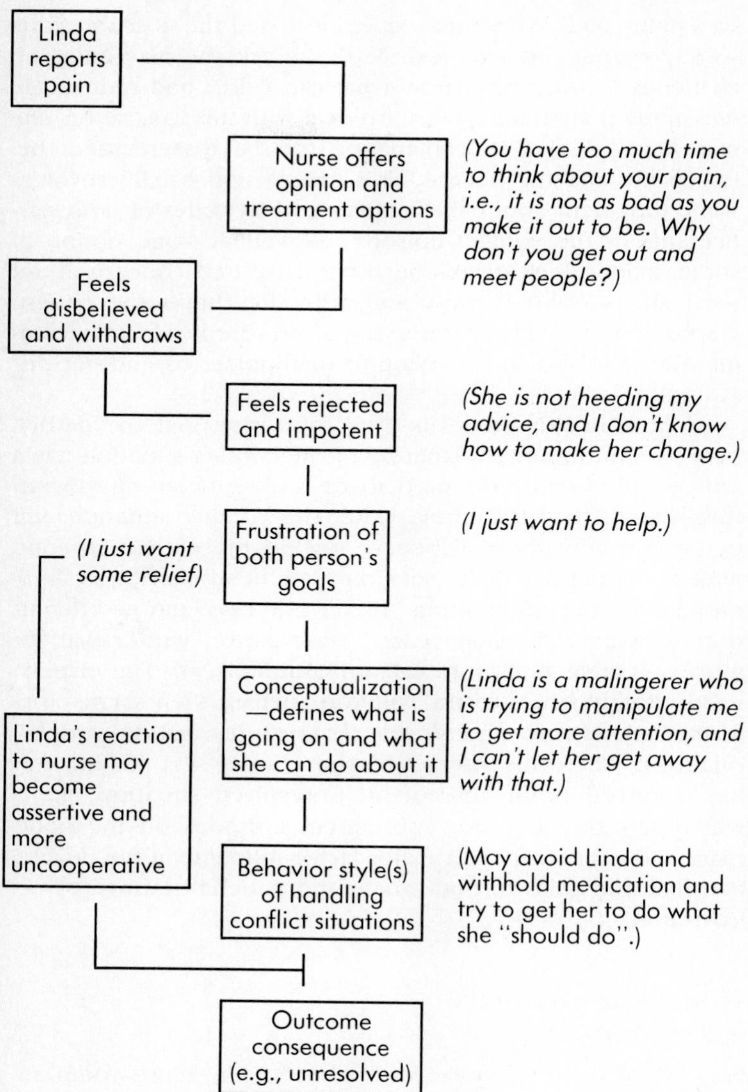

FIGURE 16-5. One conflict event.

used to examine the situation between Linda and the nurse previously outlined in Figure 16-2. Briefly, from the perspective of the nurse, the conflict episode was produced when she was frustrated in her attempts to carry out her role, that is to be the caregiver and provide pain relief for Linda. When Linda's pain failed to be relieved or improved the nurse's efforts were thwarted. In response to this block she may have felt challenged in her role (now what can I do?) and reduced in her status (I am inadequate). To deal with this frustration, she may have created an explanation for the disagreement between her and the patient. This explanation usually involves some judgment about the motives and attitudes of both participants in the conflict episode, as well as some notion of some action alternatives—her own frustrated concern about what she should do now and why she thinks the patient responded as she did. "I'm trying to prevent her from becoming addicted and she is trying to manipulate us and get our attention."

Central to this model is the proposition that the participant's definition or explanation of the conflict situation has a critical influence on the participant's subsequent behavior. In this regard, how the nurse views the conflict situation will determine how she will behave toward the patient to cope with the situation. If she sees the patient's behavior as "manipulative and undermining" of her role expectations (definition of issues) she may react by avoidance, withdrawal, or more assertive behaviors (action alternatives). The patient subsequently reacts to this behavior, which then serves as a further stimulus for the nurse's response (escalation or deescalation). When this interaction stops, some sort of outcome has occurred (joint agreement, unresolved situation, etc.), which sets the stage for subsequent episodes on the same issue and is likely to be a major factor influencing the degree to which the goals of both nurse and patient continue to be frustrated.

Steps of Conflict

Frustration

Most of us are familiar with some of the more common issues from which conflicts arise, such as disagreements, denial of a request, violation of an agreement, active interference with some goal or activity, competition for scarce resources, ignoring of one's feelings, reducing of one's status, and so on. The source of the frustration of the nurse in the previous example may be her feeling of helplessness in not being able to help Linda and solve her problem.

Definition of the Situation

According to the basic premise of the model, the most important step in this conflict episode is the participants' explanation for why they are responding to the issue as they are, because it follows that this explanation will influence the methods the participants will use to handle the conflict. Further, it is apparent that there must be a variety of definitions for any given situation. If this is so, then what factors influence the individual's explanation? Thomas[31] suggests that it is our investment in the issue, including the degree of our concern and its importance to us, plus our knowledge of the complexity of the issue, that influence our definition. In this regard, then, awareness of the concerns of the other person involved as well as awareness of one's own concerns would make subsequent cooperation more likely. For example, if the nurse explains the conflict episode as occurring because "Linda becomes frightened when her analgesics are wearing off and we don't know how to reassure her" (awareness of the concerns of both parties), as contrasted with a more self-centered concern, "Linda is on that buzzer every 3 hours demanding her next dose even before it all wears off," then treatment approaches could be expected to be quite different.

Related to this aspect of self-concern is the insight or perspective that the nurse is able to bring to the issue. At one extreme, she may think only of the specific issue contested, "Linda wants her medication right on schedule"; "she couldn't possibly hurt that much"; "it isn't time yet". In contrast, she could identify more basic concerns that are responsible for both of their behaviors—"I have been too busy to get Linda's pain medication on time and she has become fearful that she won't get it when she really needs it." When participants have a perspective on the concerns underlying an issue, the probability of reaching a solution that is agreeable to both parties increases.[31] Contributing to the perspective that we bring to the pain management situation are our knowledge, beliefs, and attitudes about pain and its management.

Common mistakes made in responding to a pain problem are to respond to persistent pain sufferers as if their pain were acute, as if the pain had a specific demonstrable cause and a defined treatment. Similarly, there is a popular belief that the severity of the injury equals the severity of the pain and that the severity of the pain equals the amount of disability. Given that some persistent pain problems have no definable beginning and that many have no observable course, lesion, or impairment to associate with the amount of reported pain, it is easy to see how conflict can arise and how resolution may be impossible. When the personal, social, and emotional concerns that underlie the pain complaint are viewed as less acceptable or respectable than demonstrable physical concerns, they may be unrecognized or ignored. On the other hand, if the nurse brings a perspective that is more comprehensive, given her knowledge and awareness of the issues, more explanations can be generated and more options for management become available.

The notion of importance of the conflict issue also appears to have some bearing on how easily the conflict may be resolved. When the conflict is defined as involving specific people, related to a single concrete issue and an isolated incident, then resolution is possible. However, issues that are treated as matters of principle and that involve multiple actors and/or established patterns are not easily resolved short of war! For example, if the situation is defined as a difference of opinion between Linda and the nurse over the timing of her next dose of analgesia needed to maintain her comfort, then the intervention can be simple and straightforward. In contrast, consider the same data with a different definition. Linda is seen as a malingerer trying to manipulate the staff into altering her dosing schedule because she is believed to be becoming addicted to her drugs.

Behavior

Based on the explanation or definition of the situation that each participant has developed, each participant then engages in behavior vis-à-vis the other designed to cope. Accordingly, each person adopts various tactics to satisfy his or her concerns and to alter the other person's behavior to what they see as possible in the situation.

According to Thomas,[31] there are five basic approaches to the conflict situation. These include competitive, collaborative, avoidant, appeasing, and compromising tactical behaviors. Competitive and collaborative behaviors are those most likely to be used when the issues are judged to be important to a person. Competitive tactics also are called bargaining tactics, and collaborative tactics are called problem-solving tactics. Although bargaining tactics are designed to deal with demands and risks ("If you don't start learning to live with your pain, you could become a drug addict"), collaborative tactics are designed to increase mutual interest by finding alternatives that satisfy the concern of both participants ("what strategies can you use to help distract you from your pain?").

Alternatively, appeasing and compromising approaches seek to achieve some peaceful coexistence ("You can do whatever you want to do") or common ground ("I will give you your medication before bedtime, but you will have to walk around the ward three times during the evening"). Avoidant tactics reflect indifference to the concern of either participant and are an example of withdrawal or isolation.

The more one attends to the concerns of the other, the more cooperative is the encounter. The less attention one gives to the other's concerns, the more uncooperative is the encounter. The most uncooperative position is the win-lose power struggle. The conflict of interest seems to be total, and the only outcomes possible are total satisfaction and total frustration. "Even if she sits on her call bell all night, she still gets her Tylenol only every 4 hours as long as I'm around!" Alternatives are unlikely to be generated and definitions of the situation will tend to become simpler with a more narrow perspective.[31] In contrast, the collaborative and appeasement positions achieve their ends cooperatively, the former through a problem-solving process in which both persons' concerns are satisfied, and the latter through a process of appeasement that achieves a type of "peaceful coexistence."

Behavioral Reaction

During the course of negotiation with the patient, the nurse's methods may change as a reaction to the patient's behavior. Such changes are frequently described in an escalation/deescalation dimension. Escalation usually describes an increase in the level of conflict and might involve increasing hostility and/or competitiveness between the nurse and patient, which result in coercive tactics and decreasing trust. For example, nurses or patients may use the threat of "reporting" the other to the doctor for some expected punishment. The patient may telephone the physician herself and the nurse subsequently may be chastised by the physician and required to alter her position. The patient, on the other hand, may be threatened with early discharge or having her drug supply "cut off".[12]

On the other hand, deescalation may occur if, after hearing the patient's arguments, the nurse reevaluates her definition of the situation and preferred alternatives. She may change her position in regard to late doses when she realizes the physiological consequences or indeed the professional consequences that this produces, that is, a medication error. Reevaluation, however, is fostered in a climate of open communication and trust and with the use of persuasive rather than coercive tactics, in short, by collaboration and problem solving. In this regard, the nurse needs to recognize that the patient's behavior is in part a response to her own behavior. Hence her approach to Linda (bargaining) and her distrust of Linda's report and motives were reinforced by generating the predicted behavior in the patient; Linda's further pain complaints and withdrawal were seen as evidence of addictive behavior. If Linda felt the nurse was distrustful of her report of pain, she would fight her on every issue and actually might prod her into fighting/arguing. Depending on her level of trust or suspicion toward Linda, the nurse looks for different things. If suspicious of Linda's motives, she is attentive to signs of resistance, hostility, and conflict of interest—which she is then more likely to find. With this bias, she underestimates the commonalities between them and may miss the patient's cooperative overtones and signs of good will.

Outcome

The final stage in the process model is the outcome of the conflict event. At the time when the interaction between the participants ends (nurse goes off duty and Linda goes to bed), not only is there some type of explicit or tacit agreement: "You will not get any medication from her," but there are also "leftover" feelings resulting from their responses to the way they behaved toward each other (distrust, anger, hurt). It is proposed that both the type of agreement (resolved, unresolved, indifference, contained) and the participants' perceptions of what went on during the conflict (bargained, compromised, avoided, problem solved) constitute the ingredients that will nourish the relationship for subsequent interactions.

The quality of the resolution for both parties (whose concerns were addressed and with what effect) will determine what the "aftermath" is like.[31]

◆ SUMMARY

We have proposed that some of the problems in pain management experienced by both the patient and nurse can be explained by a process model of conflict. An assumption in our approach is that a more abstract description of the factors that are involved in a conflict episode would reveal its complexity and would expand the options considered acceptable. This broader choice of options should lead to more satisfactory treatment and relief of pain.

Specifically we have used the conflict model to explore the interactions between a chronic pain sufferer and nurse when either one or the other or both were distressed. Under these conflictive conditions, the usual approaches taken were inadequate or resistant to the desired outcome. In short, the patient and nurse both did not know how to deal with the problem of concern—pain. Implicit was the strong demand to help the patient with the pain problem as soon as possible. In this "worst-case" scenario, possible interactions and outcomes were depicted when narrow or one-dimensional frameworks or conceptualizations of "pain" were used. The inadequacies of these frameworks were revealed in their inability to offer an "opening" or opportunity to provide more meaningful definitions or alternate approaches.

In addition, we have tried to provide an understanding of the responses of the pain sufferer and those who relate to him through a background of beliefs, attitudes, and attributions. The effect of various approaches to thinking on the characterization of different styles of behavior was explored in the conflict model. The functional or dysfunctional consequences for both parties in the interaction were similarly discussed.

Further, we attempted to develop the theme that no single framework or model of thinking and no single style of acting or interacting with the patient can be used successfully in all situations.

Finally, and most important, we assumed that all individuals can learn to be more conscious and deliberate about how they think and interact.

REFERENCES

1. Austin KL, Stapleton JV, and Mather LE. (1980). Multiple intramuscular injections: a major source of variability in analgesic response to meperidine. *Pain 8,* 47-62.
2. Bellissimo A and Tunks E. (1984). *Chronic pain: the psychotherapeutic spectrum.* New York: Praeger.
3. Benner P and Wrubel J. (1989). *The primacy of caring: stress and coping in health and illness.* Don Mills, Ontario: Addison-Wesley Publishing Company.
4. Beyer J, DeGood DE, Ashley LC, and Russell GA. (1983). Patterns of post-operative analgesic use with adults and children following cardiac surgery. *Pain 17,* 71-81.
5. Brodwin PE and Kleinman A. (1987). The social meaning of chronic pain. In Burrows G, Elton O, and Stanley G (eds), *Handbook of chronic pain management.* Amsterdam: Elsevier Science Publishers.
6. Cartwright PD. (1985). Pain control after surgery: a survey of current practice. *Ann R Coll Surg Engl 67,* 13-16.
7. Cohen FL. (1980). Post-surgical pain relief: patients' status and nurses' medication choices. *Pain 9,* 265-274.
8. Copp LA (ed). (1985). *Recent Advances in Nursing: Perspectives on pain.* New York: Churchill Livingstone.
9. Crook J, Rideout E, and Browne G. (1984). The prevalence of pain complaints in a general population. *Pain 18,* 299-316.
10. Crook J, Tunks E, Rideout E, and Browne G. (1986). Epidemiological comparison of persistent pain sufferers in a specialty pain clinic and in the community. *Arch Phys Med Rehab 67,* 451-455.
11. Crook J, Tunks E, Kalaher S, and Roberts J. (1988). Coping with persistent pain: a comparison of persistent pain sufferers in a specialty pain clinic and in a family practice clinic. *Pain 34,* 175-184.
12. Davis MS and van der Lippe RP. (1968). Discharge from hospital against medical advice: a study of reciprocity in the doctor-patient relationship. *Soc Sci Med I.*
13. Donovan M, Dillon P, and McGuire L. (1987). Incidence and characteristics of pain in a sample of medical-surgical inpatients. *Pain 30,* 69-78.
14. Duff R, and Hollingshead A. (1968). *Sickness and society.* New York: Harper and Row Publishers, p. 116.
15. Fagerhaugh SZ and Strauss A. (1977). *Politics of pain management: staff-patient interaction.* New York: Addison-Wesley Publishing Company.
16. Faherty BS and Grier MR. (1984). Analgesic medication for elderly people post surgery. *Nurs Res 33,* 369-372.
17. Fisch R, Weakland J and Segal L. (1982). *The tactics of change: doing therapy briefly.* San Francisco: Jossey-Bass Publishers.
18. Fordyce WE. (1976). *Behavioral methods for chronic pain and illness.* St. Louis: Mosby.
19. Jacobs R. (1983). Psychological aspects of chronic pain. *J Natl Med Assoc 75*(4), 387-391.
20. Keeri-Szanto M. (1979). Drugs or drums: what relieves post-operative pain? *Pain 6,* 217-230.
21. Lazare A. (1973). Hidden conceptual models in clinical psychiatry. *N Engl J Med 288*(2), 345-350.

22. Mechanic D. (1978). *Medical sociology,* (ed 2). New York: The Free Press.
23. Moore ME, Berth SN, and Naypaver A. (1984). Chronic pain: inpatient treatment with small group effects. *Arch Phys Med Rehab 65*(7), 356-361.
24. National Institutes of Health Consensus Development Conference Statement. (1986). *The integrated approach to the management of pain 6*(3).
25. Reuler J, Gerard D, and Nardone D. (1980). The chronic pain syndrome: misconceptions and management. *Ann Intern Med 93,* 588-596.
26. Rosenstiel A and Keefe F. (1983). The use of coping strategies in chronic low back pain patients: relationship to patient characteristics and current adjustment. *Pain 17,* 33-44.
27. Scarry D. (1985). *The body in pain.* New York: Oxford University Press.
28. Sternbach RA. (1974). *Pain patients: traits and treatments.* New York: Academic Press.
29. Sternbach R (ed). (1978). *The psychology of pain.* New York: Raven Press.
30. Taenzer P, Melzack R, and Jeans ME. (1986). Influence of psychological factors on post-operative pain, mood and analgesic requirements. *Pain 24,* 331-342.
31. Thomas KE. (1976). Conflict and conflict management. In Dunnette M (ed), *Handbook of industrial and organizational psychology.* Chicago: Rand McNally, 889-935.
32. Tunks E. (1978). A client-centered approach to rehabilitation of patients with chronic pain. Abstract, *Second World Congress on Pain,* Montreal, Quebec.
33. Turk D, Meichenbaum D, and Genest M. (1983). *Pain and behavioral medicine.* New York: The Guilford Press.
34. VonKorff M, Dworkin S, LeResche L, and Kruger A. (1988). An epidemiological comparison of pain complaints. *Pain 32,* 173-183.
35. Weis OF, Sriwatanakul K, Alloza JL, Weintraub M, and Lasagna L. (1983). Attitudes of patients, house staff, and nurses toward post-operative analgesic care. *Anaesth Analg 62,* 70-74.
36. Weir R, Roberts J, Crook J, Browne G, and Barnes W. (1990). Predictors of analgesic administration in the first 48 postoperative hours. *Can J Nurs Res* 22, 61-72.

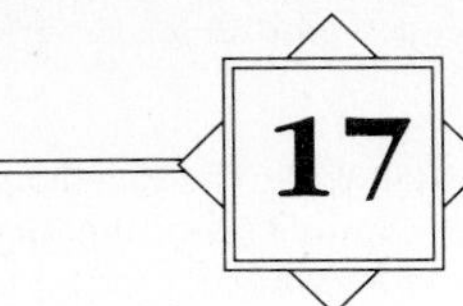

The Pain of Arthritis

Susan M. Wright

◆ NURSING CARE OF PATIENTS WITH ARTHRITIS PAIN

There are approximately 37 million people in the United States who suffer from arthritis in one of more than 100 forms. Traditionally, arthritis is considered a disease of the joints. However, diseases that fall under the classification of arthritis can affect the connective tissue, soft tissue, and other organ systems. The classic form of arthritis is rheumatoid, a systemic inflammatory disease with primary manifestation in the small joints. The most common form of arthritis is osteoarthritis. It occurs as the result of a degenerative process, either as a normal part of the aging process or through injury or excessive stress on a joint. These are two very different disease entities in terms of their pathology and etiologic processes. However, the most pressing concern for the overwhelming majority of arthritis patients is pain. Pain is frequently the symptom for which an individual with arthritis seeks medical treatment, and pain in the arthritis patient can contribute significantly to morbidity. This chapter will address the problems related to pain in the arthritis patient, and current research treatment strategies for arthritis pain.

◆ PAIN AND THE PROCESS OF ARTHRITIS

Pain can be classified into three broad categories: acute pain, chronic pain of malignant origin, and chronic pain of nonmalignant origin.[99] People with arthritis and related conditions may experience any or all of these types of pain. The pain of arthritis is most often multifocal. In one sample of patients with arthritis, more than 90% reported at least moderate pain over the previous month.[53] One half to two thirds of patients with rheumatoid arthritis rank pain as their most important symptom.[41,82] Pain is also a major determinant in perceptions of health by both the patient and physician,[40,56] and pain is strongly related to functional impairment and the development of disability.[33,53]

Arthritis pain can occur as the result of a local or systemic inflammation, or as the result of a degenerative process. For example, rheumatoid arthritis is considered a systemic disease that results in severe inflammation in multiple joints and other organ systems. Any connective tissue may be affected, along with the reticular framework that connects and supports the organ, the soft tissues, and even the blood cells and bone marrow.

Osteoarthritis is a localized degenerative response from wear and tear on the joint, which primarily affects weight bearing joints. Although inflammation and degeneration are separate but related processes, degeneration can result from inflammation. The exact relationship between the two processes is not known. Both are normal bodily functions. Degeneration, a normal part of the aging process, seems to be accelerated in the case of arthritis or rheumatologic disease. There is initially breakdown of the joint cartilage followed by bony destruction characterized by bone spurs along the marginal aspects of the joint.

Clinically, the relationship between pain and inflammation is unclear. The response varies greatly by both disease and by individual. For example, the person with rheumatoid arthritis may or may not experience more pain than the person with osteoarthritis. In the latter, the patient often has significant swelling without pain. Whereas, in crystal-induced inflammation, that is, gout, the patient will usually experience excruciating pain.[15] Whatever the relationship, it is almost always the pain that motivates the individual to seek medical help.

The inflammatory response can be a systemic or localized problem, affecting connective tissue such as the bones, joints, ligaments, tendon, and cartilage. Inflammation may result from infection, crystal deposition, antigen-antibody complex deposition and/or trauma. In the joint, there is vascular engorgement of the synovial membrane, interstitial edema and tissue infiltration by plasma cells, lymphocytes and macrophages. The resultant edema and tissue engorgement may stimulate nociceptors in the joint capsule or the surrounding tissue, which results in pain.[115] The rat version of chronic inflammatory arthritis is currently the most widely accepted animal model for chronic pain.[22] In rats with adjuvant arthritis, substance P, a pain transmitter, was found in increased concentrations around the dorsal cord, roots and ganglia.[69] Capsaicin, the substance that makes hot peppers hot, also depletes substance P from sensory neurons. When rats with arthritis were given injections of capsaicin into joints, they showed less evidence of pain.[9,22] Other research indicates that the nervous system also plays a significant role in arthritis.[70] Pain perception in the arthritis patient is not a singular entity, but is the result of involvement of multiple systems. It is possible that the pain is a more significant contributor to disease morbidity than the inflammation or related factors.

In summary, a patient with arthritis may have acute flares of inflammation that may trigger acute bouts of pain and at the same time may have chronic pain from longstanding joint destruction. In addition, emotional factors, fatigue, and other psychosocial responses play a role in the pain of arthritis. This presents a significant challenge to the health care provider's ability to assess and treat the pain associated with arthritis.

◆ COMMON DISEASES OF ARTHRITIS

The most common diseases in the arthritis family include rheumatoid arthritis, osteoarthritis, systemic lupus erythematosus fibrositis, and ankylosing spondylitis. All of these attack connective tissue at one or more levels and are considered to be within the realm of rheumatologic disease. Table 17-1 illustrates the major characteristics of the most common arthritic diseases.

The pain of arthritis can be significantly disabling. One third to one half of these patients describe the sensory aspect of their pain as throbbing, shooting, tender, or sharp. It appears that these are consistent regardless of disease severity.[13,21] However, for the affective component of the pain, as assessed by the McGill Pain Questionnaire, there is greater variability in descriptions (see Chapter 4). For example, inpatients with more severe arthritis used more intense affective responses, although not as often as outpatients.[13]

Each specific disease entity within the family of arthritis diseases involves some variations in the patterns of pain. In

◆ **Table 17-1**
Common arthritic diseases

	RA	OA	SLE	AS	Fibrositis	Gout
Sex	F > M	F = M	F > M	M > F	F > M	M > F
Age at onset	Childhood; young adult	Middle-age	Young adult	Young adult	Young adult	Variable
Distribution						
Small joints	+ + +	+ +	+	–	–	+ +
Large joints	+	+ + +	+	+ +	–	+
Spine	+ (Cervical)	+ (Lumbar)	–	+ + + (All)	–	–
Sacroiliitis	–	–	–	+ + +	–	–
Muscles	+	–	+	–	+ + +	–
Multiple system	+ + +	–	+ +	+	+?	+ (Renal)
Characteristics						
Serology	Rheumatoid factor	–	???	HLA-B27	–	Uric acid
Inflammatory	+ + +	±?	+ +	+ +	+?	+ +
Stiffness	+ + +	+ + +	+?	+ + +	–	–
Swelling	+ + +	+	–	–	–	+ +
Trigger points	–	–	–	–	+ + +	–
Fatigue	+ +	–	+ +	+	+ + +	–

(Data from Campbell et al., 1983; Gibson, 1985; McCarty, 1979; Primer on Rheumatic Diseases, 1989; Ruoff, 1980; Wolfe, 1984.)
RA, rheumatoid arthritis; OA, osteoarthritis, SLE, systemic lupus erythematosis; AS, ankylosing spondylitis.

rheumatoid arthritis, the pain tends to vary throughout the day. It is worse in the morning and with movement after long periods of inactivity. It is multifocal, chronic, and usually progressive. In osteoarthritis, the classic symptom is pain on use of the affected joint. Pain in the early stages is relieved with rest, but later the pain occurs at rest and at night, thus becoming a significant problem.[126] The pain and subsequent limitations in mobility are usually chronic and necessitate physical, psychological, and social adjustments for the individual. In systemic lupus erythematosus, fatigue can be a major factor in lupus and can make it more difficult to cope with pain. The pain of lupus can be acute or chronic and may be progressive and severe. In fibrositis the pain is diffuse and multifocal. It is also associated with severe fatigue. In fact, some believe that people with fibrositis may experience stage 3-4 (non-REM) sleep disturbances.[92] Clinically, many of the symptoms of fibrositis are similar to those of chronic sleep deprivation, symptoms that include diffuse muscular pain.[91,116] The physical evidence for the pain associated with fibrositis is not clear, and there is debate about its origin, whether psychological, biological, or both. Fibrositis patients experience more pain in the torso and large joints, while patients with rheumatoid arthritis experience more pain in the peripheral joints, especially the hands and feet. The intensity of the pain is the same for both groups.[65] The pain of fibrositis is multifocal, diffuse, and less localized to the joints. The hallmark symptom is specific trigger point tenderness.[41,65] Fibrositis has the potential to be more disabling than rheumatoid arthritis. The pain of ankylosing spondylitis varies according to the stage of the disease. In early stages, sacroiliac and low back pain are present and are usually relieved by movement. In the middle phase, pain varies but includes significant morning stiffness. In the later stages, the morning stiffness and pain at rest are gone, but the patient may experience significant joint pain and muscle spasms in the spine secondary to postural changes.[16,46,107]

These are five of the most prevalent types of arthritis. There are over 100 different clinical entities, among them psoriatic arthritis, Reiter's syndrome, Sjögren's syndrome and polymyalgia rheumatica. Pain is a factor in each and is sometimes the most significant effect of the disease. Any type of arthritis carries with it the potential for pain. The characteristics of that pain will vary between diseases and between individuals with the same disease. This variation necessitates accurate and comprehensive assessment so that the pain can be treated with maximum effectiveness.

◆ CLINICAL ISSUES RELATED TO ARTHRITIS PAIN

There are several key issues or clinical concerns with respect to dealing with the person with pain secondary to rheumatologic disease. The pain is usually chronic, multifocal, and often severe, undertreated, and/or mistreated. Of major concern is the inability or unwillingness of health professionals to treat the pain associated with arthritis. The pain of arthritis, as in other diseases, is often considered a "side effect" of the disease process. Not until recently has it been acknowledged that pain may be a major contributor to the morbidity of the disease.

A recent study demonstrates that the potential for morbidity from pain was well demonstrated in rats with adjuvant arthritis, the animal model for chronic inflammatory arthritis. The investigators selectively cut the spinothalamic tract of rats with arthritis to eliminate nociceptive input from the affected extremities without affecting motor control. When compared to the group of rats with arthritis with normal nociception, rats with pain lost more weight and were less active. When pain was factored out of the model, the severity of the arthritis alone did not make a significant contribution to either weight loss or activity.[25] Other researchers have suggested that pain from arthritis is a significant contributor to functional disability, disease activity and perceived health status.[53] Kazis, Meenan, and Anderson[56] found that pain made a highly significant contribution toward explaining both the patient and physician estimates of overall health assessment, medication usage, and the prediction of both subsequent disability and subsequent pain.

Pain may be the single most important determinant of health status in people with rheumatologic disease. Pain is a multidimensional concept, which interacts with and is affected by a number of variables. These variables become the clinical issues when developing a plan of care for the patient with arthritis pain. Because arthritis is a chronic illness, usually accompanied by chronic pain, many of these variables will factor into the patient's overall well being. Some of the primary factors to consider when dealing with pain are fatigue, sleep disturbance, depression and functional impairment, with work disability as a subset of that problem.

Fatigue

Fatigue can be a major problem for people with arthritis. It can be a prodromal symptom of increased inflammation, a direct result of the pain, and can stem from the fact that some arthritis is often a systemic illness. If there is one key variable in arthritis on which everything else hinges, it is energy, or lack thereof. Fatigue alters one's perception of pain significantly, often turning a tolerable level of pain into something intolerable. Psychologically, more physical and mental energy may be needed to cope with the task of living with pain on a daily basis. Also, the pain is often accompanied by anxiety, increased muscular tension and autonomic nervous system arousal, which results in greater demand for energy and thus, greater subsequent depletion in energy. Therefore managing fatigue is often a more significant challenge than managing the actual pain.

Several researchers have focused on teaching the management of fatigue by teaching people with arthritis pain energy conservation measures.[38,43,77] Energy conservation measures include learning to pace activities, taking frequent short rests, and stopping before the pain reaches an intolerable level. When patients with rheumatoid arthritis followed the recommendations of an energy conservation program they improved on measures of pain, anxiety, and depression.[77] In a related study, patients with rheumatoid arthritis found pain, depression, and fatigue to be significant limiting factors in their ability to carry out the day's activities. When this group was taught energy conservation, 67% improved on measures of pain, 83% experienced less fatigue (as measured by an activity record), and 47% were more physically active than they were before the program.[38] In another experimental study, 15 of 25 people with rheumatoid arthritis were given a workbook intended to teach them standard energy conservation behaviors. The results of this study were equivocable but suggested that people who adopted energy conservation behaviors had an improvement in physical activity. There were no significant differences in pain in any of the groups.[43] In general, these findings support a relationship between pain and fatigue in people with arthritis and demonstrate that energy conservation balanced with physical activity is an important approach to consider in developing a treatment plan for the person with arthritis pain.

Sleep Disturbance

Related to the issue of fatigue in people with arthritis is the issue of sleep disturbance. In the animal model, rats with adjuvant arthritis showed marked variations in sleep anatomy including increased fragmentation, increased non-REM sleep, a loss of normal diurnal variations, and a general slowing of EEG activity.[64] People with rheumatoid arthritis showed increases in awake time and an increase in non-REM sleep when monitored in a sleep laboratory.[78,90] Sleep physiology, pain, and mood symptoms have also been studied in people with osteoarthritis. Two groups of patients with osteoarthritis of the hands were assessed, those with and without morning symptoms. The primary difference between the two groups was an increased frequency of myoclonic leg jerks in the group with morning symptoms. This disorder resulted in a fragmented sleep pattern, resulting in decreased mood, more pain and tenderness, and decreased grip strength.[89]

The problem of sleep disturbance among arthritis patients may be of particular importance in people with fibrositis, a disease in which some believe that sleep disturbance is one of the primary pathogenic features. Fibrositis patients demonstrate non-REM disturbance, sleep fragmentation, and alpha and delta wave disturbances.[92-94] It is also interesting to note that in normal people under laboratory conditions, prolonged sleep deprivation can result in a temporary musculoskeletal pain syndrome similar to fibrositis.[91] Future pharmacologic research may focus on drugs like benzodiazepines, which may help in improving sleep quality as well as relieving musculoskeletal symptoms.[95] If sleep is identified as a problem, fatigue is likely to accompany it and thus may have significant consequences in terms of pain.

Depression

Depression is another phenomenon that occurs, often with, although is not specific to, the pain of arthritis. The literature reports a wide range for incidence of depression in people with chronic pain and/or arthritis, from 10% to 83%.* Depression is thought to increase one's perception of pain. In general, depressed rheumatoid arthritis patients report significantly more pain than their nondepressed cohorts.[34,129]

It is possible that fatigue, sleep disturbance, and depression act in a type of synergistic relationship, which can markedly change one's perception of pain. Depression is associated with sleep disturbance, usually lack of sleep, which in turn would exacerbate the fatigue. In addition, a decrease in activity increases fatigue in the long-run. The patient's world becomes smaller and smaller, which is, in the worst case, limited to just his or her own body and mind. As one's attention draws inward like this, it entraps the individual in a vicious cycle, making this pain difficult to treat.

Functional Impairment and Work Disability

The ability or inability to move is a primary clinical issue in the treatment of arthritis pain. Limitations in the ability to move lead to major disability in people with arthritis, and pain is a contributing factor in limiting movement. Lack of movement leads to various levels of functional impairment. People with arthritis also experience stiffness, inflammation, swelling, and actual destruction of tissues in and around the joints, making it a challenge to decide which combination of these factors contribute more to functional impairment and disability.

The relationships among functional impairment, pain, and other measures of disease activity and severity suggest higher correlations between functional impairment and pain than between either active joint count or morning stiffness, both measures of disease activity.[53] Pain does not seem to be related to any of the objective disease indices.[49,53] In a predictive equation that includes pain, functional impairment, disease indices, coping strategies, and affective states, joint swelling and both state and trait anxiety are the most reliable predictors of pain, accounting for about half of the variance in a multiple regression equation.[49] Other studies corroborate the conclusion that pain bears no significant relationship to either functional impairment or disease severity.[101,118]

Work disability, a specific form of functional impairment, is

* References 3, 8, 34, 59, 111, 128.

a concern in people with arthritis pain. Researchers have attempted to construct models of work disability, to identify which factors contribute to it most significantly. In some studies, disease factors, such as pain, were less important in determining work disability than workplace characteristics and social factors.[48,98,127] A later study of women with rheumatoid arthritis found physical disability to be a more important determining factor than workplace, age, or family factors.[110] Flor and Turk[33] attempted to predict disability and pain from cognitive variables related to the degree of control individuals felt they had over their pain state. None of the disease related variables explained either pain levels or disability. However, there was a significant relationship between the control one felt over the pain and the amount of pain and disability one experienced. Minimal or no linear relationship existed between functional impairment, indices of disease, and the patient's perception of pain. Currently, long-term arthritis treatment programs are often directed at increasing functional capacity, on the assumption that as function increases and pain behaviors decrease, the subjective experience of pain also decreases. If no direct relationship between pain and function exists, I suggest that the focus of treatment needs to change to include relief of pain.

Additional Factors

Additional factors such as social support,[2,101,123] meaning of the pain,[76,96] personality characteristics,[75,104] and meteorological factors[28,61,102] may all make some contribution to both the development and course of arthritis pain. One also has to consider the effect arthritis pain can have on overall quality of life.

Burckhardt[12] developed and tested a model that included support, attitudes, self-esteem, and internal control of health as mediating factors. Age, severity of pain, sex, severity of impairment, social network, and socioeconomic status were the input factors. None of the input variables showed a significant effect on quality of life, including pain. However, pain was found to contribute significantly to a negative attitude about the disease. Mediating variables such as an internal locus of control and a positive self-esteem were found to modulate or buffer that effect. In a related study, Laborde and Powers[62] studied life satisfaction in osteoarthritis patients.

Better life satisfaction was associated with better health perception, an internal locus of control, and less pain. In patients with rheumatoid arthritis, Lambert[63] found pain to be the single best predictor of psychological well-being. However, it accounted for only 8% of the variance in a regression model. Again, this reinforces the complexity of the relationship between pain and other factors related to arthritis.

It is a popular myth that people with arthritis get used to pain as the disease progresses. Research does not support this. It appears that when the pain is present, it can be just as detrimental after 30 years as it is after 30 days. However, what does appear to be true is that people learn how to work around the pain. They learn energy conservation measures, they plan activities for periods when they know they will be relatively pain-free, they learn to avoid places and situations that may exacerbate their pain. An internal locus of control may be an important mediating variable. Though still a point of debate, it appears that people who are willing to take some control, responsibility, and accountability for managing their pain may have less morbidity than those who don't.

Pain in arthritis, as in any disease, is a complex problem. There is no magic formula to predict the amount of pain any individual will have. If there is a common theme here, it is that pain is not well predicted by any variable and that pain can have a significant effect on psychological and physical well-being. The key factors in direct relation to pain are fatigue, sleep disturbance, depression, lack of social support, and other affective and psychosocial variables. In fact, the trend seems to indicate that the attention in treatment is on the wrong place—attention is paid to laboratory values and the amount of swelling before it is given to the pain. As with other types of pain, arthritis pain should be treated on an individualized basis, based on accurate assessment and awareness of the pertinent clinical issues.

◆ ASSESSMENT

The debate between the subjective and the objective, the idea that seeing is believing rather than believing is seeing, and the quest for an objective source to measure pain is rooted to the very framework of the medical model and, in the case of pain, imparts a belief that the patient is an unreliable source. In reality, probably neither patient self-report nor assessment of objective indicators is sufficient. It is likely that a combination of assessment methods will yield more information about the patient and will lead to improved care. It is within that framework that the following section reviews the assessment of arthritis pain from a multidimensional perspective, including simple and complex tools for self-report of pain quality, location, and intensity, as well as behavioral, functional, and affective factors related to pain.

Although many have tried, there is currently no universal predictor of pain in people with arthritis, or with any condition, for that matter. The pain experience is complex and will vary between individuals. In the medical community, the focus on diagnosis and assessment leans toward "objective" measures for pain. For arthritis, these objective measures include joint counts, swelling and redness ratings, standard x-ray examinations, and more recently, thermography. The assumption is that the degree of redness and swelling in a joint is directly correlated to the intensity of the pain. However, there is little, if any, correlation between physical findings and the pain experienced by people with arthritis.

Ongoing, accurate assessment is very important to determine response to treatment and developing a dynamic, individualized plan of care. The kind of assessment the arthritis patient should receive will depend on several factors: whether the pain is acute or chronic, whether the origin is known or unknown, whether functional impairment is present, and whether the cognitive or affective functioning is affected. The assessment may range from simple self-report to multidimensional or complex measures, which may also include functional and/or affective state components.

Self-Report Measures

Simple assessment of arthritis pain focuses on the symptoms and may take one of several forms, for example, rating scales and body diagrams. Verbal and visual rating scales, such as the categorical, numerical, or visual analogue, provide measures of pain intensity and related concepts (see Chapter 4). The visual analogue scale (VAS)[114] has been used with rheumatoid arthritis patients and found to have a high degree of reliability and validity.[17] The VAS can be measured and scored to the nearest millimeter and therefore may be more sensitive than either a numerical or categorical scale. This factor is more important in research than in the clinical setting although there are high correlations between the 10 point numerical scale and the VAS.[20,31] The two may be interchangeable and selection generally depends on patient and/or researcher preference.

One needs to consider that the pain may differ from one area of the body to another and that the same person may have two very different kinds of pain simultaneously. The addition of a pictorial model of the body may help patients to clearly mark the area(s) of their pain. However, these tools measure only one dimension of the pain experience, usually intensity and arthritis pain is often multifocal and multidimensional.

Multidimensional Measures

Multidimensional pain assessment broadens the information data base and may include subjective instruments like the McGill Pain Questionnaire (MPQ)[86] and the Brief Pain Inventory (BPI)[26] for the measurement of pain. A detailed description of multidimensional assessment is found in Chapter 4.

The MPQ has been tested in people with arthritis and was reported to discriminate people with arthritis from those with other painful conditions. This study found that words such as gnawing, aching, exhausting, and annoying were characteristics of arthritis patients and represented primarily the affective component of pain.[32] However, in two later studies, the majority of patients used words like throbbing, shooting, tender, and sharp to describe the sensory aspects of their pain. They also showed greater variability in the descriptions of the affective component of the pain.[13,21] In some studies, the MPQ differentiated between some types of arthritis, specifically fibrositis and rheumatoid arthritis, based on the specific selected adjectives but not on measures of intensity or number of words chosen.[65] Wagstaff, Smith, and Wood[120] also demonstrated the ability of the MPQ to discriminate among three types of arthritis correctly about two thirds of the time. Although it appears that the MPQ can offer insight into the quality of arthritis pain, the implications for practice are unclear. Perhaps they could serve as an adjunct to diagnosis in the early part of the disease process. The implications in later stages are less clear. If clinicians and researchers could learn about individual or group patterns of pain over time, these data could be used in a more concrete manner, that is, to predict an exacerbation.

The BPI offers additional insight into the effects of pain on daily life, which can be very helpful in discharge planning and identification of patient-family related needs. The BPI has been used just as successfully, albeit less frequently than the MPQ in people with arthritis pain.[53] Studies have found significant variability in the degree of correlation between pain measures in people with arthritis, especially between the MPQ and the VAS.[108,109,132] One recent study suggests that correlations between measures may be higher and less variable in light of more demonstrable pathology (as in rheumatoid arthritis). Thus correlations are lower and more variable when there is little or no demonstrable pathology (as in fibrositis).[70,103] Again, the clinical implications for this are unclear at this time, but perhaps as researchers and clinicians learn more about the pattern of arthritis pain, these implications will become clear.

In some major arthritis centers, behavioral assessment is utilized as part of the pain assessment. Some may consider behavioral assessment to be an objective measure of pain. However, it may be more useful and effective to view behavioral assessment as a useful adjunct to a comprehensive assessment but the assessment should not be confused with or substituted for the patient's self-report of the pain experience. Proponents of behavioral observation claim several advantages over subjective measures of pain. There may be significant measurement error involved in repeated use of rating scales, and they may not be sensitive to changes over time.[29,57] In addition, the patients report of pain may be confounded by the presence of anxiety and/or depression and, theoretically, behavioral observation excludes those variables. However, in clinical practice it is evident that depression and anxiety affect behavior as well as self-report.

A number of studies have examined the relationship between behavioral assessment, the patient's report of pain, disease activity, and disease severity. Indices of disease severity and activity include x-ray examinations, grip strength, joint count, and sedimentation rate, and physical behaviors, which are included in the behavioral assessment of pain, include grimacing, rigidity, bracing, or guarding. These behaviors are observed and quantified. Studies, primarily from one group of researchers, have found a relationship between pain behaviors and overall disease activity as well as physician pain estimates. The relationship between the patients' subjective assessment of pain and their pain behaviors was not reported.[5,6] Total pain behavior scores were statistically able to differentiate rheumatoid arthritis from low back pain subjects as well as the depressed and nondepressed pain-free subjects.[9] However, Hagglund et al.,[49] in a nearly identical sample, found no relationship between disease activity, disease severity, and the patient's report of pain. There is no clear consensus as to the exact nature of the relationship between pain behaviors and subjective pain assessment.[81] Behavioral assessment may be a worthwhile edition to a comprehensive assessment. If there is a discrepancy between the patient's perception of pain and the behavioral score, one should examine why this discrepancy exists.

The last significant factor to consider in the comprehensive assessment of the patients with arthritis pain is their functional status. A number of instruments have been developed for this singular purpose: the Arthritis Impact Measurement Scales (AIMS),[84] the Functional Status Inventory (FSI),[54,55] and the Health Assessment Questionnaire (HAQ).[36,37] The AIMS has nine subscales measuring aspects of physical, social, and mental health status, including pain and depression. The FSI measures dependence, pain, and difficulty experienced in the performance of activities of daily living. The HAQ measures performance in the activities of daily living focusing on difficulty and physical assistance needed to complete tasks. All have comparable reliability and validity.* With respect to pain, the AIMS has a specific subscale, the FSI includes pain as a dimension of mobility, and the HAQ includes a visual analogue scale. In comparison with each other, with respect to the measurement of arthritis pain, the AIMS had the highest relative efficiency, the most sensitivity, and produces a more global assessment.[74]

Affective assessment usually focuses on one or more of three states: depression, anxiety, and fatigue, all of which can have significant effects on the perception of pain. There are many instruments used to assess these variables. None is preferred for use in people with arthritis. Some functional status inventories, specifically the Arthritis Impact Measurement Scales and the Health Assessment Questionnaire, include sub-

* References 4, 36, 52, 58, 73, 83, 85, 106.

scales for depression, anxiety, and fatigue. They may not be sensitive enough to detect variations in the level of depression or anxiety over time, but they are useful as screening tools.

In summary, the assessment of the patient with arthritis pain should be a multidimensional approach to a multidimensional problem. This will always include an assessment of pain intensity using one or more rating scales, the patient's perception of pain, and the patient's self-report. It is important to understand the patient's experience and the implications for living with pain every day. Multidimensional assessment may include assessment of disease parameters, behavioral observation, and functional assessment. The assessment should be tailored to meet the needs of the individual patient.

◆ TREATMENT OF THE PAIN OF RHEUMATOLOGIC DISEASE

Pharmacological Treatment

The primary mode of treatment is pharmacological. Pharmacological treatment of arthritis pain has two primary aims:

1. To reduce inflammation and/or modulate the autoimmune response, thereby indirectly modulating the pain.
2. To directly modulate the pain response.

However, based on the current medical paradigm, the primary emphasis in treating arthritis pain is aimed at decreasing inflammation. A secondary benefit of that is a decrease in pain.

Pharmacological treatment of the pathogenesis of arthritis and treatment of the pain associated with the arthritis are two distinct but related issues. This discussion will focus on the latter. In the treatment of arthritis pain, there are three broad categories of drugs in use today:

1. Analgesics, both peripheral and central acting.
2. Antiinflammatory drugs with analgesic properties.
3. Adjunctive drugs, primarily the use of antidepressants.

Pure analgesics, consist of two groups, peripheral and central acting. The primary objective in the use of these medications is to provide pain relief for the patient. Acetaminophen is a relatively safe peripheral agent, which can be used at minimal risk to the patient with arthritis. However, in prolonged use, both liver and renal function should be assessed, because there can be a significant degree of toxicity associated with the chronic use of acetaminophen. In addition, one must be aware of the interactive effects of acetaminophen with other medications being taken by the patient with arthritis. For example, methotrexate is now being used as a third-line therapy for rheumatoid arthritis. Since methotrexate therapy is associated with significant liver toxicity, it is important for these patients to know the amount of acetaminophen they are taking.

The use of opioid analgesics for acute management of arthritis pain should be guided by the same principles as those for the use of opioids for a patient with acute pain (see Chapter 7). The long-term use of opioid analgesics in patients with arthritis and other types of chronic nonmalignant pain is a growing area of research, albeit controversial. Initial studies in people with chronic nonmalignant pain (not necessarily arthritis pain) suggest that given strict guidelines, it is possible to use opioids safely over years.[105] It is likely that clinicians are operating under incorrect and unnecessary fears of addiction and tolerance, fears that, in the next few years, will be proven unfounded through currently active research. If pain, independent from the disease, can contribute significantly to morbidity, then managing pain in addition to managing the disease may significantly decrease morbidity. Long-term opiate therapy is one way to approach the problem, and it deserves serious consideration.

Nonsteroidal antiinflammatory agents (NSAIDs) comprise the second major class of drugs used to manage pain in people with arthritis (see Chapter 7). The exact mechanism of analgesia in antiinflammatory drugs, such as ASA, ibuprofen, and indomethecin, is not known. It is believed that they block pain impulse generation in the peripheral chemonociceptors, specifically, prostaglandins, which are found in inflammatory exudate, and sensitize the receptors to stimulation. NSAIDs inhibit the synthesis of prostaglandin in the periphery.[51,125] It has also been suggested that NSAIDs alter immune cell function and inhibit exudate activation and cell migration into synovial membranes.[45] In addition, studies using a rat model for chronic arthritis pain suggest that some NSAIDs may also have a central analgesic action by inhibiting prostaglandin synthesis in the brain.[100] There is currently no way to predict which drug will work best in any given patient. The treatment is empirically based, which requires the health care provider to be aware of the pain and to assess it accurately and consistently. The primary concern with NSAIDs is the potential for these drugs to produce gastrointestinal side effects. Erosion, severe bleeding, and death are the most serious consequences of NSAID use, and nausea or stomach upset are the least serious and more common of the side effects.

The use of adjunctive analgesia, particularly tricyclic antidepressants (TCAs), is gaining popularity for the treatment of pain associated with rheumatic disease. It is possible that the relationship between pain, depression, and sleep is neurochemical, specifically through the neurotransmitter serotonin. Serotonin plays a role in regulation of mood and sleep physiology. It is probably not a coincidence that antidepressant medications that inhibit the reuptake of serotonin are effective in the treatment of arthritis pain. However, research shows the effect of TCAs on various types of arthritis pain to be equivocable, though there are more favorable than unfavorable reports.* Any analgesic effect appears to be independent of the effect of depression. Tricyclic antidepressants may act by reinforcing the central serotonergic system and inhibiting descending pain impulses.[66] Some suggest that the use of NSAIDs and TCAs concurrently in people with arthritis has an additive analgesic effect, more than the sum of either one alone.[113]

Nonpharmacological Treatment

Nonpharmacological intervention is generally aimed at directly modulating the pain response and at improving functional status with or without altering pain. These may include traditional treatments such as exercise and energy conservation strategies, biofeedback, relaxation therapy, ice and heat, or less traditional treatments such as hypnosis or massage (see Chapter 8). These treatments may be categorized as those that are based on cutaneous stimulation, psychoeducational, or cognitive approaches as outlined in Table 17-2.

Cutaneous Stimulation

Cutaneous stimulation can take the form of transcutaneous electrical nerve stimulation (TENS), ice, heat, massage, and the application of topical ointments. The Gate Control Theory (see Chapter 2) provides the most rational and clinically useful base from which to understand these interventions. A sum-

* References 19, 35, 39, 42, 47, 119.

◆ **Table 17-2**
Nonpharmacological treatments for arthritis pain

Type	Intervention
Cutaneous stimulation	Transcutaneous electrical nerve stimulation
	Ice
	Heat
	Massage
	Topical ointments (counter-stimulation)
Psychoeducational/cognitive	Thermal biofeedback
	Relaxation/guided imagery
	Hypnosis
	Arthritis self-help instruction
	Energy conservation training
Mechanical	Adaptive aids
	Splints
	Rest

mary of the current state of their use in arthritis pain follows.

TENS in the treatment of arthritis and many other types of acute and chronic pain has been the subject of much research over the past several years. The mechanism of analgesia in TENS is unknown, although it has been suggested that small diameter nociceptive nerve fiber input is inhibited through the large diameter stimulation promoted by TENS. TENS has been successful in relieving acute pain secondary to rheumatoid and osteoarthritis.[11,60,72,79] Some suggest that the mechanism of analgesia in TENS is related to the endogenous opioid system. However, the analgesia is not always reversed by naloxone.[50]

In the rat model of acute pain, TENS was shown to decrease intraarticular fluid pressure, volume, and leukocyte count in inflamed joints.[71] Bruce et al[11] suggest that TENS in combination with cognitive therapy may be useful in reducing pain, but some of that evidence has suggested that the treatment combination was associated with a decline in grip strength. However, their sample was very small, and further research is needed. From a clinical point of view, TENS for arthritis pain meets with varying approval. Often, it may be effective in relieving pain, but because the pain is usually multifocal, TENS becomes cumbersome and more trouble than it is worth. In addition, patients may gain immediate relief from TENS, but as time progresses, they achieve less pain relief. However, the issue of tolerance from TENS is still a point of debate.

Heat, ice, massage and/or the application of topical ointments provide other forms of cutaneous stimulation, all of which serve as a counterirritant to the pain. Documented research support for their use in arthritis pain is sparse but indicates some positive findings. Although heat is cognitively preferable to the patient, ice generally leads to more pain relief and more muscle relaxation.[24,67,68] Rubbing alcohol and water in equal portions can be mixed and frozen in airtight bags or surgical gloves to produce a "slushy" mixture, which can be molded to better fit the patient's joint. Massage with or without the application of topical ointments (usually containing menthol) appears to be effective in relieving pain and increasing joint range of motion.[121,124] Massage, in the form of a back rub, is clearly an independent nursing action, which, of late, has lost its meaning. Perhaps a return to the basics should be considered.

Psychological/Cognitive Strategies

Psychological, psychoeducational, and cognitive strategies include a wide variety of treatments, among them relaxation training, hypnosis, biofeedback, social support, and cognitive therapy (see Chapter 8). There is a wide range of research in this area, with great variations in complexity and quality of the studies. Comparisons and generalizations are difficult since operational definitions of the actual treatments generally differ from study to study. In addition, replication is virtually nonexistent.

In general, thermal biofeedback either alone or in combination with relaxation training has been effective in decreasing pain and pain behaviors and in increasing functional ability in people with arthritis, specifically rheumatoid arthritis.[1,10,14,27,88] In a related study Domangue et al[30] reported significant decreases in self-reported pain, anxiety, and depression, as well as significant increases in plasma beta-endorphin levels following hypnotherapy in people with arthritis. However, as with TENS, hypnoanalgesia is not always reversed by naloxone, an opiate antagonist, suggesting that another mechanism for analgesia exists besides or in addition to the endogenous opiates.[44]

Psychoeducational intervention strategies may also include counseling, group sessions, and/or a structured arthritis self-management course. The arthritis self-management course has the most consistent operational definition.[77] This community-based patient education course is designed to improve the overall knowledge about arthritis and enhance self-care practices. Knowledge, exercise, and relaxation training are key components to this course. A meta-analysis of 15 studies using these interventions, including the self-management course, indicates a 16% greater improvement in pain in treated over untreated groups of people overall. This improvement was in addition to the pain relief obtained by medications alone.[97] Through an alternative self-management program, Bradley et al[10] demonstrated a significant reduction in pain behavior, disease activity, and trait anxiety. Others have used group therapy with some success.[117] In general, it appears that these programs meet several objectives. First, they provide a structured environment for information exchange. Second, they shift the responsibility and control of the disease from the health care worker to the patient, who assumes a more active role and third, they provide social and emotional support. These factors are all important in the overall management of a chronic disease such as arthritis.

◆ SUMMARY

The impact of multidisciplinary treatment in the management of arthritis pain cannot be underestimated. As many have said, the pain of arthritis is complex. It is more than the nociception caused by the inflammatory response, more than the depression, more than the fatigue, and more than the medical diagnosis. In many, and perhaps most, of the cases, the degree of pain bears little relationship to the aforementioned variables. In general, a multimodality, multidisciplinary approach to treatment is necessary to effectively manage this problem. From a research perspective the study of a multidimensional treatment plan presents a significant challenge. In a controlled study, it is difficult to assess which part or parts is most effective. However, it is also becoming clearer to health care providers that it is this multidimensional approach that is most effective, especially in arthritis pain, when the pain is usually chronic and often severe. As clinicians and researchers become more skilled in assessing and documenting pain and the patient's response to that pain, the directions for treatment and research will become clearer. If one treats the patient empirically, as an individual, a plan will develop that allows for ongoing assessment, treatment, evaluation, and revision as needed.

REFERENCES

1. Achterberg, J., McGraw, P., and Lawlis, G. F.: Rheumatoid arthritis: A study of relaxation and temperature biofeedback training as an adjunctive therapy, *Biofeedback and Self Regulation 6*:207-223, 1981.
2. Affleck, G., et al: Social support and psychosocial adjustment to rheumatoid arthritis: Quantitative and qualitative findings. *Arthritis Care and Research 1*(2):71-77, 1989.
3. Anderson, L., et al: Rheumatoid arthritis: Review of psychological factors related to etiology, effects and treatment, *Psychological Bulletin 98*:358-387, 1989.
4. Anderson, J. J., Firschein, H. E., and Meenan, R. F.: Sensitivity of a health status measure to short-term clinical changes in arthritis, *Arthritis and Rheumatism 32*(7):844-850, 1989.
5. Anderson, K. O., et al: Prediction of pain behavior and functional status of rheumatoid arthritis patients using medical status and psychological variables, *Pain 33*:25-32, 1988.
6. Anderson, K. O., et al: The assessment of pain in rheumatoid arthritis: Validity of a behavioral observation method, *Arthritis and Rheumatism 30*(1):36-43, 1987a.
7. Anderson, K. O., et al: The assessment of pain in rheumatoid arthritis: Disease differentiation and temporal stability of a behavioral observation method, *Journal of Rheumatology 14*(4):700-704, 1987b.
8. Blumer, C., Heilbronn, M. Biological markers for depression in chronic pain, *The Journal of Nervous and Mental Diseases 170*:425-428, 1982.
9. Bervoets, K., Colpaert, F. C.: Respiratory effects of intrathecal capsaicin in arthritic and non-arthritic rats. *Life Sciences 34*:2477-2483, 1984.
10. Bradley, L. A., et al: Effects of psychological therapy on pain behavior of rheumatoid arthritis patients, *Arthritis and Rheumatism 30*(10): 1105-1114, 1987.
11. Bruce, J. R., et al: Pain Management in rheumatoid arthritis: Cognitive behavior modification and transcutaneous neural stimulation, *Arthritis Care and Research 1*(2):78-84, 1988.
12. Burckhart, C. S.: The impact of arthritis on quality of life. *Nursing Research 34*(1):11-16, 1985.
13. Burckhart, C. S. The Use of the McGill Pain Questionnaire in assessing arthritis pain. *Pain 19*:305-314, 1984.
14. Burke, E. J., et al: The adjunctive use of biofeedback and relaxation training in the treatment for severe rheumatoid arthritis: A preliminary investigation, *Clinical Biofeedback and Health 8*:28-36, 1985.
15. Calin, A.: Pain and inflammation, *The American Journal of Medicine* 9-16, September 10, 1984.

16. Calin, A.: Pathogenesis of ankylosing spondylitis: The state of the art, *British Journal of Rheumatology 27*(suppl II):106-109, 1988.
17. Callahan, L. F., et al: Quantitative pain assessment for routine care of rheumatoid arthritis patients, using a pain scale based on activities of daily living and a visual analog pain scale, *Rheumatoid Arthritis 30*(6):630-636, 1987.
18. Campbell, S. M., et al: Clinical characteristics of fibrositis: A "blinded" controlled study of symptoms and tender points, *Arthritis and Rheumatism 26*:817-824, 1983.
19. Carette, S., et al: Evaluation of amitriptyline in primary fibrositis, *Arthritis and Rheumatism 5*:655-659, 1986.
20. Carlsson, A. M.: Assessment of chronic pain. I. Aspects of the reliability and validity of the visual analogue scale, *Pain 16*:87-101, 1983.
21. Charter, R. A., et al: The nature of arthritis pain, *British Journal of Rheumatology 24*:53-60, 1985.
22. Colpaert, F. C.: Evidence that adjuvant arthritis in the rat is associated with chronic pain, *Pain 28*:201-222, 1987.
23. Colpaert, F. C., Donnerer, J. and Lembeck, F.: Effects of capsaicin on inflammation and on the substance P content of nervous tissues in rats with adjuvant arthritis, *Life Science 32*:921-928, 1983.
24. Cooling more effective, *Aches and Pains 3*(37), 1982.
25. Dardick, S. J., Basbaum, A. I., and Levine, J. D.: The contribution of pain to disability in experimentally induced arthritis, *Arthritis and Rheumatism 29*(8):1017-1022, 1986.
26. Daut, R. L., Cleeland, C. S., and Flanery, R. C.: Development of the Wisconsin Brief Pain Questionnaire to assess pain in cancer and other diseases, *Pain 17*:197-210, 1983.
27. Denver, D. R., et al: Behavioral medicine: Biobehavioral effects of short-term thermal biofeedback and relaxation in rheumatoid arthritis patients, *Biofeedback and Self Regulation 4*:245-246, 1979.
28. Dequeker, J., Wuestenraed, L.: The effect of biometeorologica factors on Ritchie Articular Index and pain in rheumatoid arthritis, *Scandinavian Journal of Rheumatology 15*:280-284, 1986.
29. Dixon, J. S., Bird, H. A.: Reproducibility along a 10 cm vertical visual analogue scale, *Annals of Rheumatic Disease 40*:87-89, 1981.
30. Domangue, B. B., et al: Biochemical correlates of hypnoanalgesia in arthritic pain patients, *Journal of Clinical Psychiatry 46*:235-238, 1985.
31. Downie, W. W., et al: Studies with pain rating scales, *Annals of Rheumatic Disease 37*:378-381, 1978.
32. Dubisson, D., Melzack, R.: Classification of clinical pain descriptors by multiple group discriminant analysis, *Experimental Neurology 51* 480-487, 1976.
33. Flor, H., Turk, D. C.: Chronic back pain and rheumatoid arthritis: Predicting pain and disability from cognitive variables, *Journal of Behavioral Medicine 11*(3):251-265, 1988.
34. Frank, R. G., et al: Depression in rheumatoid arthritis, *The Journal of Rheumatology 15*(6):920-925, 1988a.
35. Frank, R. G., et al: Antidepressant analgesia in rheumatoid arthritis, *The Journal of Rheumatology 15*(11):1632-1638, 1986.
36. Fries, J., Spitz, P. W., & Young, D. Y. (1982). The dimensions of health

outcomes: The health assessment questionnaire, disability and pain scales. *The Journal of Rheumatology, 9*(5), 789-793.

37. Fries, J. F., et al: Measurement of patient outcome in arthritis, *Arthritis and Rheumatism 23*:137-145, 1980.
38. Furst, G. P., et al: A program for improving energy conservation behaviors in adults with rheumatoid arthritis, *The American Journal of Occupational Therapy 41*(2):102-111, 1987.
39. Ganvir, P., Beaumont, G., and Seldrup, J.: A clinical trial of clomipramine and placebo: Adjunctive therapy in arthralgia, *Journal of Internal Medicine and Research 8*:60-66, 1980.
40. Gaston-Johansson, F., et al: A comparative study of pain description, emotional discomfort and health perception in patients with chronic pain syndrome and rheumatoid arthritis, *Scandinavian Journal of Rehabilitation Medicine 17*:109-119, 1985.
41. Gibson, T., Clark, B.: Use of simple analgesics in rheumatoid arthritis, *Annals of Rheumatic Disease 44*:27-29, 1985.
42. Glick, E. N.: A clinical trial of Tofranil in osteoarthritis, *Journal of Internal Medicine and Research 4*(suppl 2):20-22, 1976.
43. Gerber, L., et al: Patient education program to teach energy conservation behaviors to patients with rheumatoid arthritis: A pilot study, *Archives of Physical Medicine and Rehabilitation 68*:442-445, 1987.
44. Goldstein, A., Hilgard, E. R.: Failure of the opiate antagonist naloxone to reverse hypnotic analgesia, *Proceeds of the National Academy of Science 72*:2041-2043, 1975.
45. Goodwin, J. S. Immunologic effects of nonsteroidal anti-inflammatory drugs, *The American Journal of Medicine* 7-15, October 15, 1984.
46. Good, A. E. The pain of ankylosing spondylitis, *The American Journal of Medicine 80*(suppl 3A):118, March 24, 1986.
47. Gringas, M.: A clinical trial of Tofranil in rheumatic pain in general practice, *Journal of Internal Medicine and Research 4*:(suppl 2), 41-49, 1976.
48. Haber, L. Disabling effects of chronic disease and impairments, *Journal of Chronic Disease 24*:469-487, 1971.
49. Hagglund, K. J., et al: Predicting individual differences in pain and functional impairment among patients with rheumatoid arthritis, *Arthritis and Rheumatism 32*(7):851-858, 1989.
50. Hansson, P., et al: Influence of naloxone on relief of acute oro-facial pain by transcutaneous electrical nerve stimulation (TENS) or vibration, *Pain 24*:323-329, 1986.
51. Harris, E. D.: Evaluation of pathophysiology and drug effects on rheumatoid arthritis, *The American Journal of Medicine,* 56-61, October 31, 1983.
52. Harris, B. A., et al: Validity of self-report measures of functional disability, *Topics in Geriatric Rehabilitation 1*(3):31-41, 1986.
53. Hodes, R.: Pain, functional impairment and rheumatoid arthritis An initial inquiry, *PRN Forum: A Newsletter for the Pain Research Nurse 2*(2):1-2, 1983.
54. Jette, A. M.: Functional capacity evaluation: An empirical approach, *Archives of Physical Medicine and Rehabilitation 61*:85-89, 1980a.
55. Jette, A. M.: Functional status index: Reliability of a chronic disease

evaluation instrument. *Archives of Physical Medicine and Rehabilitation 61*:395-401, 1980b.

56. Kazis, L. E., Meenan, R. F., Anderson, J. J.: Pain in the rheumatic diseases: Investigation of a key health status component, *Arthritis and Rheumatism, 26*(8):1017-1022, 1983.
57. Keefe, F. J. Behavioral assessment and treatment of chronic pain: Current status and future directions, *Journal of Consulting and Clinical Psychology 50*:896-911, 1982.
58. Kirwan, J. R., Reeback, J. S.: Stanford health assessment questionnaire modified to assess disability in british patients with rheumatoid arthritis, *British Journal of Rheumatology 25*:206-209, 1986.
59. Kramlinger, K. G., et al: Are patients with chronic pain depressed? *American Journal of Psychiatry 140*:747-749, 1983.
60. Kumer, V. N., Redford, J. B.: Transcutaneous nerve stimulation in rheumatoid arthritis, *Archives of Physical Medicine and Rehabilitation 63*:595-596, 1982.
61. Laborde, J. W., Dando, W. A., and Powers, M. J.: Influence of weather on osteoarthritics, *Basic Science and Medicine 23*(6):549-554, 1986.
62. Laborde, J. M., Powers, M. J.: Life satisfaction, health control orientation, and illness-related factors in persons with osteoarthritis, *Research in Nursing and Health 8*:183-190, 1985.
63. Lambert, V. A.: Study of factors associated with psychological well-being in rheumatoid arthritic women, *Image: The Journal of Nursing Scholarship 17*(2):50-53, 1985.
64. Landis, C. A., Levine, J. D., and Robinson, C. R.: Decreased slow wave and paradoxical sleep in a rat chronic pain model, *Sleep 12*:167-177, 1989.
65. Leavitt, F., et al: Comparison of pain properties in fibromyalgia patients and rheumatoid arthritis patients, *Arthritis and Rheumatism 29*(6): 775-781, 1986.
66. Lee, R., Spencer, P. S. J.: Antidepressants and pain: A review of the pharmacological data supporting the use of certain tricyclics in chronic pain, *Journal of Internal Medicine and Research 5*:(suppl 1), 146-156, 1977.
67. Lehmann, J. F., de LaTeur, B. J.: Diathermy and superficial heat and cold therapy. In F. J. Kottke, C. K. Stillwell & J. F. Lehmann (eds) *Kruzen's Handbook of Physical Medicine and Rehabilitation,* 1982a, Philadelphia, W. B. Saunders.
68. Lehmann, J. F., de LaTeur, B. J.: Cryotherapy. In J. F. Lehmann (Ed) *Therapeutic Heat and Cold* (ed. 3), 1982b, Baltimore, Williams & Wilkins.
69. Lembeck, F., Donnerer, J., and Colpaert, F.: Increase of substance P in primary afferent nerves during chronic pain, *Neuropeptides 1*:175-180, 1981.
70. Levine, J. D., et al: Hypothesis: The nervous system may contribute to the pathophysiology of rheumatoid arthritis, *Journal of Rheumatology 12*(3):406-411, 1985.
71. Levy, A., et al: Transcutaneous electrical nerve stimulation in experimental acute arthritis, *Archives of Physical Medicine and Rehabilitation 68*:75-78, 1987.
72. Lewis, D., Lewis, B., and Sturrock, R. D.: Transcutaneous electrical nerve

stimulation in osteoarthritis: Therapeutic alternative? *Annals of Rheumatic Disease 43*:47-49, 1984.

73. Liang, M. H., Jette, A. M.: Measuring functional ability in chronic arthritis: A critical review, *Arthritis and Rheumatism 24*(1):80-86, 1981.
74. Liang, M. H., et al: Comparative measurement efficiency and sensitivity of five health status instruments for arthritis research, *Arthritis and Rheumatism 28*(5):542-547, 1985.
75. Lichtenberg, P. A., Skehan, M. W., and Swensen, C. H.: The role of personality, recent life stress and arthritic severity in predicting pain, *Journal of Psychosomatic Research 28*:231-236, 1984.
76. Lipowsky, Z. J.: Physical illness, the individual and the coping process, *Psychiatry Medicine 1*(4):91-101, 1970.
77. Lorig, K., et al: Outcomes of self-help education for patients with arthritis *Arthritis and Rheumatism 28*:680-685, 1985.
78. Mahowald, M. W., et al: Sleep fragmentation and daytime sleepiness in rheumatoid arthritis, *Sleep Research 16*:487, 1987.
79. Mannheimer, C. Lund, S., and Carlsson, C. A.: Effect of transcutaneous electrical nerve stimulation (TENS) on joint pain in patients with rheumatoid arthritis, *Scandinavian Journal of Rheumatology* 7:13-16, 1978.
80. McCarty, D. J.: (Ed.) Arthritis and allied conditions: A textbook of rheumatology, 1979, Philadelphia, Lea & Febiger.
81. McDaniel, L. K., et al: Development of an observation method for assessing pain behavior in rheumatoid arthritis patients, *Pain 24*: 165-184, 1986.
82. McKenna, F., Wright, V. Pain and rheumatoid arthritis, *Annals of Rheumatic Disease 44*: 805, 1985.
83. Meenan, R. B., et al: Outcome assessment in clinical trials: Evidence for the sensitivity of a health status measure, *Arthritis and Rheumatism 27*(12):1344-1352, 1984.
84. Meenan, R. F., Gertman, P. M., and Mason, J. H.: Measuring health status in arthritis: The arthritis impact measurement scales, *Arthritis and Rheumatism 23*:146-152, 1980.
85. Meenan, R. F., et al: The arthritis impact measurement scales: Further investigations of a health status measure, *Arthritis and Rheumatism 25*(9):1048-1053, 1982.
86. Melzack, R. The McGill Pain Questionnaire: Major properties and scoring methods, *Pain 1*:277-299, 1975.
87. Melzack, R., Wall, P: Pain mechanisms: A new theory, *Science 150*:791-799, 1965.
88. Mitchell, K. R.: Peripheral temperature autoregulation and its effect on the symptoms of rheumatoid arthritis, *Scandinavian Journal of Behavioral Therapy 15*:55-64, 1985.
89. Moldofsky, H., Lue, F. A., and Saskin, P. Sleep and morning pain in primary osteoarthritis, *The Journal of Rheumatology 14*(1):124-128, 1987.
90. Moldofsky, H., Lue, F. A., and Smythe, H. A.: Alpha EEG sleep and morning symptoms in rheumatoid arthritis, *The Journal of Rheumatology 10*:373-379, 1983.
91. Moldofsky, H., Scarisbrick, P. Induction of neurasthenic musculoskeletal pain syndrome by selective sleep stage deprivation, *Psychosomatic Medicine 38*:35-44, 1976.

92. Moldofsky, H., et al: Musculoskeletal symptoms and nonREM sleep disturbance in patients with "Fibrositis Syndrome" and health subjects, *Psychosomatic Medicine 37*:341-351, 1975.
93. Moldofsky, H., Tullis, C., and Lue, F. A.: Sleep-related myoclonus in rheumatic pain modulation disorder (fibrositis syndrome) and in excessive daytime somnolence, *Psychosomatic Medicine 46*:145-151, 1984.
94. Moldofsky, H., Tullis, C., and Lue, F. A.: Sleep related myoclonus in rheumatic pain modulation disorder (fibrositis syndrome), *The Journal of Rheumatology 13*:614-617, 1986.
95. Moldofsky, H., Tullis, C., and Quance, G.: Nitrazepam for periodic movements in sleep (sleep related myoclonus), *Canadian Journal of Neurologic Sciences 13*:52-54, 1986.
96. Mooney, N. E. Coping & chronic pain in rheumatoid arthritis patients: Behaviors and nursing interventions, *Orthopedic Nursing* 21-25, May/June 1982.
97. Mullen, P. D., et al: Efficacy of psycho-educational interventions on pain, depression and disability with arthritic adults: A meta-analysis, *The Journal of Rheumatology 14*(suppl 15):33-39, 1987.
98. Nagi, S.: An epidemiology of disability amoung adults in the United States, *Milbank Quarterly 54*:439-468, 1976.
99. National Institutes of Health (May 1986). The integrated approach to the management of pain: Consensus development statement, *6,* Publication Number 491-292: 41148. U.S. Department of Health & Human Services, Public Health Service, Office of Medical Application of Research, 1-28.
100. Okuyama, S., Aihara, H.: The mode of action of analgesic drugs in adjuvant arthritic rats as an experimental model of chronic inflammatory pain: Possible central analgesic action of acidic nonsteroidal antiinflammatory drugs, *Japanese Journal of Pharmacology 35*:95-103, 1984.
101. Parker, J., et al: Pain in rheumatoid arthritis: Relationship to demographic, medical, and psychological factors, *The Journal of Rheumatology 15*:433-437, 1988.
102. Patberg, W. R., Nienhuis, R. L. F., and Veringa, F.: Relation between meteorological factors and pain in rheumatoid arthritis in a marine climate, *The Journal of Rheumatology 12*:711-715, 1985.
103. Perry, F., Heller, P. H., and Levine, J. D.: Differing correlations between pain measures in syndromes with or without explicable organic pathology, *Pain 34:*185-189, 1988.
104. Polley, H. F., Swenson, W. M., and Steinhilber, R. M.: Personality characteristics of patients with rheumatoid arthritis, *Psychosomatics 11*:45-49, 1970.
105. Portenoy, R., Foley, K.: Chronic use of opioid analgesics in nonmalignant pain: Report on 38 cases, *Pain 25*:171-186, 1986.
106. Potts, M. K., Brandt, K. D.: Evidence of the validity of the arthritis impact measurement scales, *Arthritis and Rheumatism, 30*(1):93-96, 1987.
107. *Primer on the Rheumatic Diseases* (9th edition). H. R. Schumacher Jr. (Ed.) Arthritis Foundation: Atlanta, Georgia.
108. Reading, A. E.: A comparison of rating scales, *Journal of Psychosomatic Research 24*:119-124, 1980.
109. Reading, A. E.: A comparison of the McGill Pain Questionnaire in chronic and acute pain, *Pain 13*:185-192, 1982.
110. Reisine, S. T., et al: Work disability among women with rheumatoid

arthritis. The relative importance of disease, social, work, and family factors, *Arthritis and Rheumatism 32*(5):538-542, 1989.

111. Rimon, R.: Depression in rheumatoid arthritis: Prevalence by self-report questionnaire and recognition by non-psychiatric physicians, *Annals of Clinical Research 6*:171-175, 1974.
112. Ruoff, G.: The pain of osteoarthritis, *The American Journal of Medicine 80*(suppl 3A):96, March 24, 1986.
113. Sarzi-Puttini, P. S., et al: A comparison of Dothiepin versus placebo in the treatment of pain in rheumatoid arthritis and the association of pain with depression, *The Journal of International Medical Research 16*:331-337, 1988.
114. Scott, J., et al: Graphic representation of pain, *Pain 2*:175-184, 1976.
115. Smukler, N. M.: Pain perception, *Bulletin on the Rheumatic Diseases 35*:1-8, 1985.
116. Smythe, H. A.: Fibrositis and other diffuse musculoskeletal syndromes. In W. Kelley, E. Harris, S. Ruddy et al. (eds). *Textbook of Rheumatology*, 1980, Philadelphia, W. B. Saunders.
117. Strauss, G. D., et al: Group therapies for rheumatoid arthritis: A controlled study of two approaches, *Arthritis and Rheumatism 29*: 1203-1209, 1986.
118. Summers, M. N., et al: Radiographic assessment and psychological variables as predictors of pain and functional impairment in osteoarthritis of the knee or hip, *Arthritis and Rheumatism 31*(2):204-209, 1988.
119. Tyler, A. M.: Treatment of the painful shoulder syndrome with amitriptyline and lithium carbonate, *Canadian Medical Association Journal 111*:137-140, 1974.
120. Wagstaff, S., Smith, O. V., and Wood, P. H. N.: Verbal pain descriptors used by patieints with arthritis, *Annals of the Rheumatic Diseases 44*:262-265, 1985.
121. Wakim, K. G.: Physiological effects of massage. In J. B. Basmajian (Ed) *Manipulation, Traction and Massage* (ed. 3), 1985, Baltimore, Williams & Wilkins.
122. Walsh, T. D., Leber, B.: Measurement of chronic pain: Visual analog scales and McGill Melzack Pain Questionnaire compared. In: R. Melzack (Ed.), *Pain Measurement and Assessment,* 1983, Raven Press, New York.
123. Weinberger, M., Hiner, S. L., and Tierney, W. M.: Improving functional status in arthritis: The effect of social support, *Social Science and Medicine 23*(9):899-904, 1986.
124. White, J. R.: Effects of a counterirritant on perceived pain and hand movement in patients with arthritis, *Physical Therapy 53*:956-960, 1973.
125. Wolf, R. E.: Nonsteroidal anti-inflammatory drugs, *Archives of Internal Medicine 144*:1658-1660, 1984.
126. Wolfe, F.: Arthritis and musculoskeletal pain, *Nursing Clinics of North America 19*(4):565-574, 1984.
127. Yelin, E., et al: Work disability in rheumatoid arthritis: Effects of disease, social and work factors, *Annals of Internal Medicine 93*:551-556, 1980.
128. Zathiropoulos, G., Barry, H. R.: Depression in rheumatoid disease, *Annals of Rheumatic Disease 33*:132-135.
129. Zorumski, C. F., Rubin, E. H.: Psychopharmacologic and behavioral approaches to chronic arthritic pain, *Comprehensive Therapy 10*(8):35-39, 1984.

18

Patients with Idiopathic Low Back Pain: Physical Fitness as a Treatment Strategy

Sandra M. LeFort

◆ INTRODUCTION

IN HER ESSAY entitled "On Being Ill," Virginia Woolf wrote:

English, which can express the thoughts of Hamlet and the tragedy of Lear, has no words for the shiver and the headache . . . The merest schoolgirl, when she falls in love, has Shakespeare or Keats to speak her mind for her; but let a sufferer try to describe a pain in his head to a doctor and language at once runs dry."[92]

How true this is for those of us who have tried to explain our own pain to others or who have attempted to understand what pain is like for another person. Far from the stimulus-response approach to pain of a few decades ago, the present level of knowledge indicates the vast complexity of the pain experience. Pain is now known to be a highly personal, variable experience that is influenced, not only by neurophysiological mechanisms responding to sensory stimuli but also by social and cultural learning, the meaning of the situation, and other physical, psychological and cognitive factors. The puzzle becomes even more complex when pain becomes chronic. Indeed chronic pain syndrome—nonmalignant pain lasting more than 6 months from time of expected healing—is now thought to be an entity in its own right regardless of its cause.

It has been estimated that over one third of the North American population has persistent or recurrent pain problems necessitating medical intervention.[62] Low back pain provides an especially important area for research because of its high prevalence in the general population, the detrimental effects of pain and disability on the individual and his or her family's quality of life, and the high cost to society of long-term physical and psychosocial impairment that can accompany this syndrome.

The Scope of the Problem

Low back pain (LBP), the so-called nemesis of medicine and the albatross of industry, is a major health concern in the industrialized world.[69] Epidemiological studies from Scandinavia, Britain, the Netherlands, and the United States report that LBP is of epidemic proportions, significantly affecting between 50% and 90% of all individuals in the adult population at some time in their lives.[6,32,52,91] Recent medical anthropological and clinical studies have also indicated a high incidence of spinal pain in the general population of less developed nations such as Nepal and Oman.[1,2,90]

It is known that men and women are about equally affected by back pain with the peak onset between 20 and 30 years and the highest prevalence between 40 and 60 years.[27] In the age group over 55 years, however, more women report low back symptoms than men, a finding that may be related to the development of osteoporosis in the menopausal years.[16,32] It is not understood why low back pain and related disability peak in middle age.

In most cases, LBP is a self-limiting condition with a recovery rate of 70% during the first month and 90% by 2 months.[12,27,91] However, the recurrence rate is high and with each recurrence the LBP becomes more severe and long lasting.[46,48,89] As a result, individuals with back complaints are likely to experience a significant number of disability days per year and to be frequent users of health care services.[16,70] In the United States, LBP is the second most frequent reason for physician visits, the fifth most frequent cause of hospitalization, and the third ranking reason for surgical procedures.[3,4,8] Too often, the search for a cure results in problems that are worse than the original back complaint, problems such as drug dependency and unnecessary and numerous surgeries.[66]

An estimated 5% of those suffering acute episodes of LBP go on to develop chronic LBP, a condition that has generally been resistant to traditional medical management.[32] About 1% of the U.S. population is chronically disabled by back pain, and 2% of the work force has compensable back injuries each year.[3] This chronic group represents up to 85% of the cost of low back pain to society, an estimated $80 billion in the United States.[4,32] Even more significant is the human cost of chronic pain—the physical, emotional, and social consequences that occur both to the individuals who are suffering and to their families.[75]

In the United States, data from the National Center for Health Statistics indicate that impairments of the back and spine are the leading cause of activity limitation in persons with chronic conditions who are under age 45, and they are the third most frequent cause of impairment in persons aged 45 to 60 years.[52] Canadian survey data show similar trends. In 1978 and 1979 the Canada Health Survey (CHS) collected information from approximately 32,000 individuals in 12,200 households across Canada. Back, limb, and joint disorders were second only to arthritis and rheumatism as the most prevalent acute or chronic health problem for all ages, and it was the most prevalent health problem for the 15-year-old to the 64-year-old age group.[45]

Additional support for these findings was provided by the Canadian Health and Disablity Survey 1983-1984. This cross-sectional survey of over 15,000 disabled Canadians reported that the most prevalent disabling conditions of adults were chronic conditions of the musculoskeletal system. The back was affected most often in the age group 35 years to 54 years, and the reported incidence was almost equal for men and women.[86]

Since LBP tends to affect individuals in their most productive years, the effect on industry is staggering. Rowe[76] found that LBP was second only to upper respiratory infections as the cause of illness-related absence from work over the 10-year period from 1956 to 1965 in one New York plant. This was true for employees with sedentary work as well as for those with physically demanding jobs. In a Swedish study Helander (1973 as cited in Andersson et al, 1984)[6] found that from 1961 to 1971, 12.5% of all annual sickness absence days were related to low back disorders. No other disease category was responsible for a greater number of days lost from work. In Britain 25% of all working men were reported to be affected by low back disorders each year.[40]

In both Canada and the United States, the total number of claims for job-related back injuries, the average time off work, and the amount awarded in compensation payments are all increasing.[16,90] In Canada from 1972 to 1981, an average of 20% of all lost-time work injuries occurred to the back or spine.[85] In 1988 this had increased to an average of 27%.[84]

Correspondingly, compensation costs for job-related back injuries have continued to rise. For example, an estimated $788 million was awarded in 1983, compared with $690 million in 1982 for job-related back injury claims in Canada.[16] In addition, 1981 to 1983 Ontario statistics indicate that the duration of time off work for back injuries is, on the average, 40% higher than that for all other injury claims combined.[16]

The chronic and recurrent nature of back problems adds to the significance of the data. Only 50% of individuals who are absent from work for more than 6 months because of back pain will return to work. Absence of more than 1 year reduces this to 25%, and after 2 years of absence, the chances of a worker returning to productive employment are negligible.[60,68] Thus it is clear that the morbidity, disability, activity limitation, and economic cost brought about by low back pain are considerable to both the affected individual, his or her family, and to society as a whole.[52]

Etiology of Low Back Pain

Low back pain is a nonspecific symptom and a subjective experience rather than a definite diagnostic category. Generally, the individual with LBP has constant or intermittent pain that has a particularly unpleasant quality, often described as deep, aching, and burning.[64] It is usually of musculoskeletal origin and is located in the lumbar region of the spine, between the rib cage and the pelvis. Most commonly, the pain radiates from the lower back to one or both buttocks and upper thighs and is unassociated with any of the neurologic signs that indicate disk herniation, such as focal muscular weakness, asymmetry of reflexes, sensory loss in a dermatome, or specific loss of intestinal, bladder, or sexual function.[72,83] The pain, however, may occasionally radiate from below the gluteal fold to include the upper leg above the knee or may radiate to the entire limb; radiating pain to the leg may or may not be accompanied by neurologic signs.

For any given individual, the likelihood of identifying a specific cause for acute LBP is on the order of 5% to 20%.[32,36] In a Quebec study of spinal disorders, Spitzer, LeBlanc, and Dupuis[83] stated:

> The etiologic diagnosis of spinal disorders is difficult because the physical signs and symptoms often have little specificity. There is often a discrepancy between the level of pain and the loss of function, on the one hand, and the minimal physical signs on the other (p. S18, S20).

Occasionally, LBP is caused by disk prolapse or herniation or metabolic disorders such as osteoporosis. Other infrequent causes of LBP include spinal trauma, causing vertebral body fracture, congenital abnormalities, such as spondylolysis, and degenerative spinal diseases, such as spinal stenosis or osteoarthritis and inflammatory or neoplastic lesions.[33] It is noteworthy that degenerative changes of the disk and spine occur to almost everyone and exist in individuals who are totally free of back pain symptoms.[15,24] Therefore radiography that indicates a narrowing of the intervertebral disk is not diagnostic of LBP.

For the majority of individuals, the pathophysiology of their LBP is unknown, and their condition is therefore categorized as idiopathic low back pain or low back syndrome. Nachemson,[68] a respected researcher in the field for 30 years, has stated, "The only thing we can say is that it is somewhere in the motion segment that pain is elicited. Something must rupture in the acute phase, but we don't really know what" (p. 3). Although the exact offending structure remains obscure, research is focusing on the intervertebral disk, with its surrounding longitudinal ligaments and facet joints.[69] (See Figure 18-1.)

Melzack and Wall[64] have hypothesized that in many cases of idiopathic LBP, the major culprit is abnormal activity in nerve-root fibers resulting from minor changes in the surrounding vertebrae and tissues. These cumulative minor irritations might eventually produce symptoms that can be the beginning of a vicious cycle of spasm and pain. An alternative view, proposed by Sarno[77] is that pain is caused by muscular tension that activates the autonomic nervous system, causing vasoconstriction of the arterioles in skeletal muscle. Vasoconstriction could lead to relative ischemia in the muscle thereby causing pain.

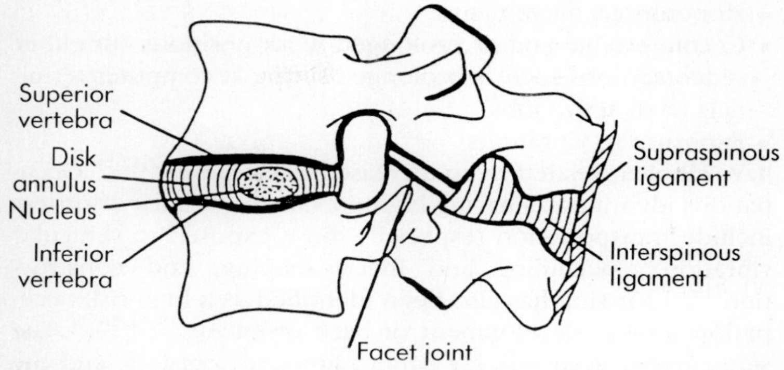

FIGURE 18-1. The basic structured unit of the spine (motion segment). (Reproduced with permission from Pope MH, Lehmann TR, and Frymoyer JW. Structure and function of the lumbar spine, 1984. In Pope MH, Frymoyer JW, and Andersson G (eds): *Occupational low back pain*, p. 6, Westport, Conn: Praeger.)

◆ PREDISPOSING FACTORS TO LBP

The factors that make some people more susceptible to idiopathic low back pain than others are beginning to be identified.[88] These risk factors include:

Physical Factors

There is a positive relationship between low activity levels and LBP.[66] Increased physical fitness and greater muscle strength and muscle flexibility appear to play a role in the prevention and recurrence of LBP episodes and in the rehabilitation of those with chronic LBP.[13,19,54,82] In animal studies moderate exercise has been found to increase the flow of nutrients into the intervertebral disk.[47] It is interesting to note that individual factors such as height, weight, body build, and limb length have not been demonstrated to have a relationship to LBP.[5]

Occupational Factors

Involvement in occupations that require:

- Heavy physical work
- Repetitive lifting in the forward bent-and-twisted position (particularly when the lifting requirements exceed the worker's physical capacity)

- Monotonous movements
- Uncomfortable and/or prolonged work positions (in either sedentary jobs such as prolonged sitting at computer terminals or in active jobs)
- Exposure to vibrations

have all been related to an increased risk of LBP.[12,32,68] Occupations identified as having high prevalence of back disorders include transportation (especially those exposed to vehicular vibration), machining and metal shaping, and construction.[16,35] Nursing has also been identified as a high-risk occupation for the development of back problems.[18,51,56,74] The static action necessary for patient lifts and transfers, and the frequent movement of equipment by nurses are thought to be factors in the high prevalence of LBP in nursing personnel.[44]

Psychological Factors

Although a number of psychological factors have been related to LBP, especially chronic LBP, the cause and effect relationship remains unclear.[78,83] For example, alterations in mood and self-esteem, as well as high anxiety, increased life stress, depression, work dissatisfaction, hypochondriasis, and somatization (focusing on bodily symptoms) have been associated with LBP.[5,32,37,78] Pathopsychological conceptual models discuss chronic LBP in terms of chronic neurosis, the pain-prone personality, masked depression, and learned helplessness. However, because most studies of the LBP population have been retrospective in design, it is not known whether these characteristics are predisposing factors to the onset of LBP or whether they are a result of the pain experience.[38] What is known is that emotional states modify the cognition of pain, and that during periods of depression and anxiety, symptoms may worsen.[72] It is also clear that psychological and social variables can serve to maintain disability.[31,90] Thus it appears that the interplay of physiological and psychological factors are involved in the experience of chronic pain and in chronic pain behavior.

Other Factors

Smoking has been found to compromise the nutrition of the intervertebral disks in preliminary animal studies[35] and has been identified as a risk factor for LBP in epidemiological studies.[35,51] In addition, it has been postulated that coughing may lead to increased intradiscal pressure and thus to increased spinal loadings resulting in LBP.[5]

Whatever the cause, the subjective experience of idiopathic low back pain involves complex neurophysiological and psychological phenomena that may create distress in the individual. If the acute experience of LBP becomes chronic, then even more complex psychological and learning factors come into play, resulting in major life disruption.

◆ TREATMENT

Nurses who work in primary care settings, occupational health settings, and in the community may be called on to examine patients who complain of back pain. A thorough history and a preliminary physical examination (see the accompanying boxes) will be required to rule out any serious

◆ ELEMENTS OF THE PATIENT HISTORY

A thorough history of the LBP patient should include:

1. The history of the LBP, previous treatments, and the response to treatment.
2. The history of the current episode, the circumstances surrounding the injury, work-related factors (such as occupation, work position, and exposure to vibration) and the pain pattern, including aggravating and relieving factors. In addition, associated factors especially sensory changes such as numbness and tingling, and changes in bladder and bowel control must be identified. These symptoms may indicate an acute surgical emergency.
   NOTE: Most patients with idiopathic LBP report that their pain is relieved by rest. If this is not the case, suspect other organic causes, and refer immediately to a physician.
3. Overall health status and other diseases.
4. Functional assessment that includes the patient's level of disability and psychological status.

Modified from "Evaluation of the worker with low back pain" by Frymoyer J and Milhous R. (1984). In Pope M, Frymoyer J, and Andersson G (eds), *Occupational low back pain* (pp. 157-184). Westport, Conn: Praeger.

◆ PRELIMINARY PHYSICAL EXAMINATION OF THE LBP PATIENT

INSPECTION	Inspect gross body movements, gait, posture, and spine (note curvature, any differences in height of the shoulders, iliac crests, and the skin creases below the buttocks).
RANGE OF MOTION	Ask the patient to walk on heels and toes (indicates intact function of L5 and S1). Within his or her range of comfort, ask patient to flex from the waist. Sit down and stabilize the patient's pelvis with your hands; ask the patient to bend laterally to the right, then to the left, and to bend backwards to test extension. To evaluate axial rotation, ask the patient to twist his or her shoulders to the right and then to the left.
PALPATION	With patient standing and putting his or her weight on the examining table, palpate spinous processes and paravertebral muscles for tenderness and spasm.
NEUROLOGIC EXAMINATION	With the patient supine, test sensation and muscle strength of both legs. Elicit ankle jerk and knee reflexes.
SPECIAL PROCEDURE	With patient supine, slowly raise the patient's relaxed leg until back pain occurs, then dorsiflex the foot. This generally increases back pain. In individuals without back pain, the hip can be flexed 90 degrees without pain. Pain behind the knees is indicative of tight hamstrings, not LBP.

Modified from *A Guide to Physical Examination* (3rd ed) by Bates B. (1983). Philadelphia: Lippincott.

disorders, such as a herniated disk, that may require immediate emergency intervention. Several publications that outline these assessments in detail are recommended for further reading.[34,65,67,83]

Despite the magnitude of the LBP problem, the advances in

diagnostic procedures, and the abundance of research and literature on the topic, little is really known about the specific causes of idiopathic low back pain and the effectiveness of treatment.[27,68] Treatment in the acute phase tends to be symptomatic in nature, aimed at reducing the level of pain, promoting healing, and maintaining function.[79] Traditional conservative treatments include a wide range of modalities. The most universal therapy is bed rest. Others include analgesics and muscle relaxants, physiotherapy, spinal manipulation, flexion and/or extension exercises, corsets and braces, traction, and educational programs that emphasize care of the back. However, evidence supporting the effectiveness of these methods is conflicting, and the usefulness of these treatments remains unclear.*

Because of the generally debilitating effects of inactivity, even bed rest is a questionable treatment. Several authors have stated that strict bed rest is not necessary for LBP unless there is significant radiation. Even in these cases, current research findings suggest that bed rest should last no longer than 2 days at a time, up to a maximum of 4 days.[14,21,83] Instead of bed rest, patients should avoid sitting (this position is the most stressful on the back), should walk around as much as they are able, and should relax by lying down at intervals.[14]

Nachemson,[68,69] Gilbert et al,[39] and others have pointed out the difficulty in studying a condition that is usually self-limiting. It may be the case that most patients would improve in the acute phase regardless of treatment modality. However, because the recurrence rate of LBP is so high, the impact of chronicity so great, and because not all patients improve with conservative therapy, treatment approaches must look beyond the immediate acute episode. This has led to a search for other forms of treatment that might prevent the cycle of recurrence and chronicity.

One area receiving renewed attention in the literature is the role of activity, exercise, and physical fitness for the LBP population.† Although physical activity has always been recommended for individuals with LBP once the acute phase was over, few studies have examined the specific effects of exercise and fitness on the LBP population.

* References 27, 39, 69, 73, 80, 83.
† References 32, 61, 68, 71, 81, 93.

◆ LBP AND PHYSICAL FITNESS

A recent survey of the literature indicates that there are a number of general conclusions that can be drawn about low back pain and physical fitness.

1. There is strong evidence that improved fitness, both aerobic fitness and muscle strength, plays a significant role in the prevention and recurrence of back injuries.*
2. Evidence suggests that individuals with LBP (either acute or chronic) who participate in physical fitness programs derive both physical and psychological benefits.†
3. Many studies of the chronic LBP population report decreased levels of self-reported pain and disability with increased activity levels.‡
4. Evidence supports the view that two major factors contribute to the development of chronicity: the disuse or deconditioning syndrome that results from inactivity[17,59] and environmental conditioning factors that encourage the sick role.[28]

Therefore physical fitness programs, by preventing deconditioning and discouraging the sick role, may be helpful to individuals with idiopathic LBP who are not improving with traditional therapies.

◆ COMMUNITY-BASED REHABILITATION PROGRAM

My recent research project studied a community-based rehabilitation program that emphasized physical fitness and improved muscle strength in the treatment of individuals with LBP who were not improving with traditional conservative therapies. The purpose of the study was to determine if changes occurred in levels of self-reported pain and disability as low back injured individuals became more physically fit.

The physical fitness program, called the *Lifestyles Program,* was conducted in a fitness facility in a medium-sized city in eastern Canada. The components of the program are presented in the accompanying box. Most individuals attended the program 5 days per week, for 1 hour each day for 12 weeks.

---

* References 13, 19, 20, 49, 50, 55, 66, 68, 69, 87, 88.

† References 10, 11, 19, 20, 29, 41-43, 55.

‡ References 7, 10, 11, 23, 25, 57-59, 61.

◆ **COMPONENTS OF LIFESTYLES PROGRAM**

1. Aerobic fitness classes (Waterfit) two times per week.
2. Strength-training sessions (Nautilus) three times per week.
3. Sauna and whirlpool (daily as desired for relaxation).
4. Nutrition counseling (optional).
5. Biweekly monitoring by physiotherapist and/or physician.

The waterfit aerobic component, designed to improve cardiorespiratory endurance and flexibility, was conducted in the swimming pool in water waist-deep to shoulder-height. The buoyancy and supportive nature of water make it an ideal environment for improving fitness, especially for those with an injury. By and large, the water exercises consisted of variations of walking and jogging lengths in the pool (with and without extra resistance) for at least 20 minutes, as well as range of motion, flexibility, and stretching exercises. A floatboard held at arms length that was pushed and pulled through the water provided extra resistance. With supervision, subjects gradually increased their speed and level of exercise in a programmed fashion, week by week. As with any aerobics program, there was an 8 to 10 minute warm-up period at the beginning of the class and a cool-down period at the end of the class. Swimming was not encouraged since it tended to aggravate low back pain for many individuals.

The use of 11 strength-training machines, manufactured by Nautilus Sports/Medical Industries, was designed to enhance the strength and endurance of specific muscle groups. Not all subjects used all machines; this depended on the nature of the injury and the stage of recovery. Individuals gradually increased the amount of weight lifted on each machine. Participants were consistently monitored by Lifestyles Program staff throughout their Nautilus sessions for correct body alignment, correct use of equipment and appropriate increases in weights. Subjects were cautioned not to continue a particular exercise if pain increased significantly.

There are unique features of this program that warrant discussion. First, although the program was individualized with close monitoring by supervisory staff, all the program components were done in a group setting. Individuals did not remain isolated but had the opportunity to make friends and acquaintances with others who had similar problems. Secondly, in contrast to conservative forms of therapy, individuals with LBP were being encouraged to leave the house, to have a social life, and to be physically active.[41,42] Thirdly, their rehabilitation was being conducted in a fitness or health promotion setting rather than in a setting associated with sickness and disability, such as a hospital. All of these factors were designed to support and reinforce wellness.

Data Collection

All individuals with idiopathic low back pain who were referred to the Lifestyles Program from May to December 1988 and who could understand English were eligible for inclusion in the study. Clients were referred to the program by either a physiotherapist or a physician as soon as possible after the expected healing time of the injury. However, long waiting periods for assessment by orthopedic specialists and/or physiotherapists delayed referral for several weeks or months for some clients.

The researcher interviewed all subjects about their pain and related disability on five occasions: the subject's initial day of orientation to the program (Day 0), and at 2 weeks, 4 weeks, 8 weeks, and 12 weeks. By taking repeated measures, changes were monitored over time and each subject served as his or her own control.

The primary measure of pain in this study was the McGill Pain Questionnaire (MPQ).[63] Because the MPQ is primarily a measure of perceived pain at the moment, a second pain questionnaire was developed by the author. It attempted to evaluate subjects' perceptions of the intensity, frequency, and duration of pain over a 7-day period (see Table 18-1). The Pain Questionnaire was always administered before the MPQ to obtain information about pain over the week, before asking about pain at the moment.

Pain-related disability was measured using the Oswestry Low Back Pain Disability Questionnaire.[26] The questionnaire, which takes less than 5 minutes to complete, is divided into 10 sections relating to different activities of daily living: personal care, lifting, walking, sitting, standing, sleeping, sex life, travelling, and pain intensity. Each section contains six statements that describe activities of increasing difficulty (see box on

◆ **Table 18-1**
Pain questionnaire

1. Are you having pain right now? Yes ___ No ___
Please mark an X at the spot that best describes your pain right now.

NO PAIN |————————————| WORST POSSIBLE PAIN

2. If you are pain free now, when did you last have pain?

3. About how often have you had pain this week?

4. In general, was your pain this week:
___Constant (never free of pain) ___ Periodic (comes and goes) ___ Brief (less than 15 min.)

5. Please mark an X at the spot that describes the *least* pain you had this week.

NO PAIN |————————————| WORST POSSIBLE PAIN

6. Please mark an X at the spot that describes the *worst* pain you had this week.

NO PAIN |————————————| WORST POSSIBLE PAIN

7. Overall how would you rate your pain this week?

0	1	2	3	4	5
no pain	mild	discomforting	distressing	horrible	excruciating

p. 496). These are scored on a scale from 0 to 5, with 5 representing the greatest difficulty. The scores for all sections are added together, doubled, and then expressed as a percentage.

In addition, a 16-item author-designed questionnaire was developed to gain information about (1) demographic characteristics, (2) the history of the low back injury, (3) other medical conditions and medications, and (4) smoking as a

◆ SAMPLE ITEMS FROM THE OSWESTRY LOW BACK PAIN DISABILITY QUESTIONNAIRE

SECTION 3 – LIFTING

___ I can lift heavy weights without extra pain.
___ I can lift heavy weights but it gives extra pain.
___ Pain prevents me from lifting heavy weights off the floor, but I can manage if they are conveniently positioned, e.g., on the table.
___ Pain prevents me from lifting heavy weights but I can manage light to medium weights if they are conveniently positioned.
___ I can lift only very light weights.
___ I cannot lift or carry anything at all.

SECTION 9 – SOCIAL LIFE

___ My social life is normal and gives me no extra pain.
___ My social life is normal but increases the degree of pain.
___ Pain has no significant effect on my social life apart from limiting my more energetic interests, e.g., dancing.
___ Pain has restricted my social life and I do not go out as often.
___ Pain has restricted my social life to my home.
___ I have no social life because of pain.

From The Chartered Society of Physiotherapy, London, England. Modified from Fairbank JC, Couper J, Davies JB and O'Brien JP. 1980. The Oswestry low back pain disability questionnaire. *Physiotherapy*, 66(8), 272.

possible predisposing factor. This was administered at program entry.

Results

Subject Characteristics

Of the 52 subjects eligible for inclusion in the study at Day 0, 50 voluntarily consented to participate. However, subjects exited the program at various times for a wide range of reasons. In all, 44 subjects completed 8 weeks in the program, and 35 subjects completed 12 weeks. In addition, one subject was dropped from the statistical analysis because of missing data. Since the statistical analyses of the data at 8 weeks and at

12 weeks revealed similar results, it was decided to report the 8-week analysis since the 8-week group included a broader range of subjects than did the 12-week sample. Thus the final sample at 8 weeks included 43 subjects.

The study subjects at 8 weeks included 26 men (60%) and 17 women (40%), all of whom had idiopathic low back pain as their primary pain problem. Ages ranged from 21 to 57 years with the majority of subjects in their mid-to-late thirties (mean age = 36 ± 9 years). Most subjects were married with children, and were receiving Workers' Compensation and/or disability benefits. Almost all the subjects were not working because of their injury but had full time jobs waiting for them. All the individuals in the study were either born or raised in Canada, and were of British or French extraction.

Most of the pain literature differentiates acute pain and chronic pain using 6 months as the marker. Using this classification, 47% (n = 20) of the sample had acute pain (pain lasting less than 6 months) and 53% (n = 23) reported chronic back pain (pain lasting more than 6 months). If, however, the differentiation between acute and chronic pain is defined as 3 months since time of injury, as some authors recommend,[83] then fully 88% of subjects (n = 38) had had pain longer than 3 months, indicating a chronic problem.

Slightly more than half the subjects (n = 22) reported that this was their first back injury, while the remainder (n = 21) had had at least one other episode of back pain. There were almost equal numbers of smokers and nonsmokers. Sixteen subjects reported other current health problems. The most common coexisting problem was cardiovascular disease.

Subjects in this study represented all occupational categories. Most common were the production processing, transportation, and scientific categories. Of special interest was the relatively large number of individuals involved in nursing—six registered nurses and five nursing assistants or nursing aides. Sixty-four percent of this group (n = 7) worked in acute care hospitals, and the remaining 36% (n = 4) worked in long-term care or home care settings. The finding that almost one quarter of the study subjects were involved in nursing was consistent with epidemiological data that have reported a high prevalence of LBP for nursing personnel in many developed countries.[18,44,51,56]

When asked what caused their injury, over 50% of subjects attributed their low back injury to a combination of lifting and twisting; this is the most frequently cited cause of back injury at the workplace.[32] Other causes of the back injury cited by subjects included "falls," "being struck" "just happened," and "other." The category "just happened" included situations such as bending over and twisting, bending and feeling something "snap," turning and coughing, or awkward positioning for a period of time while doing a job. One subject reported that pregnancy exacerbated a degenerative disk problem. Five of the seven individuals reporting the category "other" had been in car accidents.

Results of Pain and Disability Measures

The pain variables analyzed for the 43 subjects who completed 8 weeks in the Lifestyles Program included items 3 to 7 of the Pain Questionnaire (see Table 18-1), the Pain Rating Index (PRI) from the MPQ and the list of symptoms from the MPQ. When subjects were asked how frequently they had experienced pain within the past 7 days, they tended to report their answers in terms of numbers of days they had had pain rather than by specific episodes. As seen in Figure 18-2, 33 subjects (76.7%) at the initial interview reported pain every day; this decreased to 26 subjects (60.5%) by 2 weeks and stayed constant. At

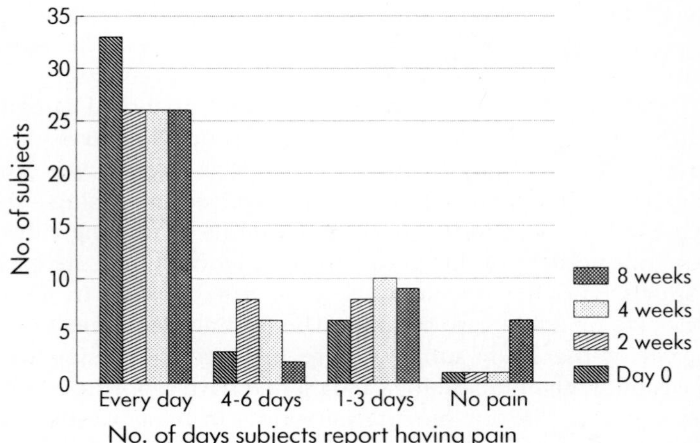

FIGURE 18-2. Frequency of pain in last 7 days (n = 43).

day 0, only 1 subject reported having had no pain in the previous week compared with 6 subjects reporting no pain at week 8. These differences were not statistically significant ($P > .05$).

Subjects were asked about the duration of their pain: had the pain episodes been constant, periodic, or brief over the past 7 days? As Figure 18-3 illustrates from day 0 to 8 weeks, there was a small but steady decline in the number of subjects who reported periodic pain, and a rise in the number of subjects reporting no pain. There was also a slight rise in the number of subjects reporting constant pain. These differences were not statistically significant ($P > .05$).

As part of the MPQ, subjects were asked about symptoms that are often associated with pain. Figure 18-4 depicts the number of subjects ($n = 43$) reporting these associated symptoms over the previous week at day 0 and at 8 weeks. All symptoms improved or stayed constant over the 8 weeks in the program. There was a statistically significant decrease in the incidence of headache ($P < .02$) and a statistically significant decrease in sleep disturbance ($P < .01$) at week 8, compared with day 0.

Scores for items 6 to 8 of the Pain Questionnaire (least pain this week, worst pain this week, and the rating index for pain this week) and the total PRI score from the MPQ were analyzed using multivariate analysis of variance (MANOVAs). Table 18-2 shows the means, standard deviations, and statistical

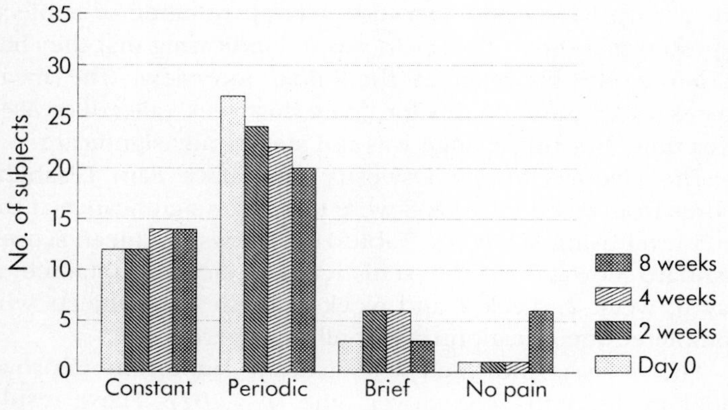

FIGURE 18-3. Duration of pain ($n = 43$).

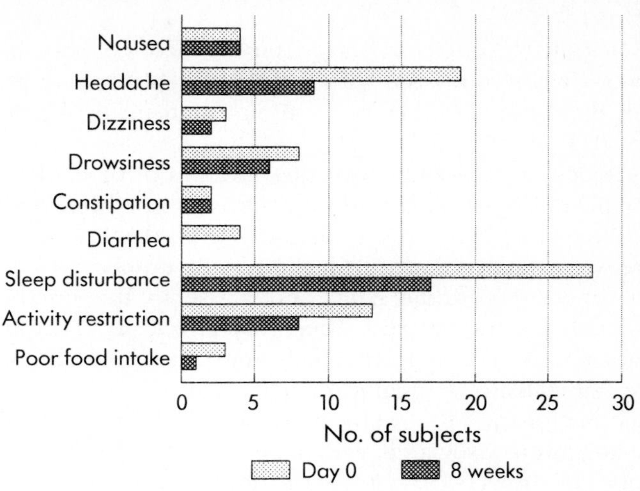

FIGURE 18-4. Symptoms associated with pain (n = 43).

significance of the pain scores at Day 0, 2 weeks, 4 weeks, and 8 weeks.

The analyses indicated a statistically significant reduction in "worst pain" scores with the largest change between week 4 and week 8 ($P < .01$). In addition, the total PRI of the MPQ showed a statistically significant reduction over the 8 weeks in the program indicating a decrease in perceived pain severity and intensity ($P < .001$). Although mean scores for "least pain this week" gradually decreased over the 8-week period, these results were not found to be statistically significant. This was not a surprising result because a large number of subjects reported that their "least pain was 0," indicating that they had pain-free periods even at the initial interview. The mean scores for the rating index for "pain this week" also decreased over time, but this change was not statistically significant.

The changes in the Oswestry Low Back Pain Disability scores from day 0 to week 8 were tested for significance at the 0.05 level using MANOVA. Table 18-3 shows the mean scores, standard deviations, and statistical significance obtained at day 0, week 2, week 4 and week 8 for the 41 subjects who completed the questionnaire at all time periods.

The analysis indicated a statistically significant improvement in disability scores over time ($P < .01$). These results demonstrated an overall improvement in the ability of subjects to perform activities of daily living.

◆ **Table 18-2**
Results of pain measures: group means (±sd), $n = 43$

Measure	Day 0	Week 2	Week 4	Week 8	Probability
Least pain this week (0-100 mm scale)	13.1 (±16.3)	13.0 (±15.6)	11.6 (± 15.8)	8.3 (±12.1)	not significant
Worst pain this week (0-100 mm scale)	68.5 (±25.2)	64.2 (±24.9)	60.0 (±26.4)	51.8 (±32.6)	$P < .01$
Pain rating this week (0-5 scale)	2.3 (±0.8)	2.1 (±0.8)	2.1 (±0.7)	1.9 (±1.1)	not significant
Pain rating index (PRI from MPQ)	21.6 (±8.9)	17.5 (±7.4)	15.8 (±7.4)	14.8 (±10.1)	$P < .001$

◆ **Table 18-3**
Results of disability measure: group means (±sd), n = 41

Measure	Day 0	Week 2	Week 4	Week 8	Probability
Disability	35.4 (±13.1)	32.3 (±13.1)	31.1 (±13.6)	29.6 (±14.6)	$P < .01$

Discussion of Pain and Disability Results

The significant changes observed in the mean "worst pain" scores and in the mean PRI scores suggest that as subjects progressed through the Lifestyles Program, the intensity and severity of their low back pain decreased. However, the pattern of pain occurrence appears not to have changed significantly for this group. In general, this group of subjects had pain just as often and for the same duration at week 8 as at day 0. This group pattern was not universal. Six individuals reported having had a pain-free week at the 8 week interview compared with 1 individual reporting a pain-free week at all previous interviews. In summary, the results suggest that for many of the 43 subjects in this study, participation in a well-monitored group physical fitness program did not aggravate low back pain, but it may have played an important role in decreasing perceived pain intensity and in improving their ability to perform activities of daily living.

Treatment programs for LBP that emphasize physical fitness and conditioning have reported results similar to those reported here. A decrease in pain intensity and an improvement in performing activities of daily living have been cited as outcomes of treatment programs for acute LBP populations,[55] as well as for chronic LBP populations.* The results of the analyses of the pain and disability measures of this study lend further support to the general proposition that increasing physical activity plays a role in reducing perceived pain for subjects with idiopathic LBP, and in improving the functional capacity of these individuals.

Clearly, the results of this study support the potentially advantageous role that improved levels of physical fitness can have for clients with idiopathic low back pain. In addition, this treatment modality may be important in preventing further injury and in reducing the chronicity of this debilitating condition.

Because of the high prevalence of LBP in the general population, the majority of nurses will at some point have contact with individuals who experience LBP. In their roles as patient educators, nurses are in a particularly important position to provide counselling about the deleterious physical and psychological consequences of inactivity and deconditioning; the

* References 10, 22, 30, 53, 57-59.

overall positive effects of keeping active once the acute phase of a low back injury is over; and about what constitutes a "safe" physical fitness program for individuals with low back pain. It is important for clients to realize that all fitness programs are not alike and nurses have a central role to play in helping patients with LBP become "wise consumers" of fitness programs.

REFERENCES

1. Anderson RT. (1987). Investigating back pain: The implications of two village studies in south Asia. In Hockings P (ed), *Dimensions of social life. Essays in honor of David G. Mandelbaum* (pp. 385-396). Berlin: Mouton de Gryter.
2. Anderson RT. (1984). An orthopedic ethnography in rural Nepal. *Med Anthropol, 8*(1), 46-59.
3. Andersson G. (August 1990). *Epidemiology of back pain.* Paper presented at the meeting of the International Back Pain Society, Glasgow.
4. Andersson G. (August 1990). *Natural history of back pain.* Paper presented at the meeting of the International Back Pain Society, Glasgow.
5. Andersson G, and Pope M. (1984). The patients. In Pope M, Frymoyer J, and Andersson G (eds), *Occupational low back pain,* (pp. 137-154). Westport, Conn: Praeger.
6. Andersson G, Pope M, and Frymoyer J. (1984). Epidemiology. In Pope M, Frymoyer J, and Andersson G (eds), *Occupational low back pain* (pp. 101-114). Westport, Conn: Praeger.
7. Aronoff GM, Evans WO, and Enders PL. (1983). A review of follow-up studies of multidisciplinary pain units. *Pain, 16*(1), 1-11.
8. Aronoff GM, McAlary PW, Witkower A, et al. (1988). Pain treatment programs: do they return workers to the workplace? *Occupational Medicine: State of the Art Reviews, 3*(1), 123-136.
9. Bates B. (1983). *A Guide to Physical Examination* (ed 3). Philadelphia: Lippincott.
10. Beekman EE and Axtell L. (1985). Ambulation, activity level and pain. Outcomes of a program for spinal pain. *Phys Ther 65*(11), 1649-1655.
11. Beekman EE, Axtell L, Noland KS, et al. (1985). Self-concept: an outcome of a program for spinal pain. *Pain, 22*(1), 59-66.
12. Berquist-Ullman M and Larsson U. (1977). Acute low back pain in industry. A controlled prospective study with special reference to therapy and confounding factors. *Acta Orthop Scand,* (Suppl 170), 1-117.
13. Biering-Sorenson F. (1984). Physical measurements as risk indicators for low-back trouble over a one-year period. *Spine, 9*(2), 106-119.
14. Boachie-Adjee O. (1988). Conservative management of low back pain. An evaluation of current methods. *Postgrad Med, 84*(3), 127-133.
15. Bogduk N. (August 1990). *Back pain—what is the lesion?* Paper presented at the meeting of the International Back Pain Society, Glasgow.
16. Bombardier C, Baldwin J, and Crull L. (1985). The epidemiology of regional musculoskeletal disorders: Canada. In Hadler NM and Gillings DB (eds), *Arthritis and Society. The Impact of Musculoskeletal Diseases* (pp. 104-117). Boston: Butterworths.

17. Bortz WM. (1984). The disuse syndrome. *West J Med, 141*(5), 691-694.
18. Buckle P. (1987). Epidemiological aspects of back pain within the nursing profession. *Int J Nurs Stud, 24*(4), 319-324.
19. Cady LD, Bishoff DP, O'Connell ER, et al. (1979). Strength and fitness and subsequent back injuries in firefighters. *J Occup Med, 21*(4), 269-272.
20. Cady LD, Thomas PC, and Karwasky MS. (1985). Program for increasing health and physical fitness of fire fighters, *J Occup Med, 27*(2), 110-114.
21. Deyo RA, Diehl AK, and Rosenthal, M. (1986). How many days of bedrest for acute low back pain? A randomized clinical trial. *New England Journal of Medicine, 315,* 1064-1070.
22. Dolce JJ, Crocker MF, and Doleys DM. (1986). Prediction of outcome among chronic pain patients. *Behav Res Ther, 24*(3), 313-319.
23. Dolce JJ, Crocker MF, Moletteire C, et al. (1986). Exercise quotas, anticipatory concern and self-efficacy expectancies in chronic pain: a preliminary report. *Pain, 24*(3), 365-372.
24. Dolce JJ and Raczynski JM. (1985). Neuromuscular activity and electromyography in painful backs: psychological and biomechanical models in assessment and treatment. *Psychol Bull, 97*(3), 502-520.
25. Doleys DM, Crocker M, and Patton D. (1982). Response of patients with chronic pain to exercise quotas. *Phys Ther, 62*(8), 1111-1114.
26. Fairbank JC, Couper J, Davies JB, et al. (1980). The Oswestry low back pain disability questionnaire. *Physiotherapy, 66*(8), 271-273.
27. Flor H and Turk D. (1984). Etiological theories and treatments for chronic back pain. I. Somatic models and interventions. *Pain, 19*(2), 105-121.
28. Fordyce WE. (1986). Learning processes in pain. In Sternbach RA (ed), *The psychology of pain* (pp. 49-65). New York: Raven.
29. Fordyce WE, Brockway JA, Bergman JA, et al. (1986). Acute back pain: a control-group comparison of behavioural vs traditional management methods. *J Behav Med, 9*(2), 127-140.
30. Fordyce WE, McMahon R, Rainwater G, et al. (1981). Pain complaint—exercise performance relationship in chronic pain. *Pain, 10*(3), 311-321.
31. Fredrickson BE, Trief PM, VanBeveren P, et al. (1988). Rehabilitation of the patient with chronic back pain. A search for outcome predictors. *Spine, 13*(3), 351-353.
32. Frymoyer JW. (1988). Back pain and sciatica. *New England Journal of Medicine, 318*(5), 291-300.
33. Frymoyer JW and Howe J. (1984). Clinical classification. In Pope M, Frymoyer J, and Andersson G (eds), *Occupational low back pain* (pp. 71-98). Westport, Conn: Praeger.
34. Frymoyer J and Milhous R. (1984). Evaluation of the worker with low back pain. In Pope M, Frymoyer J and Andersson G (eds), *Occupational low back pain* (pp. 157-184). Westport, Conn: Praeger.
35. Frymoyer JW, Pope MH, Clements JH, et al. (1983). Risk factors in low back pain. An epidemiological survey. *J Bone Joint Surg (Am), 65-A*(2), 213-218.
36. Frymoyer JW, Pope MH, Constanza MC, et al. (1980). Epidemiologic studies of low-back pain. *Spine, 5*(5), 419-423.
37. Frymoyer JW, Rosen JC, Clements BA, et al. (1985). Psychologic factors in low-back pain disability. In Urist MR (ed), *Clin Orthop* (No. 195), (pp. 178-184). Philadelphia: Lippincott.
38. Fuerstein M, Carter RL, and Papciak AS. (1987). A prospective analysis of

stress and fatigue in recurrent low back pain. *Pain, 31*(3), 333-344.

39. Gilbert JR, Taylor WD, Hildebrand A, et al. (1985). Clinical trial of common treatments for low back pain in family practice. *British Medical Journal, 291*(6498), 791-794.
40. Haber LD. (1971). Disabling effects of chronic disease and impairment. *Journal of Chronic Disease, 24*(7), 469-487.
41. Hannah TE, Hannah E, Mosher D, et al. (1988). Fitness benefits of a lifestyles programme for the rehabilitation of Workers' Compensation recipients: effects of heart rate, muscle strength, and weight. *Journal of Rehabilitation, 54*(2), 37-41.
42. Hannah TE, Hannah E, Mosher D, et al. (1988). Psychological benefits of a lifestyles modification programme for Workers' Compensation recipients. *Physiotherapy Canada, 40*(6), 10-15.
43. Hannah TE, Kozma A, Stones M et al. (1989). Effects on mood of a lifestyles program for the rehabilitation of injured workers. *J Occup Med, 31*(5), 454-457.
44. Harber P, Shimozaki S, Gardner G, et al. (1987). Importance of non-patient transfer activities in nursing-related back pain. II. Observational study and implications. *J Occup Med, 29*(12), 971-974.
45. Health and Welfare Canada & Statistics Canada. (1981). *The health of Canadians. Report of the Canadian health survey* (Catalogue No. 82-538E). Ottawa: Minister of Supply and Services.
46. Hirsch C, Jonsson B, and Lewin T. (1969). Low-back symptoms in a Swedish female population. In Urist MR (ed), *Clin Orthop* (No. 63), (pp. 171-176). Philadelphia: Lippincott.
47. Holms S and Nachemson A. (1983). Variations in the nutrition of canine intervertebral disc induced by motion. *Spine, 8*(8), 866-874.
48. Horal J. (1969). The clinical appearance of low back disorders in the city of Gothenburg, Sweden. *Acta Orthop Scand,* (Suppl No. 118), 8-73.
49. Jackson CP and Brown MD. (1983). Is there a role for exercise in the treatment of patients with low back pain? In Urist MR (ed), *Clin Orthop* (No. 179), (pp. 39-45). Philadelphia: Lippincott.
50. Jackson CP and Brown MD. (1983). Analysis of current approaches and a practical guide to prescription of exercise. In Urist MR (ed), *Clin Orthop* (No. 179), (pp. 46-54). Philadelphia: Lippincott.
51. Jensen, RC. (1987). Disabling back injuries among nursing personnel: research needs and justification. *Res Nurs Health, 10*(1), 29-38.
52. Kelsey J and White A. (1980). Epidemiology and impact of low-back pain. *Spine, 5*(2), 133-142.
53. Kleinke CL and Spangler AS. (1988). Predicting treatment outcomes of chronic back pain patients in a multidisciplinary pain clinic: methodological issues and treatment implications. *Pain, 33*(1), 41-48.
54. Kottke TE, Caspersen CJ, and Hill CS. (1984). Exercise in the management and rehabilitation of selected chronic disease. *Prev Med, 13*(3), 47-65.
55. Linton SJ, Bradley LA, Jensen I, et al. (1989). The secondary prevention of low back pain: a controlled study with follow-up. *Pain, 36*(2), 197-207.
56. Mandel JH and Lohman W. (1987). Low back pain in nurses: the relative importance of medical history, work factors, exercise and demographics. *Res Nurs Health, 10*(3), 165-170.
57. Manniche C, Bentzen L, Hesselsoe G, et al. (1988). Clinical trial of intensive training for chronic low back pain. *Lancet II*(8626-8627), 1473-1476.

58. Mayer T, Gatchell R, Kishino N, et al. (1985). Objective assessment of spine function following industrial injury. A prospective study with comparison group and one-year follow-up. *Spine, 10*(6), 482-493.
59. Mayer TG, Gatchell RJ, Kishino N, et al. (1986). A prospective short-term study of chronic low back pain patients utilizing novel objective functional measurement. *Pain, 25*(1), 53-68.
60. McGill CM. (1968). Industrial back problems: a control program. *J Occup Med, 10*(4), 174-178.
61. McQuade KJ, Turner JA, and Buchner D. (1988). Physical fitness and chronic low back pain. In Urist MR (ed), *Clin Orthop* (No. 233), (pp. 96-100). Philadelphia: Lippincott.
62. Meinhart NT and McCaffery M. (1983). *Pain. A nursing approach to assessment and analysis.* Norwalk, Conn: Appleton, Century, Crofts.
63. Melzack R. (1975). The McGill pain questionnaire: major properties and scoring methods. *Pain, 1*(2), 277-299.
64. Melzack R and Wall P. (1982). *The challenge of pain.* Middlesex, UK: Penguin.
65. Munro J and Macleod J. (eds). (1986). *Clinical Examination.* Edinburgh: Churchill Livingstone.
66. Murphy KA and Cornish RD. (1984). Prediction of chronicity in acute low back pain. *Arch Phys Med, 65*(6), 334-337.
67. Murtagh J, Findlay D, and Kenna C. (1985). Low back pain. *Aust Fam Physician, 14*(11), 1214-1224.
68. Nachemson AL. (1984). Prevention of chronic back pain: the orthopedic challenge of the 80's. *Bull Hosp Jt Dis Orthop Inst, 44*(1), 1-15.
69. Nachemson AL. (1985). Advances in low-back pain. In Urist MR (ed), *Clin Orthop* (No. 200), (pp. 266-278). Philadelphia: Lippincott.
70. Nagi SZ, Riley LE, and Newby LG. (1973). Social epidemiology of back pain in the general population. *Journal of Chronic Diseases, 26*(12), 769-779.
71. Nutter P. (1988). Aerobic exercise in the treatment and prevention of low back pain. *Occupational Medicine: State of the Art Reviews, 3*(1), 137-145.
72. Pope MH, Lehmann TR, and Frymoyer JW. (1984). Structure and function of the lumbar spine. In Pope M, Frymoyer J, and Andersson G (eds), *Occupational Low Back Pain,* (pp. 5-38). Westport, Conn: Praeger.
73. Quinet RJ and Hadler NM. (1979). Diagnosis and treatment of backache. *Semin Arthritis Rheum, 8*(4), 261-287.
74. Rossignol M, Suissa S, and Abenhaim L. (1988). Working disability due to occupational low back pain: three-year follow-up of 2,300 compensated workers in Quebec. *J Occup Med, 30*(6), 502-505.
75. Rowat K. (1983). *The meaning and management of chronic pain: the family's perspective.* Unpublished doctoral dissertation. University of Illinois, Chicago.
76. Rowe ML. (1969). Low back pain in industry. A position paper. *J Occup Med, 11*(4), 161-169.
77. Sarno JE. (1984). Therapeutic exercise for back pain. In Basmajian J (ed), *Therapeutic exercise* (ed 4), (pp. 441-463). Baltimore: Williams & Wilkins.
78. Schmidt AJ and Arntz A. (1987). Psychological research and chronic low back pain: a stand-still or breakthrough? *Soc Sci Med, 25*(10), 1095-1104.

79. Selby DK. (1982). Conservative care of nonspecific low back pain. *Orthop Clin North Am, 13*(3), 427-437.
80. Shotkin JD, Bolt B, and Norton DA. (1987). Teaching program for patients with low-back pain. *J Neurosci Nurs, 19*(5), 240-243.
81. Simmons Raithel K. (1989). Chronic pain and exercise therapy. *The Physician and Sports Medicine, 17*(3), 203-209.
82. Smidt GL, Amundsen LR, and Dostal WF. (1980). Muscle strength at the trunk. *Journal of Orthopaedics and Sports Physical Therapy, 1*(3), 165-170.
83. Spitzer WO, LeBlanc FE, and Dupuis M. (1987). Scientific aproach to the assessment and management of activity-related spinal disorders. A monograph for clinicians. *Spine, 12*(7S), S1-S59.
84. Statistics Canada. (1989). *Work injuries. 1986-1988.* (Catalogue No. 72-208). Ottawa: Minister of Supply and Services.
85. Statistics Canada and Labour Canada. (1984). *Employment injuries and occupational illnesses. 1972-1981.* (Catalogue No. L31-52). Ottawa: Minister of Supply and Services.
86. Statistics Canada and Secretary of State of Canada. (1986). *Report of the Canadian health and disability survey. 1983-1984.* (Catalogue No. 82-555E). Ottawa: Minister of Supply and Services.
87. Svensson HO and Andersson GB. (1983). Low back pain in forty- to forty-seven year old men: work history and work environment factors. *Spine, 8*(3), 272-276.
88. Troup JD, Martin JW, and Lloyd EF. (1981). Back pain in industry. A prospective study. *Spine, 6*(1), 61-69.
89. Valkenburg H and Haanen H. (1982). The epidemiology of low back pain. In White A and Gordon S (eds), *Symposium on idiopathic low back pain* (pp. 9-22). St. Louis: Mosby.
90. Waddell G. (1987). A new clinical model for the treatment of low-back pain. *Spine, 12*(7), 632-644.
91. White A and Gordon S. (1982). Synopsis: workshop on idiopathic low-back pain. *Spine,* 7(2), 141-149.
92. Woolf V. (1967). On being ill. *Collected essays* (Vol. 4) (pp. 193-203). London: Hogarth Press.
93. Wynn Parry CB and Gingras F. (1988). The assessment and management of the failed back. Part II. *Int Disabil Stud, 10*(1), 25-28.

19

Relief of Burn Pain in Adults and Children

Judith A. Knighton
Lori Palozzi

◆ INTRODUCTION

THE WORDS "burn injury" evoke the image of people experiencing unimaginable suffering. Empathetic comparisons are attempted between the pain of a scalded finger and the unbearable suffering that must be endured when large portions of a person's body are involved. Burn trauma is probably the most devastating injury one can sustain, and the accompanying pain can be prolonged, intense, and physically and psychologically draining. Treatments may compound this pain with episodes of increased intensity during procedures.

The majority of burn survivors are able to recall vivid images of their most painful experiences. Many are grateful, that for some of their recovery period, they were too sick or sedated to remember all that happened to them. Unfortunately, the memory of burn pain may endure for many months after the physical sensation of pain ceases. In providing care for these patients, the nurse may be required to contribute to that pain since treatments can be lengthy and complex. The impact of this on burn team members, particularly nurses, can be severe, necessitating the development of a repertoire of coping strategies to manage the many conflicting feelings provoked by caring for patients who are in pain. Subsequently, conflicts can arise with one's role as comfort-giver.

The complex nature of burn pain makes it very difficult to treat successfully on all occasions. There is no one strategy that works well all of the time, either with the same patient on separate occasions, or among different patients. In fact, total relief of pain may be impossible. What is helpful, however, is for patients and significant others to see committed staff implementing an organized, caring, and consistent approach to pain management.

Our clinical experiences and a review of the burn literature[27,31] reveal that very few burn units have any established pain protocols to guide their practice, although each burn unit has its own culture, including a philosophy of pain management. Within the context of a given work setting, a patient's pain must be coped with in the midst of many competing priorities and concerns. A philosophy and protocol may be more developed on a unit where pain work is highly valued.

The focus of this chapter is to provide strategies for the assessment and management of pain experienced by burn patients. A brief outline of those factors which influence burn pain and contribute to its undertreatment are presented and form the basis for understanding the complex and challenging nature of burn pain management. Because there are differences in the management of children and adults, strategies for the assessment and management of both pediatric and adult burn patients are discussed.

◆ FACTORS INFLUENCING BURN PAIN

Pain is a complex and subjective experience. Burn pain is particularly complex because of the intensity, lengthy duration, and multiplicity of contributing variables. Clinical features that influence the severity of burn injuries and related pain are the depth of the burn and the length of time since injury.

Burn Depth

The severity of a burn injury is related to the depth of the burn[9] with classifications of partial- or full-thickness as described in Table 19-1.

Some burn care providers believe that full-thickness burn wounds are painless, since the nerve endings in the dermis have been destroyed. Clinical experience is proving, however, that deep somatic pain may be present as a result of surrounding inflammation and ischemia. Also, adjacent wound edges have been found to contain many hypersensitive nerve endings. It is generally recognized that partial-thickness burn

◆ **Table 19-1**
Depth of burn injury

Description	Depth	Healing Time
PARTIAL-THICKNESS		
Superficial	Epidermis and thin portion of dermis; may include blisters	Heals spontaneously within 10 days-2 weeks
Deep	Epidermis and deep dermis; blisters	Heals spontaneously within 3-4 weeks
FULL-THICKNESS		
	Epidermis, dermis, subcutaneous tissue; may include muscle and bone	Spontaneous healing not possible; grafting necessary

wounds and donor sites are painful because of destroyed epidermis and exposed nerve endings. The clinical ramifications are that the latter patients may be overly medicated at times, while the former may receive no or woefully inadequate doses of analgesic.

Burn Phases

Clinical treatment of the burned patient is divided into three phases, each one having a specific focus related to the care of the patient. They are the emergent, acute, and rehabilitative phases. The emergent phase occurs immediately following the burn injury and lasts from a few hours to a few days following the burn. During this time the severity of the burn is determined. Fluid and electrolyte stabilization is the priority. This phase ends when the initial fluid therapy is completed and diuresis occurs.

The acute phase follows, and lasts until the partial-thickness wounds are healed, or the full-thickness wounds are covered with grafts. This phase can exist anywhere from 10 days to many months, depending on the wound depth. During this phase, priorities are to administer wound care, provide adequate nutrition, and to minimize or prevent systemic complications.

The rehabilitative phase focuses on promoting minimal scarring and maximal function to involved joint surfaces. It is also a critical time for emotionally preparing the burned patient for reintegration into society.

As the burn wound heals, there is variation in the intensity and quality of the pain experience with each patient as well as among patients.

◆ FACTORS RELATED TO THE BURN

Burn Injury

The pain associated with a burn injury can be one of the most severe and prolonged types of pain ever experienced.[8,24] Patients feel pain in the burn wound and surrounding areas, the intensity of which may be increased by movement or manipulation of the affected part.

Therapy

Many therapeutic procedures are performed over the course of the burn treatment. Hydrotherapy, wound debridement (removal of burned tissue), application of topical agents and dressings, and physical therapy constitute the painful treatments facing the patient every day. These procedures contribute to one's memory of pain and daily anticipation of the experience.

Hydrotherapy or "tubbing" is considered by many burn patients to be the most physically and emotionally exhausting aspect of recovery.[16] Patients rate their pain the highest, that is, moderate to severe to excruciating, during times of debridement, and as mild or none at times of rest.[29,41]

Pain intensity in burned children was found to vary at different times during the treatment.[41] Pain scores on a scale of 0 to 10 ranged from little pain with removal of the outer bandages, to moderate pain with application of the ointment to the wound, to severe pain with removal of the innermost gauze. Debridement was moderately to severely painful. Similar results were found by Palozzi[29] in which hydrotherapy and debridement were rated from 10 to 100 on a numerical analog scale from 0 to 100 in a group of six school-aged children. The pain behaviors observed during the treatment validated these findings. Children protested the cleansing and debriding of the burns by screaming, crying, hitting out, and attempting to escape from the nurse. Stalling tactics were employed very frequently to postpone treatments, including feigning sleep, having to use the toilet, gagging, and various bargaining offers.

The incidence of pain behaviors escalates as hospitalization continues.[8,29] Children will scream and cry harder and for longer periods and will use stalling techniques in an attempt to avoid the procedure altogether. They may exhibit varying degrees of psychopathologic behavior characterized by depression, inability to distinguish painful from nonpainful events and chronic anxiety.[3,15,39,46] It is also clear that children have the ability to use or to develop their own coping strategies to effectively deal with painful situations. Strategies such as postponement, withdrawal, and threat reduction are reported.[21,35]

Similar cases in the adult population may bring about an increased sense of frustration and helplessness, with subsequent loss of patience and verbal and physical outbursts. Such behaviors are very individual, occur at differing stages of the recovery continuum, but should be viewed as normal unless detrimental in nature. These challenging behaviors may be caused by the return of normal sensation in the wound, an increase in anticipatory anxiety before the treatment, gradual loss of energy, and effects of operant conditioning on pain response.[32,35] Few adult burn patients refuse to go for their treatments, but may try various postponement and bargaining techniques with the staff from time to time. Intubated patients may indicate their displeasure by physically striking out at personnel or providing physical resistance to attempts at moving various body parts for wound care or exercise.

Healing

The nature of healing prolongs the pain experience until the wounds are completely resurfaced. Burn pain may be less pronounced at the time of the injury, may become increasingly more intense as wound care proceeds, and may gradually subside as the wound heals. However, episodes of recurring pain are associated with tissue regeneration. During healing, pain is often compounded with intense tingling or itching sensations, which may cause more discomfort than the pain itself. When the wound is covered with a skin graft, the patient may experience a significant decrease in pain at that location, but may report an increase in pain sensation at the donor site or sites.

The prolonged separation from the home environment, which is necessary for acute burn care management, may also create feelings of loneliness, helplessness, and a sense of loss of control. These can be sources of anxiety for many, which can further increase the pain experience.[5,26]

By the time of discharge (variable, depending on the severity of the burn injury), most patients experience pain to a lesser degree than while in hospital. Some patients have little to no pain on discharge, while others have moderate discomfort. This discomfort can be related to the presence of unhealed burned areas, itchiness, musculoskeletal compromise, neuropathies, splinting, or pressure therapy.

Inability to Totally Relieve Pain

It is difficult, if not impossible, to prevent or totally alleviate the burn patient's pain. To set up such an expectation is unrealistic and potentially harmful to the establishment of trusting relationships among the burn patient, significant others, and members of the burn team.

None of the proposed strategies work well all of the time, either with the same patient on separate occasions or among different patients. It is far more realistic and helpful to emphasize one's ability or desire to decrease the patient's discomfort or to maximize his or her comfort level.

Incongruity Related to Burn Pain

Since total relief of pain is usually impossible, burn staff have been found to shift their goal to helping patients *endure* pain and to *control their expression* of it.[8] Burn patients frequently experience prejudice and inadequate pain management because burn team members perceive that the patient's complaints of pain do not match the apparent tissue damage or degree of nociception.[12,22,43] This misbelief can be countered by using current pain theory (see Chapters 2 and 3).

◆ FACTORS CONTRIBUTING TO UNDERTREATMENT

Despite mounting evidence to the contrary,[31,33] burn care professionals are consistently providing patients with inadequate dosages of medication. A number of factors contribute to this undertreatment, including fear of addiction and respiratory depression and misinterpretation of behavior. In the pediatric burn population, research indicates that children receive fewer analgesics than burned adults and that younger children receive less than older children.[31,36,37]

Fear of Addiction

Perry and Heidrich conducted a study on the incidence of postburn addiction. Their sample size consisted of 181 burn care professionals who had an average of 6 years experience with burn patients. In all, they had worked with over 10,000 hospitalized burns. There were no reports of iatrogenic addiction. The twenty two cases of addiction occurred where *all* had a history of drug abuse before the burn injury occurred.

Since major burns can have a protracted healing time, many staff express concern that opioids and other medications are ordered for too long a period of time, fearing addiction as a result. However, the majority of patients stop taking opiates when their pain stops. Most patients have no or few complaints of pain after complete scar maturation at 12 to 18 months after the burn occurs.[23]

What appears to be prevalent in burn care is confusion among the terms *addiction, tolerance,* and *dependence* (see box). Inadequate drug levels may lead the burn patient to exhibit behaviors that may be misinterpreted as psychic "drug-seeking" in nature. By virtue of a potentially protracted healing time, some burn patients cannot avoid development of drug tolerance and dependence if they have received a particular medication for an extended period of time. This is not problematic (see Chapters 7 and 12).

◆ **DEFINITION OF TERMS**

Addiction	Overwhelming involvement with obtaining drug for psychic effects
Tolerance	Given dose begins to lose its effectiveness
Dependence	Withdrawal symptoms occur when drug is not taken

◆ **ONSET OF RESPIRATORY DEPRESSION**

- 7 minutes (IV)
- 30 minutes (IM)
- 90 minutes (SC)

Concern Related to Respiratory Depression

Burn physicians and nurses frequently express concern that large doses of opioids can contribute to life threatening respiratory depression in burn patients. As with any side effect, one has to decide on which side we wish to err (see Chapter 6). Unfortunately, it is difficult to predict when respiratory depression might occur. Pharmacological and clinical research have shown that the first two doses of a medication can be the most dangerous. If respiratory depression is to occur, some guidelines have been established regarding onset and route of administration (see box). For ventilated burn patients, such a concern is not as prevalent or legitimate, since the airway is protected.

In a study of respiratory depression with meperidine usage in adults (25 to 100 mg IM), Jaffe[13] found an incidence with 0.0009% (3/3263) of patients: *50 mg* in 2 instances and *25 mg* in one instance. It is interesting to note that a dose of 25 mg is below the therapeutic range for adults. This finding illustrates that patient's responses differ, and consequently their pain assessment should be individualized. In other reports, burn patients have been known to tolerate high levels of morphine, meperidine, and fentanyl without incident. The probable reason for this phenomenon is that, as analgesic tolerance develops, so too do respiratory and somnolent effects (see Chapters 7 and 12).

Behaviors

Burn patients are often accused of using attention-seeking behaviors to gain access to pain medication. Interestingly, the PRN regimen of opioid administration may contribute to such behavior as call bell ringing, frequent visits to the nursing station, and repeated requests to the room nurse.[25] In reality burn patients do not participate to a noticeable degree in such behavior, since it tends to isolate the patient from staff, significant others, and fellow burn patients.[8] In the pediatric population, parents often use the call bell, visit the nursing station, and ask the room nurse repeatedly for pain medication for their child.

◆ ASSESSMENT OF BURN PAIN

Inappropriate assessment of a burn patient's pain level can lead to inadequate pain management, with resultant inadequate pain control. Thorough pain assessment assists practitioners in making sense of complex and differing clinical impressions. The need for accurate assessment tools becomes crucial to break this vicious cycle of increased pain leading to increased anxiety leading to increased perception of pain. Only through assessment can individualized and effective care be an outcome (see Chapters 4, 9, and 10). In burn pain management, assessment must be a cooperative function among patients, families, physicians, nurses and sometimes pharmacists, social workers, and psychiatrists.

Many variables need to be considered when assessing the burn patient's level of pain. Factors relating to the burn injury and to the response to the injury follow (see boxes). Incongruences between nurse and patient perceptions of pain need to be examined.

Factors Relating to the Burn Injury

To assess tissue damage, one needs to determine the percentage of body surface area affected and the depth of the burn. Research findings are inconsistent as to whether or not patients with more severe burns suffer more pain. However, patients with more severe burns will have to endure pain over a longer period of time.

The nature of burn treatments, including the frequency of dressing changes is important. The use of physical therapy, the approximate length of the procedure, and type of treatment (complete tubbings or showers versus room dressings) should be noted.

It is important to determine whether the central and peripheral nervous systems are intact or whether the integrity is impaired, resulting in altered sensation of pain.

Analgesics being given, including the type, dosage, route,

◆ FACTORS RELATING TO THE BURN INJURY

1. Amount and type of tissue damage
2. Nature of burn treatments
3. Integrity of central and peripheral nervous systems
4. Medication effects

frequency and effectiveness of the drug, need to be evaluated. The effectiveness of other medications received, such as anxiolytics or antipruritics, needs to be examined as well (see box and Chapters 7 and 12).

Factors Relating to the Response to the Burn Injury

The meaning that a patient attributes to the pain can influence effective management. Many patients, particularly young children, view pain as a punishment for bad behavior. This is especially important if the child or adult has caused the burn injury by engaging in mischievous or risk-taking behavior.

The patient, family, and significant other should be consulted regarding the patient's usual response to past painful stimuli. It is important to note how the patient usually expresses pain. Yelling and crying are just two ways of expressing pain. The silently terrified patient may be in as much distress, but cultural, social, or simple fatigue, helplessness, or hopelessness factors may have much more to do with pain expression than practitioners may realize or acknowledge. Cultural variation of pain and its expression need to be assessed, since it will affect each patient's view of the pain experience.

The patient may use certain coping strategies previously effective in dealing with pain. His or her willingness to learn new strategies needs to be determined as well. The child's developmental stage will influence his or her understanding of pain and ability to communicate pain verbally and to use the pain rating scales. The level of a patient's anxiety related to hospitalization and impending treatment of the burn injury can increase perception of pain. The reactions of others to the patient will influence how he or she perceives the pain experience. It is important to note whether the pain is acknowl-

◆ FACTORS RELATING TO THE RESPONSE TO THE BURN INJURY

1. Meaning of pain
2. Previous experience with pain
3. Coping strategies
4. Developmental stage
5. Reactions of others to pain
6. Anxiety
7. Cultural background
8. Perceived family support

edged or ignored, since this can have an impact on the patient's behavior. This point is particularly important for the pediatric patient since the family functions as a primary source of learning and socialization.

Parental support and comfort as perceived by the child during hospitalization will have an effect on the overall reaction to hospitalization, to treatments, and to pain. Perceived support from the spouse or significant other by the adult patient may have similar effects (see Chapter 5).

Assessment is potentially confounded by the rater's personal expectations, past experiences, and beliefs. These beliefs include expectations regarding a patient's behavior based on his or her gender, age, culture, severity, extent, degree, and location of the burn and past drug and psychiatric history, the majority of which have been found to be very unreliable pain indicators.[32]

Research by Andreasen, Noyes, and Hartford[1]; Avni[2]; Jorgenson and Brophy[14]; Klein and Charlton[18]; Marvin and Heimbach[23]; and Steiner and Clark[38] hypothesize that nonnociceptive stimuli play a major role in perception of pain. Pain behavior may then be related to numerous psychological factors such as acute anxiety, helplessness, hopelessness, depression, and acute grief reactions. Subsequent management should therefore include analgesia for pain and psychotherapy and medication for observed or reported psychological components. Choice of appropriate assessment tools to measure the psychological components involves input from both participating burn team members and the patient. Experience with such tools is rather limited at present but is becoming increasingly more prevalent. Research has commenced in the area of posttraumatic stress disorder (PTSD) and its impact on burn patients' assessment of their pain.[10] At this time, all that is known for certain is that PTSD and pain perception are linked.

Burn Team Perceptions

Inappropriate assessment of a burn patient's pain level can lead to inadequate pain management. For a patient's pain needs to be met, there needs to be congruence between nurses' and patients' perceptions. Iafrati[12] examined patients' and nurses' perceptions of pain during wound care. Nurses incorrectly assessed the patient's pain 69% of the time (overestimation 34.5%; underestimation 34.5%). Assessments similar to the patients' were made only 31% of the time. Overestimations were made most frequently by new graduates, new burn nurses, associate and baccalaureate graduates, and nurses older than 30 years of age. Underestimations were made by veteran burn nurses, diploma graduates, and nurses younger than 25 years of age. The research also indicated that perceptions of pain intensity were not significantly related to the severity, extent, or location of the burn injury, a finding corroborated by Perry, Heidrich and Ramos.[32]

Walkenstein[43] discovered similar evidence of overestimation and underestimation of burn wound pain by nursing staff. In addition, she found a positive correlation between the nurses' perceptions of the burn patients' overall pain experiences and those reported by the patients. No correlation was found concerning length of time in nursing, in particular, burn nursing. Fagerhaugh[8] declared that, in general, members of the burn team assessed pain as less severe than did the patients. Team members attributed most of the patients' feelings to anxiety. There was also no correlation found between the patient's description of pain and his or her expression and assessment.

A study of 52 hospitalized adult burn patients by Perry, Heidrich, and Ramos[32] concluded that at the worst, 84% of patients experienced severe or excruciating pain throughout their hospitalization. At the least, 66% of patients rated pain as just noticeable or none at all. In contrast, a subsequent study[31] served to highlight further assessment problems when 80% of 181 burn physicians and nurses stated that, at its worst, the burn patients' pain rating would be within the moderate range, a disturbing discrepancy.

With respect to choice of burn pain assessment tools, there are a number of appropriate unidimensional and multidimensional tools, such as verbal descriptors, visual analog scales, color, and numerical rating scales. Examples of such tools as described in Chapters 4, 9, and 10 can be very applicable to the burn patient. In addition to utilizing thorough multidimensional pain assessment tools, one must administer them to burn patients on a consistent basis. It is important to note that the effectiveness of a particular tool may vary from patient to patient and with each pain experience. Fear, anxiety, previous pain experiences, degree of fatigue, stress, and depression do affect burn patients' reactions to stimuli. Because of the complexity of burn pain assessment and management, utilization of a variety of subjective and objective measurement tools is recommended. Further research and publication of clinical findings are also encouraged.

Assessment of the Intubated Patient

There is distinct difficulty in assessing ventilated, comatose, or otherwise noncommunicative burn patients. Without the crucial subjective component, burn pain assessment is dependent on the caregivers' perceptions. Observation of the patient's facial expressions, body movements, and vital signs may be the few sources of data we have in making our assessment and planning interventions. Discussions with family and friends regarding reactions to previous painful experiences may also be explored.

Assessment of the Pediatric Patient

The method for assessing pain symptoms in children is dependent on the age and stage of development of the child and should include both pain intensity and quality where possible. The highest incidence of burns occurs in the toddler age group. With preverbal children the method for assessing pain intensity is largely observation (see Chapters 9 and 10). The nurse must look for behavioral signs that the child is experiencing pain, such as protection or withdrawal of the burned part, crying, clinging to parents, and facial grimacing, in addition to other pain behaviors specific to that child. In addition to observation, involving parents in the assessment of their child's pain is essential for the nurse to obtain information about the child's previous experiences and reactions to painful events. Although parental involvement in assessment is necessary with the preverbal child, it is also equally important with children of any age.

With the school-aged population, various pain intensity rating scales, such as the Oucher, developed by Beyer[4] and a vertical version of the numerical rating scale,[41] have been used successfully (see Chapter 10). Older children and adolescents are able to use horizontal, visual, and numerical rating scales to rate the pain intensity.[34]

Assessing pain quality is more challenging, especially with a preverbal child. Nevertheless, it is important to establish the nature of discomfort and pain to select the appropriate intervention. The older child can distinguish between feelings of pain and itchiness in the burn wound, whereas the younger child may simply tug at the dressings. The nurse must also have a good understanding of the pathophysiology of wound healing. This knowledge, in combination with the child's verbalizations and behavior, will aid in the selection of an appropriate intervention. Strategies may include use of an analgesic, antipruritic, or a noninvasive intervention such as massage or vibration.

It is crucial that the nurse complete an age-appropriate pain assessment for each child before, during, and after any invasive painful procedure such as hydrotherapy and debridement. As soon as possible after admission, this pain assessment should be documented by the nurse. This assessment will provide caregivers with baseline data, help to guide interventions for pain management, and assist in the evaluation of selected interventions.

◆ PAIN MANAGENMENT OF THE BURN PATIENT

Pain management of the burn patient is a complex issue because of the multifaceted implications of burn injuries. It is important to begin to establish a trusting relationship with the patient within the first few hours following the crisis, since this is essential to an individualized approach to pain management. The nurse should be familiar with and prepared to use a wide variety of pharmacological (see Chapters 7, 11, and 12) and nonpharmacological strategies (see Chapters 8 and 11) for pain management. Appropriate nursing interventions can be selected in collaboration with the patient and family, with rationale provided for each strategy.

With burn patients, no single strategy for pain management is a panacea. As the burn wound heals and treatment strategies change, the nurse must continually reassess the efficacy of chosen interventions. The burn care practitioner must choose strategies that best match the patient's pain. For example, during a pain assessment if a patient complains primarily of itchiness, an antipruritic as opposed to an opioid agent may be more beneficial.

Pharmacological Strategies

In the early stages of burn care, medications with the exceptions of tetanus prophylaxis should be administered via the intravenous route. The presence of hypovolemic shock makes this delivery route the most advantageous for effective pain relief. In clinical burn practice, intravenous and oral routes have been found to be effective, whereas intramuscular routes can be more painful and more difficult to access over time. In addition, intramuscular injections are particularly anxiety-provoking for children and should be avoided whenever possible.

Pharmacological approaches to burn pain management include opioids, nonopioids, antipruritics, nonsteroidal antiinflammatory drugs (NSAIDs), and anxiolytics, with some proving to be more effective at certain stages of the recovery continuum than others (see Table 19-2).

Opioid Analgesics

With respect to opioid usage, morphine sulphate (Morphine, MS Contin), hydromorphone hydrochloride or sulphate (Dilaudid), fentanyl (Sublimaze), ketalar (Ketamine), and acetaminophen with codeine (Tylenol #3, #2, and #1) can be very effective with the emergent and acute phase patient with moderate to severe/excruciating pain. Dosages required for effective pain management can be very large, given the patient's individual needs and the potential development of tolerance. Administration schedules are varied, from continuous infusion, fixed-interval doses, patient-controlled analgesia (PCA), to PRN regimens for breakthrough pain. For pa-

◆ **Table 19-2**
Pharmacological approaches to pain management

Adults	Pediatrics
OPIOIDS	
Morphine sulfate	Morphine sulfate
M.S. Contin	Codeine
Hydromorphone hydrochloride	Acetaminophen with codeine
Fentanyl	
Ketalar	
Acetaminophen with codeine	
NONOPIOIDS	
Acetaminophen	Acetaminophen
Hydroxyzine	Hydroxyzine
Diphenhydramine	
NONSTEROIDAL ANTIINFLAMMATORY DRUGS (NSAIDs)	
Ibuprofen	
Indomethacin	
ANXIOLYTICS	
Haloperidol	Clorazepate dipotassium
Diazepam	Diazepam
Hydroxyzine	

tients on ventilators, continuous infusions of morphine, with supplemental single doses of the same or another opioid before therapeutic procedures, is recommended.[28]

Clinical experience with adult burn patients shows that dosages of intravenous morphine of 2 to 6 mg q 1 to 2 h have proven effective. With children, morphine dosages are best calculated using the formula of 0.05 to 0.1 mg/kg/dose q2 to 4 h for intravenous usage.[11] These dosages are suggested guidelines derived from clinical experience, and individual titration is absolutely necessary to provide optimal relief from pain. It is important to document the efficacy of the analgesia by obtaining a pain rating one hour after administration. With children and intubated patients unable to provide a pain rating, careful observation of their behavior for pain symptoms is required.

If the type or route of medication is changed, it is imperative that the new dosage be calculated to provide the same amount of analgesia in milliequivalents of morphine. In addition to ensuring the correct dosage, the nurse must administer the medication at an appropriate time before the treatment so that the patient will experience the peak analgesic effect during wound care. It is recommended that IV morphine be administered 30 minutes before treatment. However, individual assessments need to be made regarding the optimal administration times. Documentation of medication, dosage, frequency, and efficacy is essential to promote consistency in nursing care.

Nonopioid Analgesics

Nonopioid analgesics can be effective for the minor burn injury or rehabilitative patient. They may also be useful in the management of acute period breakthrough pain (i.e., in-between fixed-time interval doses) and in combination with opioid agents. The use of nonopioid analgesics, however, is frequently ineffective for severe burn pain.

Antipruritics

Antipruritic agents, such as hydroxyzine (Atarax) and diphenhydramine (Benadryl), can be necessary to alleviate the pruritis accompanied by wound healing in the rehabilitative phase.

Nonsteroidal Antiflammatory Drugs (NSAIDs)

NSAIDs such as ibuprofen (Motrin) and indomethacin (Indocin) may also prove helpful for the rare acute/rehabilitative burn patient with mild to moderate pain generating from a muscular source.

Anxiolytics

Anxiolytics can be useful once one can assess the emotional context of the patient's pain. Clinical experience has shown that the psychiatric assessment is much enhanced by the nurse's assessment of the patient's psychological affect and behavior. These agents can enhance the effectiveness of analgesics since one's perceptions of pain are directly related to one's anxiety level. Haloperidol (Haldol) has a shorter half-life than diazepam (Valium) and has been found helpful in the management of early postburn delirium, in addition to its antianxiety properties.[24] Diazepam and clorazepate dipotassium (Tranxene) have been used with older children and adolescents in an attempt to reduce anxiety related to the impending treatment. These agents must be used with caution, since paradoxical effects have been noted with children.

Antidepressants

Antidepressants are rarely needed, except with those patients exhibiting a clearly defined case of moderate to severe depression, generally diagnosed by the burn team psychiatrist.

Nonpharmacological Strategies

The use of various nonpharmacological strategies in addition to analgesics can be effective in reducing the patient's perception of pain. As with pharmacological approaches, the appropriateness of any nonpharmacological strategy is based on an individualized assessment of the burn patient's needs. Nonpharmacological approaches that can be helpful for these patients are listed in the accompanying box.

Two principles must be followed for effective use of these techniques. First, it is important to remember that these techniques are best introduced, practiced, and implemented when the patient is not experiencing moderate to severe/excruciating pain. Introduction and practice of such techniques is best performed in a nonstressful environment. Patients can then apply such techniques in more stressful situations, such as during treatment procedures. Second, these techniques alone will not bring about pain relief. When used as an adjunct to medication, the pain perception can be reduced.

Relaxation Therapy

Strategies to promote relaxation in patients undergoing painful dressing changes involve deep-breathing and progressive muscle relaxation exercises. Some patients may have their own strategies to promote relaxation, and the nurse can encourage the use of these techniques. Research by Wernick,

◆ NONPHARMACOLOGICAL APPROACHES TO PAIN MANAGEMENT

Relaxation therapy
Distraction
Guided imagery and hypnosis
Biofeedback
Transcutaneous electrical nerve stimulation
Acupuncture
Acupressure
Ice massage
Therapeutic massage
Permission for the expression of pain
Patient involvement in treatment
Family involvement in treatment

Brantley, and Malcolm[45] explored the therapeutic use of relaxation therapy with adult burn patients. Patients were taught physical and/or psychological stress reduction techniques in two or more training sessions. Practice occurred before the implementation during burn debridement. During the treatments the patients needed to be coached for only one or two sessions. A significant improvement was noted in all variables tested, that is, unauthorized request, self-rating physical, self-rating emotional, hydrotherapy rating by patient, hydrotherapy rating by staff, compliance, nurse's rating of patient's level of anxiety, and state-trait anxiety ratings.

Distraction

Age-appropriate distraction techniques can effectively help reduce the patients' perception of pain. With younger children, providing toys for play during treatments is beneficial. Preschool and school-aged children enjoy bubble-blowing, music, singing, television, or stories read aloud. With the school-aged child, involving them in a discussion provides distraction. Adolescents also enjoy their favorite music and may benefit from engaging in conversaton. Distraction techniques aimed at reducing behavioral distress in burned children undergoing painful treatments have been documented.[7,42] Adults also benefit from the use of music, television, and engagement in conversation.

Each strategy enables the patient to lower his or her anxiety level, thereby decreasing one's pain perception and/or increasing one's tolerance to painful burn treatment stimuli. It is important to allow patients an opportunity to choose the music, television program, or topic of conversation to promote a sense of control.[40]

Imagery and Hypnosis

The use of guided imagery and hypnosis with the burn population is an area in need of further exploration. Studies have shown that the use of these strategies can be somewhat effective in pain and anxiety reduction.[6,30] The nurse can engage the patient in imagery by encouraging thoughts of pleasant experiences or events and/or focusing on a desired object.

The use of guided imagery and hypnosis with the burn population can be valuable strategies. However, implementation can be somewhat hampered by the reality of the burn unit environment, that is, high stress, traditionally treatment-oriented environment, and lack of trained personnel. A licensed hypnotist is required to perform hypnosis before or during the treatment. The limited literature identifies the efficacy of hypnotherapy with some burn patients. However, most studies are flawed with respect to design, and, as a result, no firm conclusions can be drawn regarding the feasibility or utility of hypnosis with burn patients.[17]

Biofeedback

Knudson-Cooper[20] and Kibbee[16] have used biofeedback with burn patients and report that highly motivated burn patients have been taught to relax by duplicating, on demand, those internal sensations that characteristically accompany a relaxed state. In addition, burn patients report an increased sense of control.

Massage and Vibration

Clinical experience has shown that light massage of burn wound edges, on an open wound or one covered by a dressing, may provide relief to the patient experiencing a severe itching sensation. Vibration of the patient's bed or mattress in the itchy area may also provide relief. Again, use of these techniques in conjunction with an antipruritic agent will have a maximal effect.

Other Physical Strategies

Kibbee[16] has explored the use of strategies such as transcutaneous electrical nerve stimulation (TENS), acupuncture, acupressure, and ice massage with burn patients. Moderate success in reducing pain and anxiety was reported.

Giving Permission for Pain Expression

As the patient's advocate, the nurse is in the ideal position to assist patients in acknowledging and expressing their pain. Many patients act as though it is a sign of weakness to show their pain during the treatment and fight hard not to do so. Acknowledgment of the patient's pain creates an environment in which patients are more comfortable in openly expressing their discomfort through crying or yelling.

Patient Involvement in Treatment

Involving the patient in the treatment has proven to be extremely beneficial in pain and anxiety reduction during the procedure. Based on the work of Kavanaugh,[15] the provision of maximal control and predictability during dressing changes will help to reduce psychopathologic behavior observed in burned children. Nurses can accomplish this by giving both children and adults as much choice as possible regarding treatments. Decisions around which dressing to remove, what body part to wash first, and where to begin physiotherapy and debridement permit patients some input into care planning. To further maximize control, children and adults can be allowed and encouraged to participate in their care as much as possible. Children as young as age 2 can usually assist with some aspect of the treatment. School-age children report less pain when they are involved in doing their treatment.[29] Patients can help to remove outer dressings and old ointment from the wounds, wash their body and hair and help wrap the new bandages.

Parental Involvement in Treatment

In addition to patient involvement with treatments, research has shown that many parents are desirous, to varying degrees, of being directly involved in their child's care, including wound care and other painful procedures.[44] Encouraging parents' participation during their child's treatment can be a valuable strategy in helping to reduce the child's painful experience. As with other strategies, the nurse must carefully assess the child-family relationship to determine the appropriateness of this strategy. Giving the parents a choice regarding the degree of their involvement is fundamental, as is thorough preparation of the parents for the experience.

—

The authors have observed an important benefit from the utilization of these nonpharmacological techniques. Nurses express increased self-esteem and satisfaction from involving patients more directly in their own care, and from being a caregiver who helps the patient manage his or her discomfort as opposed to being the one who inflicts the pain. Patients and families benefit similarly from an increased sense of involvement and control.

—

The burn nurse should manage each patient's pain individually, using a variety of approaches. It is important not to give up if a strategy does not seem to be effective the first time.

◆ SUMMARY

Nursing staff can be the burn patient's strongest advocates with respect to effective pain management. They are the ones who are most frequently involved in performing painful burn treatments over what may be a prolonged period of time.

However, problems do exist and obstacles stand in the way of overall effective burn pain management by nursing staff. Burn pain is difficult, if not impossible, to completely alleviate. Incongruities exist between burn patients and their caregivers regarding perceptions of pain. Lack of knowledge regarding the complex issue of burn pain and its management makes the work difficult and, at times, frustrating. This issue is further exacerbated by the high-stress, high-tech level that is prevalent in burn units. Nurses can and do make a difference in pain management for the burn survivor. Increased knowledge, application of the pain assessment process, and articulation of such findings can do much to facilitate the nurse's role as provider of both comfort and care. The nurse should incorporate both pharmacological and nonpharmacological approaches when attempting to alleviate the burn patient's pain. It is only through the use of effective pain management techniques that the nurse can improve the burn patient's quality of life.

REFERENCES

1. Andreasen NJ, Noyes R Jr, and Hartford CE. (1972). Factors influencing adjustment of burn patients during hospitalization. *Psychosom Med, 34,* 517-525.
2. Avni J. (1980). The severe burns. *Adv Psychosom Med, 10,* 57-77.
3. Bernstein NR. (1976). *Emotional care of the facially burned and disfigured.* Boston: Little Brown.
4. Beyer JE. (1984). *The oucher: a user's manual and technical report.* Evanston, Ill: The Hospital Play Equipment Company.
5. Choinière M, Melzack R, Rondeau I, et al. (1989). The pain of burns: characteristics and correlates. *J Trauma, 29,* 1531-1539.
6. Crasilneck HB, Stieman JA, Wilson BJ, et al. (1955). Use of hypnosis in the management of patients with burns. *JAMA, 153,* 103-106.
7. Elliot C and Olson R. (1983). The management of children's distress in response to painful medical treatment for burn injuries. *Behav Res and Ther, 21,* 675-683.
8. Fagerhaugh SY. (1974). Pain expression and control on a burn care unit. *Nurs Outlook, 22,* 645-650.
9. Feller I and Archambeault-Jones C. (1973). *Nursing the burned patient.* Ann Arbor, Mich: Braun-Brumfield, Inc.
10. Friedman J. (1989). *Burn patient nightmares/sleep disturbances: treatment with doxopin.* Paper presented at the 21st meeting of the American Burn Association, New Orleans.
11. Hospital for Sick Children Drug Formulary (1991).
12. Iafrati NS. (1986). Pain on the burn unit: patient versus nurse perceptions. *J Burn Care Rehab, 7,* 413-416.
13. Jaffe, J.H. (1980). Drug addiction and drug abuse. In Gilman A and Goodman LS (eds), *The pharmacological basis of therapeutics* (pp. 535-584). New York: Macmillan.
14. Jorgenson JA and Brophy JJ. (1975). Psychiatric treatment modalities in burn patients. *Current Psychiatric Therapies, 15,* 85-91.
15. Kavanaugh C. (1983). A new approach to dressing change in the severely burned child and its effect on burn related psychopathology. *Heart Lung, 12,* 612-619.
16. Kibbee E. (1984). Burn pain management. *Critical Care Quarterly, 7,* 54-62.
17. Kimball KL, Drews JE, Walker S, et al. (1987). The use of T.E.N.S. for pain reduction in burn patients receiving Travase. *J Burn Care Rehabil, 8,* 28-31.

18. Klein RM and Charlton JE. (1980). Behavioural observation and analysis of pain behaviour in critically burned patients. *Pain, 9,* 27-40.
19. Knighton JA. (1982). *Becoming the parent of a burned child.* Unpublished master's thesis. University of Toronto, Toronto, Ontario.
20. Knudson-Cooper MS. (1981). Relaxation and biofeedback training in the treatment of severely burned children. *J Burn Care Rehabil, 2,* 102-109.
21. Kueffner M. (1975). Passage through hospitalization of severely burned isolated school-age children. In Batey M (ed), *Communicating nursing research: critical issues in access to data, 7,* 181-197.
22. Loeser JD. (1980). A definition of pain. *Medicine, 7,* 3-4.
23. Marvin JA and Heimbach DM. (1984). Pain management. In Fisher SF and Helm PA (eds), *Comprehensive rehabilitation of burns.* (pp. 311-329). Baltimore: Williams & Wilkins.
24. Marvin JA and Heimbach DM. (1985). Pain control during the intensive care phase of burn care. *Crit Care Clin, 1,* 147-157.
25. McCaffery M and Beebe A. (1989). *Pain: clinical manual for nursing practice.* St. Louis: C.V. Mosby.
26. Moyer MM. (1989). The use of patient-controlled analgesia for burn pain. In Funk SG, Tomguist EM, L. Archer-Coppe, et al. (eds), *Key aspects of comfort: management of pain, fatigue and nausea.* New York: Springer.
27. Orgain C, Marvin JA, and Heimbach DM. (1979). *Explaining pain management practices.* Paper presented at the 11th meeting of the American Burn Association, New Orleans.
28. Osgood PF and Szyfelbein SK. (1990). Management of pain. In Martyn JAJ (ed), *Acute management of the burned patient.* (pp. 201-216). Philadelphia: WB Saunders.
29. Palozzi L. (1990). *The burned child's experience of pain associated with hydrotherapy, debridement and dressing application.* Unpublished master's thesis. University of Toronto, Toronto, Ontario.
30. Patterson D, Quested KA, and Boltwood MD. (1987). Hypnotherapy as a treatment for pain in patients with burns: research and clinical considerations. *J Burn Care Rehabil, 8,* 263-268.
31. Perry S and Heidrich G. (1982). Management of pain during debridement: a survey of U.S. burn units. *Pain, 13,* 267-280.
32. Perry S, Heidrich G, and Ramos E. (1981). Assessment of pain by burn patients, *J Burn Care Rehabil, 2,* 322-326.
33. Porter I and Jick H. (1980). Addiction rare in patients treated with narcotics. *N Engl J Med, 302,* 123.
34. Ross DM and Ross SA. (1988). *Childhood pain: current issues, research and management.* Baltimore: Urban Schwartzenberg.
35. Savedra M. (1977). Coping with pain: strategies of severely burned children. *The Canadian Nurse, 73,* 28-29.
36. Schecter N, Allen D, and Hanson K. (1986). Status of paediatric pain control: a comparison of hospitalized analgesic usage in children and adults. *Pediatrics, 77,* 11-15.
37. Schnurrer J, Marvin JA, and Heimbach DM. (1985). Evaluation of paediatric pain medications. *J Burn Care Rehabil, 6,* 105-107.
38. Steiner H and Clark WR, Jr. (1977). Psychiatric complications of burned adults: a classification. *J Trauma, 17,* 134-143.
39. Stoddard F. (1982). Coping with pain: a developmental approach to treatment of burned children. *Am J Psychiatry, 139,* 736-740.
40. Stoddard FJ. (1990). Psychiatric management of the burn patient. In

Martyn JAJ (ed), *Acute management of the burned patient.* (pp. 256-272). Philadelphia: WB Saunders.

41. Szyfelbein SK, Osgood PF, and Carr DB. (1985). The assessment of pain and plasma beta-endorphin immunoactivity in burned children. *Pain, 22,* 173-182.
42. Tarnowski K, McGrath M, Calhoun M, et al. (1987). Paediatric burn injury: self-versus-therapist-mediated debridement. *J Pediatr Psychol, 4,* 567-579.
43. Walkenstein M. (1982). Comparison of burned patients' perception of pain with nurses' perception of patients' pain. *J Burn Care Rehabil, 2,* 233-236.
44. Watt-Watson J, Everenden C, and Lawson C. (1990). Parents' perceptions of their child's acute pain experience. *Journal of Pediatric Nursing, 5,* 344-349.
45. Wernick RL, Brantley PJ, and Malcom R. (1980-1981). Behavioural techniques in the psychological rehabilitation of burn patients. *Int J Psychiatry Med, 10,* 145-150.
46. Woodward J. (1959). Emotional disturbances of burned children. *British Medical Journal, 18,* 1009.

Appendix A

◆ **PATIENT CARE STANDARDS**

Alteration in Comfort:

Acute pain related to cancer
Definition: Verbal report and presence of severe discomfort

Characteristics

1. Communication of pain descriptors (verbal or coded)
2. Guarded behavior; protective
3. Self-focusing
4. Narrowed focus
5. Distraction behavior (moaning, crying, pacing)
6. Restlessness
7. Facial mask of pain
8. Alteration in muscle tone
9. Autonomic response (↑ HR, ↑ BP, ↑ RR)
10. Behavior (fear, anxiety)

Etiologies – Acute Pain related to

Tumor – Nerve compression or direct invasion
Blood vessel or lymphatic obstruction
Visceral obstruction

Reprinted with permission from the Nursing Department, Dana Farber Cancer Institute, Boston, Mass. (A more complete set of standards used to guide cancer pain management is available from: Dana Farber Cancer Institute, Nursing Education Department, 44 Binney Street, Boston, MA 02115.)

Musculoskeletal metastasis, pathological fractures
Effusions
Therapy—Chemotherapy
Mucositis/stomatitis
Radiation
Proctitis, skin burns, esophagitis
Surgery
Postoperative pain

Outcome Criteria

During hospitalization patient will:

1. Describe intensity and quality of pain, meaning of pain, location of pain, and factors that increase or decrease the pain.
2. Verbalize relief of pain.
3. Maintain normal bowel elimination pattern.
4. Experience no side effects of drug therapy given to relieve pain (little or no nausea or vomiting, dysphoria, sedation).
5. Assess his or her pain by stating the place, amount, interactions (things that make pain worse) and neutralizers (things that makes it better) (PAIN).

Nursing Orders/Collaborative Interventions

1. Perform baseline pain assessment on admission, identifying the following:
    a. Location of the pain(s). May diagram on front/back view of body.
    b. Quality/intensity of pain on numeric scale of 0 to 10 (0 = none, 10 = worst pain patient can imagine). If unable to use numeric scale, use word descriptor scale (none, mild, moderate, severe, excruciating). *Identify the scale being used, and consistently document the same.*
    c. Duration of the pain (when did it start?, sporadic or continuous?, does it occur in a pattern?).
    d. Associated symptoms (nausea, anorexia, fatigue).
    e. Usual relief measures taken.
    f. Changes in roles/relationships.
    g. Mood.
    h. Physical limitations.

i. Past and present pain experience and coping styles.
j. Patient's perception of causes/meaning of the pain.
k. Sleep patterns.
l. High risk indicators based on potential for developing acute pain. (Based on previously mentioned causes of acute pain in the cancer patient).

Acronym for Quick Assessment[2]

P: Place
A: Amount (0–10) – now, at worst, at best
I: Interactions – what makes it worse?
N: Neutralizers – what makes it better?

2. Implement measures to modify the patient's pain experience, including physiologic and behavioral responses.
   a. Administer analgesia.
   b. Minimize environmental stimuli.
   c. Offer or provide relaxation training.
3. Collaborate with members of the health care team to formulate a pain management plan for the patient.
4. Implement measures to reduce the following side effects of analgesics:
   a. Altered bowel function.
   b. Nausea and vomiting.
   c. Disturbed sleep patterns.
   d. Respiratory depression.
   e. Altered cognitive functioning.
5. Implement pain regimen teaching plan and evaluate progress.

Source of Documentation

Nursing assessment on admission
Nurses' notes
Flow sheets
Pain regimen teaching plan

REFERENCES

1. Chapman CR, Syrjala K, and Sargur M. (May 1985). Pain as a manifestation of cancer treatment. *Semin Oncol Nurs, 1(2),* 100-108.
2. Donovan, M. (May 1985). Nursing assessment of cancer pain. *Semin Oncol Nurs, 1(2),* 109-108.
3. Foley K and Coyle N. (May 1985). Pain in patients with cancer: profile of

patients and common pain syndromes. *Semin Oncol Nurs,* 1(2), 93-99.
4. Holland JC. (1982). *Psychological aspects of cancer.* In Holland JC and Frei E (eds), *Cancer Medicine,* (pp. 1175-1203). Philadelphia: Lea and Febiger.
5. McCaffery, M. (1979). *Nursing management of the patient with pain,* Philadelphia, Toronto: JB Lippincott.
6. McCaffery M and Beebe A. (1989). Pain: a clinical manual for nursing practice. St. Louis: Mosby–Year Book, Inc.
7. Seery R and Coyle N. (1986). *Pain,* in *Standards of Oncology Nursing Practice.* pp. 433-442. New York: John Wiley and Sons.
8. Willoughby S. (1985). *Pain.* In McNally JC, Stair JC, and Somerville ET (eds), *Guidelines for cancer nursing practice.* pp. 78-84. Orlando: Grune and Stratton Co.
9. Ziegfeld C (ed). (1987). *Core curriculum for oncology nursing.* Philadelphia: WB Saunders Co.

Appendix B

◆ Pain Regimen Teaching Plan

	Explained initials/date	Demonstrated initials/ date	Comments
Patient outcomes 1. Patient will identify pain medication(s) and state two facts about the medication(s).			
2. Patient/family member will state knowledge of pain regimen: a. dose, frequency, route.			
b. common side effects and how to manage them.			
c. non-invasive measures being used.			

Continued.

◆ Pain Regimen Teaching Plan—cont'd

	Explained initials/date	Demonstrated initials/ date	Comments
3. Patient/family member will describe bowel regimen: a. note individual regimen here.			
b. if no BM × 2 days, notify physician; time limit may be modified based on patient's usual habit.			
4. Patient/family member will identify coping strategies for dealing with pain: a. list techniques used in hospital, i.e., distraction, medication, PMR, visualization.			
b. list any resources provided, i.e., pamphlets, tapes, etc.			

5. Patient/family member will identify symptoms to report to physician: a. increased pain, unrelieved with present regimen.			
b. change in mental status (lethargy, mental clouding, disorientation, hallucinations).			
c. constipation > 2 days.			
d. inability to take (po) oral pain medications due to nausea, vomiting, stomatitis.			

Appendix C

◆ Behavioral Intervention Teaching Plan

	Explained initials/date	Demonstrated initials/ date	Comments
Patient outcomes Patient will identify three techniques available for use: 1. breath control exercises			
2. music relaxation with guided imagery (GI)			
3. progressive muscle relaxation with GI			

4. others:			
Patient will identify ways in which he or she may utilize the above: 1. pain management			
2. anxiety management			
3. nausea management			
4. insomnia relief			
Patient will demonstrate effective use of relaxation to modify discomfort and anxiety during treatment. (this will be measured by patient's verbal report, vital signs, and posturing)			
Comments/additional information			
Written information given to patient			
Individual PMR/GI tape			
Significant other included in teaching			

Index